THE ROUGH GUIDE to
Men's Health

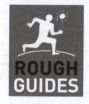
ROUGH GUIDES

www.roughguides.com

Credits

The Rough Guide to Men's Health

Editors: Lois Wilson, Pat Gilbert, Jo Kendall
Layout: Fit4Life Media
Picture research: Sarah Bentley,
Christopher Lewis/RunCity Images
Proofreading: Jason Freeman
Production: Gemma Sharpe

Rough Guides Reference

Editors: Kate Berens, Ian Blenkinsop, Tom Cabot,
Tracy Hopkins, Matthew Milton, Joe Staines
Director: Andrew Lockett

Publishing Information

This second edition published January 2013 by
Rough Guides Ltd, 80 Strand, London WC2R 0RL
11 Community Centre, Panchsheel Park, New Delhi 110017, India
Email: mail@roughguides.com

Distributed by the Penguin Group:
Penguin Books Ltd, 80 Strand, London WC2R 0RL
Penguin Group (USA), 375 Hudson Street, NY 10014, USA
Penguin Group (Australia), 250 Camberwell Road, Camberwell, Victoria 3124, Australia
Penguin Group (New Zealand), 67 Apollo Drive, Mairangi Bay, Auckland 1310,
New Zealand
Rough Guides is represented in Canada by Tourmaline Editions Inc.,
662 King Street West, Suite 304, Toronto

Printed in Singapore by Toppan Security Printing Pte. Ltd.

© Lloyd Bradley, 2013
408 pages; includes index

A catalogue record for this book is available from the British Library

ISBN 13: 978-1-40936-263-0

1 3 5 7 9 8 6 4 2

THE ROUGH GUIDE to
Men's Health

by
Lloyd Bradley

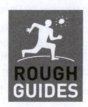

www.roughguides.com

Acknowledgements

The author would like to thank the following, without whom this book would not have been possible: all at Fit4Life Media and RunCity; Derek Yates, Lois Wilson, Pat Gilbert, Jo Kendall, Sarah Bentley, Christopher Lewis and Jason Freeman; Gideon, Sarah, Sarah, Lili and Sandra aka *The Rough Guide to Men's Health*'s panel of experts; Effua Baker, Russell Fairbrother, Pete Muir and Steve Perrine; Ruth Tidball, Andrew Lockett and Peter Buckley; Joel Chernin and Nina Sharman; Simon Kanter, Paul Simpson and Mark Ellingham; Diana, George & Elissa Bradley.

About the author

Lloyd Bradley was classically trained as a chef, is a regular marathon runner and was formerly Health & Fitness editor at *GQ* magazine and Consultant Editor at *Men's Health* and *Runner's World* magazines. He is also the author of *The Rough Guide to Running* and has written several books on music.

Picture credits

All illustrations and graphics supplied by DK Images; except pp. 39, 47, 59, 81, 135 and 350, drawn and supplied by Derek Yates

All other photography supplied by RunCity Images, except: pp. 29, 40, 41, 45, 51, 157 and 247, supplied by DK Images; p.75 cdrin/Shutterstock, p.171 nito/Shutterstock, p.207 Luis Louro/Shutterstock; p.266 Kodda/ Shutterstock, p.291 Goodluz/Shutterstock.

All other photography supplied by RunCity Images; except, supplied by DK Images

Cover credits: front cover designed by Diana Jarvis; back cover image Russell Sadur © Dorling Kindersley; inside front cover image © Corbis.

Contents

Contents

Why worry?

Why indeed? You've done alright so far. But wouldn't you like to do better? In truth, men's health is generally less a matter of worry and more a case of having a few concerns. While it would be daft to assume that the hectic twenty-first century lifestyle we lead is going tokill us, it would be equally misguided to think we can live to our fullest potential without putting a bit of effort into how we do it. And if you've got as far as picking this book up and opening it you are probably almost as aware of this as we are.

Welcome to *The Rough Guide to Men's Health*

You are holding in your hands a book that aims to get you fitter and healthier and improve your performance in just about every area of your life. A book that doesn't assume there's necessarily anything wrong with you in the first place, just that, unless you're a professional athlete with a team of psychiatrists and a relationship counsellor with a 24-hour call-out service, everything about you could function considerably better if it all had a bit of a tune-up. Most people could eat better; most people could improve the efficiency of their exercise regime; most people would like to make their relationship run smoother; would like to do better at work; would like better sex; firm up the old midriff; enjoy their holidays to the absolute max; and so on. Which is where we come in: to help you get that bit more out of whatever situations you are probably quite happy with at the moment.

Also, to start from the standpoint that there could be nothing criminally unhealthy in your lifestyle at the moment allows us to add to your life rather than take away. Too many health books – notably men's health books – devote so much energy to telling you what you shouldn't be doing, they immediately alienate potential readers. Here at the *Rough Guide to Men's Health*, we're fairly

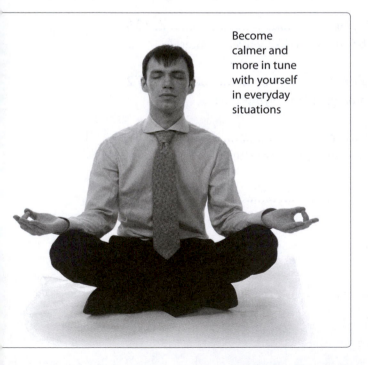

Become calmer and more in tune with yourself in everyday situations

certain we know what it is you get up to and, provided it's in moderation, there's not a great deal of point in us telling you to stop it – cigarette smoking, cocaine, heroin and unprotected sex are about all we draw an unequivocal line through. The idea here is to carry on enjoying yourself, but do so from a standpoint of being able to handle it as you do, and recover quickly afterwards. We want you to live forever, rather than die in the attempt.

How it all works

The *Rough Guide to Men's Health* won't be coming at you like a medical dictionary or targeting specific areas of your body and trying to scare you with all that could go wrong with them. Our approach is we look at the various areas of your life, then look at how they could be maximized, made easier or just kept safe. The first section, **Whatever, Whenever, Wherever**, deals exactly with those situations in a series of chapters with titles like, "At work", "On holiday", "In the

bedroom", "In the kitchen", "In later life", then discusses how your maximum health and fitness would improve each aspect of them and help you avoid problems up ahead. The chapter will then explain how to achieve this optimum state. But it does so in a combination of running text, quick tips and bite-sized information panels, allowing you to take something away from each page regardless of how much time you may be able to give it at that moment. And because we know that you'll retain this knowledge better if you understand the theories behind it, we don't neglect the background science and medical-type diagrams, but we do our best to keep them separate from the rest of the book.

Section two is **Fit For Life**, which takes a longer term and less lifestyle-specific view of your health and fitness. One chapter, "A man for all seasons", takes you through life decade by decade, letting you know what you may have to look forward to – pros as well as cons – and how you can continue to live the best life you can whatever it might

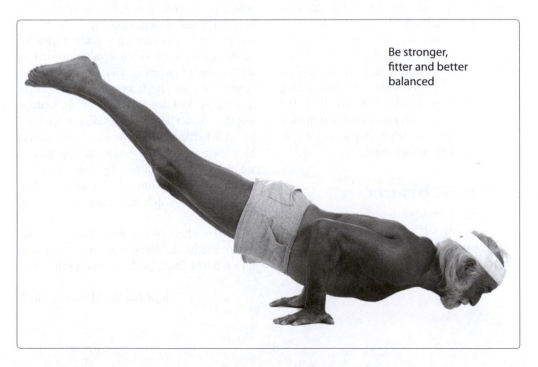

Be stronger, fitter and better balanced

throw at you. In another chapter, "Looking after Number One", the simple question posed is, Why do so many men leave it so late before going to the doctor? We detail how to get round all those excuses and then how to make sure you get the best out of it when you get there. While the final chapter in that section, "Improve your performance", is devoted to getting the best out of the advice the book has already given you, as that is the only way you are going to get the best out of your life.

The final section, **Reference**, pretty much does what it says on the tin. The main part of it is a straightforward guide to common complaints, how to spot them, what to do and how to prevent them coming back. It also carries a symptoms grid chart that allows you to find out what you might have, based on what symptoms you are showing. This takes so much of the guesswork out of diagnosing yourself, and isn't a service you'll find in too many other men's health books. Then lastly, there is a comprehensive directory of further reading, useful websites and interesting organizations, which also contains a list of the most commonly used alternative therapies, a brief explanation of what they are, and how to find out more about them.

The best brains

Of course I couldn't have done too much of this by myself, and I had the support, advice, words of wisdom and perpetual good humour of the most eminently qualified

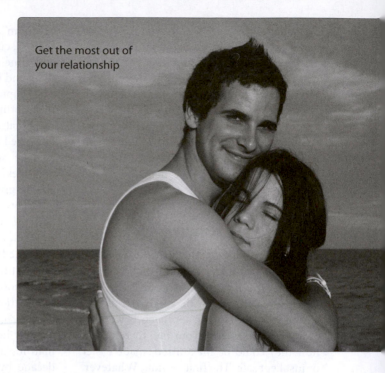

Get the most out of your relationship

Panel of Experts. One of London's top personal trainers; the editor of *Scarlet*, the world's most readable sex magazine; a GP with a busy urban practice; a member of the British Dietetic Association and the Nutrition Society; and a practising psychiatrist who, for seven years, has provided on-site counselling for the *I'm a Celebrity… Get Me Out of Here!* contestants, so she is certainly no stranger to hard work. They are, respectively, Gideon Remfry, Sarah Hedley, Dr Liliana Risi, Dr Sarah Schenker and Dr Sandra Scott, so let's give them a nice big round of applause as we meet them individually (see opposite) and find out why the *Rough Guide to Men's Health* has so much oestrogen on its Panel of Experts.

Then when you've done that, enjoy the rest of the book, drink more water and look forward to a fitter, healthier and livelier life.

Lloyd Bradley (London, 2013)

Meet the panel

The *Rough Guide to Men's Health* panel of experts advised on much of the book, and contribute directly with their words of wisdom in the expert advice boxes and the larger grey quote boxes throughout. You'd be advised to pay close attention to what they are saying. And if you're wondering why there are so many women advising on men's health, it's because they always seem to know what's best for us. Except when it comes to lifting heavy weights, obviously.

Sarah Hedley

Sarah is a writer and editor specialising in health, beauty and celebrity culture. She has appeared as a social commentator on shows including *The Oprah Winfrey Show, How to Look Good Naked, Richard & Judy* and the *BBC News*, as well as occupying the role of TV agony aunt on various TV series.

Her fifteen years' of experience also include contributing editor roles on some of the world's biggest magazines, including *Maxim* and *Cosmopolitan*, and she's enjoyed resident columnist tenures with both *The Sun* newspaper in the UK and *Men's Fitness* in the US. Currently, she lives with her husband in Dubai, where she is writing her next book and dreaming of one day owning a dog.

Dr Sarah Schenker

Our second Sarah graduated in Nutrition from the University of Surrey with a State Registration in Dietetics. After gaining three years clinical experience at St. Thomas' Hospital in London and the John Ratcliffe Hospital in Oxford, she gained her PhD in Human Nutrition from the University of Oxford and the Institute of Food Research in Norwich. Sarah then joined the British Nutrition Foundation where she worked as a nutrition scientist. Sarah now combines her sports nutrition work (consulting for

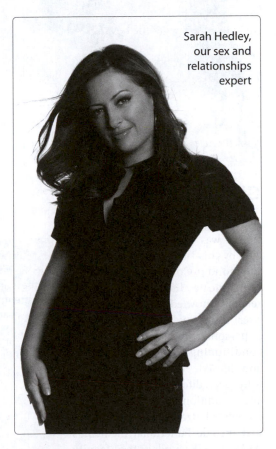

Sarah Hedley, our sex and relationships expert

football clubs including Tottenham and Chelsea) with a busy media career. She appears regularly on Channel 5's *Live with Gabby* and writes for a number of scientific journals – as well as for newspapers, popular magazines and websites.

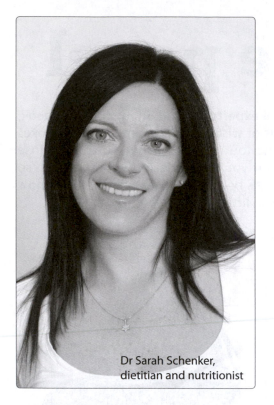

Dr Sarah Schenker,
dietitian and nutritionist

Gideon Remfry

Gideon's passion for health and fitness was ignited from an early age by his fantastic Judo coach Raymond Coulthurst, leading him into a lifetime pursuit of related knowledge. He now has over twenty years experience as a personal trainer, strength and conditioning coach, educator and lifestyle modulator. He is a fully accredited UKSCA strength and conditioning coach and has completed training programmes that include Functional medicine's AFMCP UK under the faculty of the IFM; PIPC3; Biosignature modulation; Chek (Institute of Advanced Exercise Education); and pre- and post-natal training. He applies his coaching experience

and tools such as physiological assessments, lab-testing, lifestyle, nutrition and training information gathering, to establish a therapeutic partnership between patient and practitioner. Gideon has written for various publications such as *Men's Health*, *Women's Health*, *Vogue*, *Red*, *GQ*, and regularly contributes articles to *Men's Fitness* magazine.

He also featured as the resident trainer on the first series of the TV show *Britain's Top Model*. Gideon is based exclusively at KX members club in South Kensington, London, where he builds and co-ordinates individual lifestyle packages and manages the fitness team. He is currently training as a naturopathic nutritionist.

Dr Sandra Scott

Sandra trained as a psychiatrist at the Maudsley Hospital in South London. Her work has included family therapy, cognitive behavioural therapy, parent/child work and acute adult psychiatry. She has worked in the UK on both *Celebrity Big Brother* and *Big Brother*s 2, 3, 4 and 5, and provided

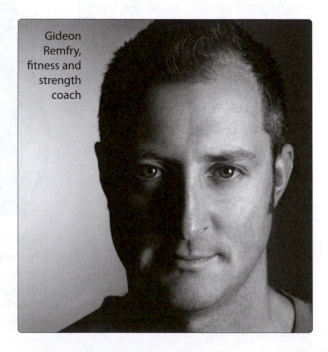

Gideon Remfry, fitness and strength coach

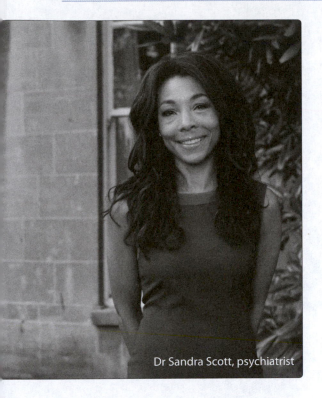

Dr Sandra Scott, psychiatrist

Dr Liliana Risi

Liliana is a South African sociologist and General Practioner with an Msc in Sexual health. She set up the research programme for Marie Stopes International – the UK's leading provider of sexual and reproductive healthcare – and has published research into what changes people's behaviour. She contributed to the establishment of a gardening scheme for patients with chronic health problems, and is a great believer in mindfulness-based practice – the ability to pay deliberate attention to one's experience from moment to moment.

She is now the GP Cancer and Palliative/ End of Life Care Clinical Lead for the Tower Hamlets GP Commissioning Group. She is interested in promoting a non-medical approach to the end of life. This means normalising the dying process in discussions with her patients and her colleagues to develop advanced decisions as part of proactive care and a good death.

psychological support for three series of *Hell's Kitchen*. Sandra also worked on BBC1's *Tomorrow's World Special, Lab Rats*, where she took six volunteers and put them through scientific experiments designed to explore the human condition.

For eleven years she has been taking trips out into the Australian jungle to counsel the celebrities for *I'm A Celebrity ... Get Me Out Of Here!* She oversaw the filming and was on hand for any crisis that arose on the ground-breaking Channel 4 documentary *Boys Alone*, which followed ten eleven- and twelve-year-old boys living unsupervised for five days and nights, dealing with issues of friendships and group dynamics between them. She has written for a number of publications and was a regular contributor to *The Times Education Supplement, Marie Claire* and *The Daily Mail*. Sandra is currently working on her third series of E4's *Tool Academy*.

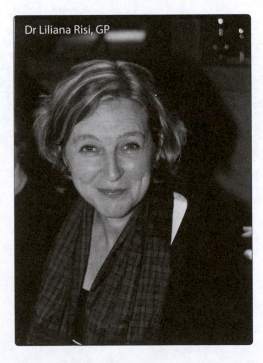

Dr Liliana Risi, GP

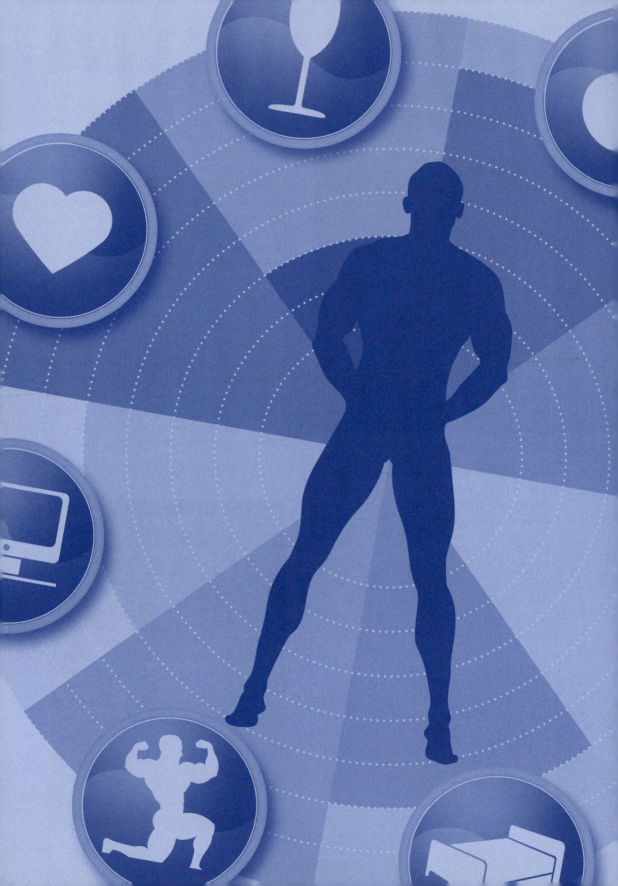

PART 1
WHATEVER, WHENEVER, WHEREVER

In the kitchen & on the run

There's a reason healthy eating has never been higher up on the social agenda: the reality is that many of us are getting significantly less nutrition from our food than in days gone by. This is due to a combination of the time pressures of our twenty-first-century lifestyle, the low priority given to education about food in school and the demand for (and supply of) cheap food across the developed world. However, it's still not that difficult to eat your way to better health, and the difference it makes will be instantly noticeable.

Cheap food, low value

Why we eat is very straightforward. We need to provide calorific fuel to power our muscles; and to provide our bodies with the necessary nutrients (in the form of vitamins and minerals) to function, repair ourselves and ward off infections. We expend calories through physical effort and nutrient reserves are used up as our bodies go about their regular business. We feel hungry when we require more calories or nutrients, prompting us to eat to replenish the levels. Thus everything stays evenly balanced and in perfect working order. Or at least that's the theory.

In practice, over the last couple of decades, the time that should be spent on eating healthily every day has gone the way of a good night's sleep – it's seen as time that could be spent doing something much more exciting. The attendant demand for quick, easy, grab-and-go food has led to an industry boom in the production of processed ready meals, takeaways and snacks. These products often sacrifice nutritional content for greater volume, bulking themselves up with sugar, salt and trans fats.

As a result, it's surprisingly easy to be very well fed yet remain undernourished, often without realizing it. You might feel full yet be functioning well below your best, and a poor

F

Fact: In the twenty-first century, single men between the ages of 20 and 35 have been statistically shown to have worse diets, in terms of lack of nutrition and number of damaging ingredients, than any other demographic on both sides of the Atlantic. While this might not appear to be doing them too much harm – at that age, the metabolism tends to be super efficient – these bad habits are storing up trouble for later life.

How it all works: nourishment

By the time food leaves the stomach, it has been reduced to a thick oozing liquid called chyme. This allows it to pass easily into the small intestine, which is where the absorption into the system of ninety percent of its nutrient content takes place. Nutrients are separated from the waste product and taken up by the millions of microscopic tendril-like projections – villi – that line the small intestine's internal walls, allowing them to pass through into the bloodstream. Once in the bloodstream they are delivered to the liver which stores, processes and controls their release into the system, once again via the bloodstream, to whatever organ requires them. The liver also regulates the flow of sugar into the bloodstream and filters out any toxins – this is why the liver is so affected by excess alcohol consumption, as the body sees that as a poison to be removed.

The first stage of the small intestine is the duodenum, where the chyme is mixed with bile and pancreatic juice fed in by the liver and pancreas, respectively. These liquids will neutralize stomach acid to allow the digestive enzymes to function more efficiently. The iron, calcium and folic acid content of the food is transferred into the bloodstream through the duodenum walls, but the majority of nutrient absorption takes place further down the intestinal tract at the very end of the duodenum and in the second section of the small intestine, the jejunum.

Once in the jejunum, the process is known as "active absorption" because it uses energy to select what is needed from the chyme, hence feelings of drowsiness after a big meal. In this central section, protein, fat and the fat-soluble vitamins A, D, E and K are absorbed through the walls, and carbohydrate is broken down into glucose and glycogen to be stored in the liver or the muscles or burned immediately for energy.

In the third section of the small intestine, the ileum, the digestion process started in the previous sections will be completed, and any vitamin B12 will be absorbed. Also, any excess bile will be taken back into the system and returned to the liver for reprocessing.

What is left then passes into the large intestine, where it is dried out and, as the water is removed, the water-soluble B (all except B12) and C vitamins are absorbed into the system. They are not taken to the liver, but directly to the tissues or organs in which they will be utilized. This means the body has no storage capability for these vitamins and therefore they need to be taken every day.

1. Food is taken in through mouth
2. Food is broken down in stomach
3. Food is further broken down by bile and pancreatic juice
4. Nutrients are extracted and moved to the liver via the bloodstream
5. From the liver, nutrients are distributed around the body
6. Waste matter is passed on to the colon

Portions or servings?

In the UK, according to the Food Standards Agency, the five portions of fruit and veg a day guideline refers to 80g helpings. In spite of this, most food labels give nutrition advice per 100g.

In the US, a "serving" is one medium-sized fruit; half a cup of raw, cooked, frozen or canned fruits or vegetables; 6 fl oz (170ml) of one hundred percent fruit or vegetable juice; half a cup of cooked, frozen or canned beans or peas; or one cup of raw leafy vegetables.

diet can leave your immune system severely compromised. It's low nutrition that is at the root of so many of today's inexplicable and almost unquantifiable ailments – those times when we feel "just sort of stressed out" or "a bit under the weather" or are susceptible to any illness going around.

So much of today's food is padded out with "empty calories" – calories that provide a top-up of fuel when we start to flag, but very few nutrients. These empty calories make us feel hungry again almost immediately. It's

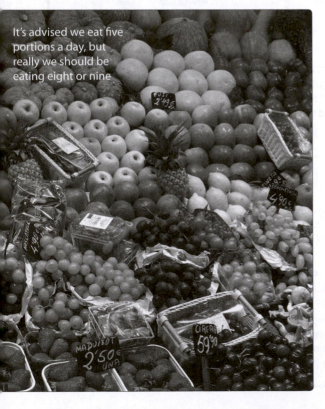

It's advised we eat five portions a day, but really we should be eating eight or nine

more than likely that you will actually need little of this extra fuel. The excess ends up on our bodies as fat, affecting the heart and the blood-sugar levels.

There is also the long-term psychological effect these changed eating habits are having on us. We are now paying less and less attention to the whole notion of eating as a pleasurable family or social activity – we regularly skip breakfast, snatch lunch on the run, or eat dinner off our knees. As a result, everything to do with food becomes devalued and we are even less likely to take it seriously. The unequivocally salty or sugary taste of so much processed food compromises our appreciation of flavour, undermining the important, pleasurable emotional experience of eating.

It's one of the ironies of modern life that cooking has never been so trendy – witness the number of cookery shows on TV and the level of fame achieved by some actually quite ordinary chefs. Yet we're eating worse food than we ever have. The Western world is undergoing an obesity crisis, while levels of both heart disease and type 2 diabetes (both diet-related), are soaring. In spite of all the sway of the celebrity apron-wearers and the "food porn" cookery shows, we seem to care less about what we eat and how we eat it.

However, with a little attention to forward planning, it's incredibly easy to turn your eating habits around. Even if you are already off the junk food, you can still get more out of how you eat, whether you think you can cook or not.

Six significantly damaging dietary habits you may not realize you have

Habit	How it can affect you
Eating too much	Restaurant portions and pre-packaged servings have increased considerably in size during the last decade or so, so it is very easy to be overeating without thinking you are consuming any more than you have always done.
Eating at strange times	Random eating habits, or constant grazing, usually go hand in hand with food of poor nutritional value, simply because it is convenience, rather than routine, defining what you are eating. All too often that means processed snacks, junk food and cheese.
Confusing the issues of nutritional health and weight loss	There are plenty of men who aren't noticeably porky and who assume they are eating well simply because they are not putting on weight. This isn't necessarily the case. An increase in nutrition levels will considerably boost their feeling of general well-being and raise the immunity capabilities of their bodies.
Substituting nutrition via food for supplements	Satisfying your nutritional needs through a balanced diet will always be much more beneficial than eating rubbish and popping vitamin pills. Good food affects you in all sorts of ways other than simply supplying vitamin A or fibre and it's this holistic, rather than targeted, approach to nutrition that the body needs to stay truly healthy.
Believing what it says on the tin	Far too much food sloganeering is relative rather than subjective. Simply announcing something to be "a healthier option" is meaningless. Healthier than what? A tub of lard? "30% fat free!" can simply be a way of spinning "70% fat!". Always read the whole of the label.
Misunderstanding nutritional guidelines	There are many conflicting eating plans and reportedly scientific pieces of dietary advice out there. Beyond basic guidelines such as can be found in this book, it will be impossible to find out what is precisely right for you without getting yourself checked out by a professional.

What's a well-balanced diet?

It has often been said that a good diet needs to incorporate the five major food groups (cereal, dairy, meat, fruit, vegetables). When this theory was first put forward, around fifty years ago, it suited practically everybody. These days, however, a significant proportion of the Western population don't eat meat, and there are growing numbers that feel better off without dairy. Thus the idea of defining a good diet by actual foods is looking distinctly outdated; it makes much more sense to talk about what *you* need to provide for *your* body.

The basic building blocks of a healthy diet are carbohydrate, fibre, protein and fat (see below), which need to be supplemented with the micronutrients of vitamins and minerals. As long as this is all in place, what food you obtain these from is simply a matter of personal choice.

Water works

Despite the best efforts of the bottled water industry to flog us H_2O, it's still not unusual for men not to drink enough water during the course of the day. In the Western world, in the twenty-first century, we should be drinking at least two litres per day. Keeping your water levels replenished is absolutely vital, as around seventy percent of your body is water and making sure it stays that way means everything else has the correct environment within which to function.

We lose water through sweat, urination, vapour escaping out of our mouths, and through our eyeballs. Yet it has to keep flowing to make sure everything moves around our system as it should and that waste is removed. So water needs to be constantly topped up. In fact, when you think you feel hungry it is more likely you are actually thirsty and in the initial stages of dehydration, so taking regular drinks will go a long way to stopping you snacking between meals.

Don't try to quench your thirst with fizzy or sugary drinks, or even fruit juice, and definitely not beer, as these will not provide the water that your thirst is telling you your body needs – it could result in your drinking more of them in an attempt to stave it off. Drink more water if the weather is warm or you have been exerting yourself physically – or if you have a cold, as coughing, sneezing and blowing your nose will use up fluid reserves. One good habit to get into is to take a large drink of water as soon as you wake up in the morning, as your body will have been drying out while you slept.

The purpose of a good diet is to supply you with enough energy to go about your daily business, the substances needed for cell growth, repair and healing, and the defences to fight off infection or guard against harmful bacteria. Obtaining the nutrients we need through diet can also go a long way to prevent serious conditions such as arthritis, osteoporosis or heart disease occurring later in life, and eating correctly can even prevent or counteract depression. At the same time, a healthy diet won't offer too much of anything that could have a detrimental effect, like fat, sugar or salt. Eating correctly is what your body has evolved to expect. As soon as you do, therefore, your all-round feelings of well-being will increase.

Carbohydrates

Carbohydrates are metabolized into blood glucose to become the body's primary source of energy, and exist in our diet in two forms: simple and complex. The former are also known as simple sugars, and include fructose (the natural sugar found in fruit), sucrose (refined table sugar) and lactose (milk sugar). Maple syrup, corn syrup and honey are also included in these groups. If it is refined, sugar is straightforward calorific energy, offering nothing else in the way of nutrition (empty calories, in other words).

Because sugar is converted quickly into glucose to power the body, sugar rushes are swift and palpable. The downside is they get used up just as suddenly, resulting in an equally dramatic crash. Simple carbs should be taken on by eating fruit, rather than through the refined sugar found in so much processed food. At least that way

Expert advice: "It's important to vary the fruit and veg you eat. Too many people just eat the stuff they like, day in, day out, and think that will do. It's better than nothing, but it won't give you the range of nutrients you need." Dr Sarah Schenker

Micronutrients: the vitamins and minerals

Nutrient	Found in	What it does	How deficiencies can affect you
Vitamin A	Liver, fish oil, tomatoes, leafy green veg, oranges	Promotes strong bones and teeth, good eyesight and healthy skin	Spots, acne and itching; poor night vision
Vitamin B1 (thiamine)	Whole grains, nuts, beans, liver, eggs	Supports the metabolization of carbohydrate	Muscle fatigue as the carbs aren't able to fuel them efficiently
Vitamin B2 (riboflavin)	Eggs, liver, brown rice, leafy green veg, brewer's yeast	Aids digestive process; repairs tissues; helps adrenalin production	Mouth sores; fatigue as energy is not released from food properly
Vitamin B3 (niacin)	Liver, poultry, nuts, beans	Metabolizes carbohydrate and fat; produces sex hormones; maintains the nervous system	Fatigue and a low sex drive
Vitamin B12	Liver, red meat, poultry, dairy, eggs	Aids the nervous system; produces red blood cells in bone marrow	Fatigue and anaemia due to low red blood cell count
Vitamin C	Citrus fruit, kiwi fruits, blackcurrants, strawberries, green veg	Boosts the immune system; promotes healthy teeth, gums and bones	Fatigue; bad teeth and swollen, sore or bleeding gums
Vitamin D	Fish oils, eggs, liver	Regulates calcium being used for bone growth	Liver and kidney problems and possible osteoporosis
Vitamin E	Vegetable oil, leafy green veg, nuts, meat	Protects red blood cells	Fatigue and anaemia
Folic acid	Leafy green veg, egg yolk, whole grains, nuts	Produces red blood cells	Anaemia
Calcium	Dairy, sardines and whitebait (because you eat the bones), eggs, leafy green veg	Builds bones and teeth; promotes muscle movement and cell function	Brittle bones and muscle and nerve problems
Magnesium	Nuts, whole grains, soy beans, dairy	Builds bones and teeth; aids the nervous system	An increased likelihood of kidney stones
Iron	Leafy green veg, nuts, whole grains, liver, meat	Transports oxygen to the red blood cells and, with them, to the muscles	Anaemia and chronic fatigue
Zinc	Meat, whole grains, seafood	Aids the prostate gland and sperm production; lowers blood pressure	Hair loss, reduced appetite and fatigue
Chromium	Red meat, dairy, leafy green veg	Acts as a catalyst to many different enzymes	High blood pressure, fatigue, reduced fertility

Recommended daily allowances

	Man 20–29 years old	30–39	40–49	50+
Energy	2800kcal	2500kcal	2500kcal	2300kcal
Protein	58g	55g	55g	58g
Fibre	24g	24g	26g	28g
Carbohydrate	350g	330g	330g	280g
Fat (rec. amount of saturates)	95g (30g)	95g (30g)	95g (30g)	85g (27g)
Salt (rec. amount of sodium)	6g (2.4g)	6g (2.4g)	6g (2.4g)	6g (2.4g)
Vitamin A	1000mcg	1000mcg	1000mcg	1000mcg
Vitamin B1 (thiamine)	1.5mg	1.4mg	1.4mg	1.2mg
Vitamin B2 (riboflavin)	1.7mg	1.6mg	1.5mg	1.4mg
Vitamin B3 (niacin)	19mg	18mg	17mg	16mg
Vitamin B12	3.0mcg	3.0mcg	3.0mcg	3.0mcg
Vitamin C	60mg	60mg	60mg	60mg
Vitamin D	10mcg	7.5mcg	5.0mcg	5.0mcg
Vitamin E	10mcg	10mcg	10mcg	10mcg
Folic acid	400mcg	400mcg	400mcg	400mcg
Calcium	750mg	750mg	750mg	800mg
Magnesium	300mg	300mg	300mg	300mg
Iron	10mg	10mg	10mg	10mg
Zinc	10mg	10mg	10mg	10mg
Chromium	500mcg	500mcg	500mcg	500mcg

A calorie is the energy needed to raise the temperature of one gram of water by ten degrees Celsius.

A kilo calorie (kcal or C) is 1000 calories. It's what's used on food packaging to denote the amount of energy provided.

A milligram (mg) is a thousandth of a gram.

A microgram (mcg) is a millionth of a gram.

Good chol, bad chol

Not all cholesterol is the devil on a dish – in fact, it is vital to keep the body functioning. Manufactured by the liver, cholesterol falls into two categories: low-density lipoprotein (LDL) and high-density lipoprotein (HDL). For a harmonious balance, the body requires a 75/25 percent split.

Both do the job of transporting nutrients around the system via the bloodstream, but HDL (known as "good cholesterol") is returned to the liver for reprocessing once it has delivered its load, while LDL ("bad cholesterol") is of a low enough density to penetrate the surface of the artery walls, establish a hold and start building up deposits. The less-flexible HDL particles actually play a big part in keeping the arteries from clogging up by knocking LDL off the inner surfaces.

It is only an excess of LDL that is a potential killer – clogged arteries mean high blood pressure and increased risk of heart disease. But because we cannot regulate which type our bodies produce, it's safest to cut down on any cholesterol-producing fat.

they will be accompanied by the nutrients in the fruit.

Complex carbohydrates are found in whole grains, vegetables, pulses and fruit, and exist as sugars that include starches and fibre as part of their molecular make-up. Fibre is an absolutely crucial part of our diet, as it is the part of the plant that is not broken down during the digestion process. This permits it to move through our system, helping to keep the internal walls of the intestines clear – a kind of scouring pad effect. It will also retain water to deliver to the colon to keep faeces soft, and attract some of the chemicals that create cholesterol and remove them from the system. In doing this fibre prevents constipation, regulates cholesterol and is believed to reduce the risks of bowel and stomach cancer by clearing out accumulative hazardous waste. Potatoes, wholewheat pasta and bread, cereals and beans are great sources of fibre-rich complex carbohydrate.

Protein

Protein is vital to build new tissue and is therefore essential for growth and to repair damage to the body. It is made up of amino acids that are either synthesized within the

Mythbuster: tea and coffee have no place in a healthy eating plan

You don't need to give up tea and coffee entirely to be more healthy, but if you're drinking half a dozen cups a day you ought to cut down. Too much coffee, especially after a meal or when taking a vitamin supplement, can impede the absorption of minerals into the system – particularly iron. This means that behind the instant caffeine buzz you will actually be contributing to longer-term fatigue. Also, to use tea or coffee, particularly with sugar or with a sugary or carb-loaded snack, as a quick pick-me-up may well be allowing you to ignore any underlying nutrition-related causes of your lack of energy during the day. You will find that once you start eating properly you'll have so much more vigour that you'll no longer need all that caffeine. If you are considering giving up tea and coffee, phase it out gradually over two or three weeks, as going cold turkey will lead to bad headaches; also make sure you are eating right to offset the inevitable tiredness.

Fact: The only eating plan that will work is the eating plan you stick to. There is no point in devising yourself such a spartan regime that it becomes impractical to integrate into your life, meaning you either can't go along with it or you resent it so much it won't last long. Go for something that will disrupt your lifestyle as little as possible.

body (nonessential amino acids) or have to be introduced through the diet (essential). Of the dietary protein, all animal protein – found in meat, fish, poultry, eggs and dairy – contains the essential amino acids, as do all soy bean products. But every other example of vegetable protein – whole grains, leafy green veg, nuts and pulses – will only contain some. Therefore vegans can only meet their complete protein needs from eating combinations of foods. It's known as mutual supplementation, and dictates that beans, nuts and wholegrain cereals need to be combined with brown rice to tick all the protein requirement boxes, just as brown rice, whole wheat and nuts need to be supplemented with beans.

Protein deficiency is almost unheard of in developed countries, although convalescents will often need to increase their protein intake beyond the "recommended daily allowance" as it will be in greater demand by the body's healing process.

Fats

Fat is the other good source of calorific energy, but in such a concentrated form that it is very easy to unwittingly overbalance your personal "calories consumed/calories expended" equation with too much fat. There is far too much fat in the American and, increasingly, the British diet, which is making obesity such a problem. Ideally, no more than 25 percent of your daily calorific intake should come from fat, and even less if you have a tendency towards weight gain.

Some fat is crucial to an efficiently functioning system as it is turned into cholesterol in the liver, which promotes cell growth and hormone manufacture, and transports the fat-soluble vitamins A, D, E and K around the bloodstream. Dietary fat takes on four different forms, each of which affects the system in a slightly different way. Saturated fats are the mainstay of cholesterol production – notably "bad" LDL cholesterol (see box on the previous page)

Sell by? Use by? Best before?

These date stamps are not legally required or regulated as part of food labelling, and are there as recommendations rather than tablets of stone:

Sell by is from the manufacturer for the shop's guidance, advising it on the latest it should be on sale. As far as consumers are concerned there will be a few more days – perhaps even a week – left in the product.

Best before indicates at which point the product will start to deteriorate and no longer be at its finest in terms of flavour or texture.

Use by is the product's expiration date and it should not even be kept, let alone eaten, beyond this point. Throw it out.

B

Best investments in your larder:

Garlic

Whether it actually wards off vampires is moot, but garlic will help you in so many other ways it's no wonder it was once believed to have super powers. Garlic boosts the immune system, is a powerful anti-fungal agent, reduces blood cholesterol, assists with blood sugar management and lowers blood pressure. Peel each clove, chop finely and add to food for a kick of warm flavour.

Salmon

Very high in omega-3, the essential fatty acid that raises HDL cholesterol and protects against heart attacks by reducing blood clotting. For a really quick and easy meal, buy some slamon fillets, lightly brush with oil, squeeze a lemon over them and grill.

Black pepper

Use it freshly ground – you should be able to smell the oil being released – and it will help your blood circulation, which also acts as a digestive aid, meaning it will help you get more out of the food that it is added to. Mill over food either at the cooking stage or at the table. Or both.

Spinach and kale

The most nutritiously efficient vegetables, they are practically bursting with vitamins A, C and K, plus they have a very high iron, potassium,

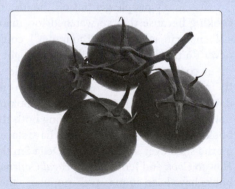

magnesium and folate content. Steam very briefly or eat raw in a salad.

Sweet potatoes

Nutrition-wise, these are higher performing potatoes as they are a fantastic source of vitamin C, carotenoids, potassium and fibre. Wash, but don't peel, and bake or steam exactly as you would a regular potato.

Olive oil

By far the best oil to use, it is so loaded with monounsaturated fats, it works to lower LDL cholesterol. It has a lower burning point than vegetable oil, so don't use it for frying – not that you were going to fry anything anyway.

Broccoli

Masses of vitamins C and A, folic acid and the carotenoids that boost your immune system and protect your cells against "free radicals", molecules that underlie the ageing process, which can lead to cancer. Lightly steam or cut into small florets and eat raw.

Bilberries

A super-performing food that will help reduce the strain on your heart as it eases blood circulation by reducing clotting and clearing deposits from your blood vessel walls. Eat raw or use in the occasional treat pie or muffin.

Tomatoes

An excellent source of vitamins A and C, and rich in lycopene – the chemical that is believed to lower the risk of prostate, lung and stomach cancer. Eat raw in salads, use as a base for stews or soups, or brush with oil, season with salt and pepper and grill.

Walnuts

The superstar of the nut world, walnuts are rich in monounsaturated fats and omega-3 fatty acid. Walnuts also contain chemicals that keep the artery walls clear, lower the risk of gallstones and help the brain function. Eat them as a snack or chop and add to salads.

Don't eat that, eat this!

Avoid in your diet	Include in your diet
Boiled vegetables	Steamed or roast vegetables
Bottled flavourings/sauces	Fresh herbs and spices
Potatoes	Sweet potatoes
Coffee	Green tea
Butter	Low-fat olive oil spread
Fried fish	Steamed fish
White flour products	Wholemeal flour products
Carton juice	Fresh squeezed juice
Fried eggs	Poached eggs
Chips	Jacket potatoes
Sweets	Dried fruit
Fried meat	Grilled meat
Crisps	Nuts
Lager	Red wine

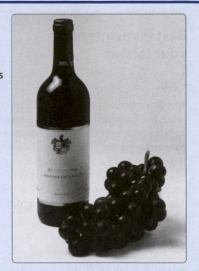

– and are found mainly in meat, dairy and poultry. It is recommended that saturated fats make up less than half of your fat intake. Polyunsaturated fats, found in corn, soy bean and sunflower oils, will actually lower your overall blood cholesterol level, but this is not such a good idea because it also causes your "good" HDL cholesterol levels to drop. Polyunsaturated fat should also be less than half of your fat consumption. Monounsaturated fat is the good guy, as it reduces harmful LDL cholesterol without affecting HDL levels. Olives and olive oil are a rich source of monounsaturated fat, as are nut and vegetable oils. This type of food should make up the majority of your fat consumption.

Trans fat, also known as hydrogenated fat or hydrogenized oil, has risen to great prominence in processed foods recently, especially in the US, and is an acknowledged killer. It is the product of polyunsaturated fats that have been treated with hydrogen to harden the oils in order to make them go further in food manufacture as margarine or shortening. Its potentially deadly side effect is that it will send the LDL concentration in your bloodstream through the roof, while reducing HDL levels.

Food containing trans fats should be avoided at all costs.

Reclaim your kitchen

The basis of any healthy eating plan is having as much control as possible over what is on your plate. The best way to achieve this is to prepare it yourself. If your idea of cooking is microwaving a ready meal, you'll be pleased to discover that the secret of doing it yourself is to keep things simple.

Too many people get put off the idea of cooking because they've watched too many TV chefs in action and thought, "I could never do that". Or, worse still, they bought a tie-in cookery book, attempted a couple of the recipes, which have either gone wrong during the preparation or turned out looking nothing like the picture – meaning both the book and the culinary aspirations have stayed on the shelf ever since. It's why Delia Smith's *How to Cook* and Jeff Smith's *Frugal Gourmet* books have been so massively popular – they don't assume an existing expertise.

Both authors explain the "why" as well as the "what" of food and cookery, and impart a fair amount of the theory behind how it all works. This is far more important than page after page of beautifully photographed recipes, as the key to all cookery is knowing what will happen to a piece of food when you do something to it. It's this basic understanding that will leave you far more likely to get into it. Plus it will allow you to keep things interesting, as you'll have the knowledge to make up your own dishes.

Once you get into the kitchen and start cooking there are keys to keeping it simple. Start off by using ingredients that you already have, because you know you're going to like them and you'll be familiar with what preparation they need. Or only buy new stuff you know you will use again once you've

T *Tip: Wash, under running water, any non-peelable fruit or vegetable you are going to eat raw. You have no idea where it's been, who's handled it and how much pesticide residue remains on its surface.*

opened the jar – nothing leads to resentment in the kitchen quicker than having to buy a big jar of capers and only ever using a teaspoon of them before eventually throwing them away. In the beginning, until you become sure of yourself, adorn food as little as possible, as this will bring out its natural flavour as much as it will save you time and trouble.

Food hygiene

Avoid cross-contamination of cooked and raw food Don't allow them to come into contact with each other on the work surface or in the fridge; use different cutting boards to prepare each; and wash knives and utensils immediately after contact with raw meat, fish or poultry.

Wash your hands after handling raw meat, fish or poultry Do this immediately, as you can transfer bacteria to fridge door handles, work surfaces or your clothes.

Clean up as you go along Keep a sink full of water (so hot you should barely be able to keep your hands in it) for washing up in and so you can wipe down work surfaces frequently.

Keep your fridge cold enough Below 5°C (41°F).

Make sure reheated food is *thoroughly* reheated Do this even if you are in a hurry, as it's all too easy to heat it to a point at which the centre is warm enough for bacteria to multiply but not hot enough to kill them.

Make sure frozen food is fully thawed before you start cooking If it isn't this could interfere with the time it takes to cook and it may not be done all the way through.

Don't put hot food in the fridge It will cause the fridge to work too hard to maintain the correct internal temperature, thus overloading it and affecting the temperature controls. Also the hot food will warm up whatever else is in there.

Cover everything not in use Either in the fridge or on the work surface, as you never know what might be in the air in your kitchen.

Store raw meat, fish and poultry at the bottom of the fridge It will be cooler down there and will also remove the possibility of blood dripping on to any other foods.

Wash your hands before you start touching food You'd be amazed at how many people don't.

B

Best investments in the kitchen:

Steamer

Steaming vegetables rather than boiling them makes sure you keep as much of the water-soluble vitamin B and C content as possible. It also reduces the likelihood of the food overcooking and going limp and tasteless. Steamers are available as self-contained electrical units or traditional models that need to be put on the stove.

Blender

Smoothies, fruit shakes and pured vegetable soups should be part of your healthy eating plan, therefore a blender with a capacity of at least a litre is a must. Look for a model with pulse as well as continuous speeds.

Wok

Used carefully, this large, round-sided pan will allow you to stir-fry platefuls of vegetables without oil or any water, which will retain the maximum vitamin content and cook to a lovely crispness.

Juicer

From a nutritional point of view, juice you've squeezed yourself beats juice from a carton

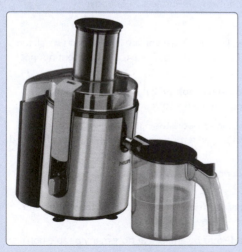

hands down: a juicer is a must. Although a citrus press is a good start, a juice extractor will allow you to blend some very tasty and highly beneficial drinks.

Kitchen roll

We all like fried food and nobody expects you to give it up totally; however, before you put it on your plate, put it on a paper towel to blot up the excess oil.

Sharp knives

Having decent kitchen knives will make cooking much easier and therefore much more pleasurable, which means you're likely to do more of it. Knives that fit your hands and perform specific functions are a must, and keeping them sharp reduces the risk of you cutting yourself as you will have to use less pressure.

Good-quality roasting tray

A tray that distributes heat evenly and doesn't stick will make roasting vegetables a joy. Buy one that can double as a grill pan, with ridges on the bottom to drain fat away from the food.

Coarse-grinding pepper mill

As soon as peppercorns are cracked they start to lose their flavour and nutrients, therefore grind them directly into/over your food to maximize flavour and benefit.

Airtight containers

If you are going to cook in advance or prepare snacks to keep in the fridge you will need to store them. Buy containers that can be used in both the freezer and the microwave for maximum efficiency.

Pastry brush

When grilling – or even frying – food, brush it with oil rather than pouring it on or, worse still, pouring it into the pan. Using a brush can cut around eighty percent from your oil usage.

What's in a name?

If a food product mentions an ingredient as a discrete, stand-alone part of its name – strawberry yoghurt – it must have actual strawberries in it. If, by contrast, it calls itself strawberry-flavoured yoghurt it doesn't need to have any strawberries in it, but the flavouring must have come from the fruit itself. Strawberry- flavour yoghurt, however, can derive its taste from anything, provided it ends up approximating the taste of strawberries. Should the yoghurt have a picture of strawberries on the label, it doesn't have to actually contain the fruit, but the flavour must be derived from it rather than from chemicals. Remarkably, fish or meat that announces itself as "smoked" doesn't have to have been near a fire; it only needs to have been treated in some way to make it taste smoky.

Similarly, a food's country of origin could well be different from the country of processing, yet it may be labelled in reference to the latter: a British pork pie doesn't have to have been made with British pork. It's usually good practice to disregard such terms as "Traditional", "Selected" or "Country"; they are essentially meaningless.

It's always better to cook with a dry heat – on the grill or in the oven – rather than boiling or frying, as they will either dissolve a fair amount of the nutrient content or see it absorb unacceptable levels of fat. Then make sure you cook food for as short a time as possible, as this will preserve flavour, nutrients and texture – if you can eat it raw, do so. Shop regularly and carefully, to make sure what you start off with is as fresh as possible. Don't keep food for too long, even if it's in the fridge, always pay careful attention too the date stamps and use common sense as to when to throw out fresh produce.

But I don't have time to cook healthy food

Of course you do. If you've got time to put a frozen pizza in the oven you've got time to roast a tray of vegetables. If you've got time

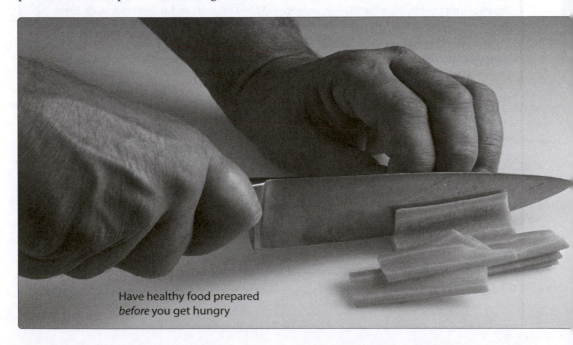

Have healthy food prepared
before you get hungry

to open a carton of juice you've got time to squeeze a grapefruit. If you've got time to fry up a Full English, you've got time to knock up a bowl of broccoli soup. If you've got time to meander around the supermarket picking out ready meals, you've got time to stroll through a street market choosing fresh fruit and veg. And you'll get better banter from the stallholders than you will from the checkout operators. True, cooking from scratch will take more time than convenience food – that's why it's called convenience food – but look upon it as a bit of time spent now to allow you much more time later, as you will surely live longer.

The thing to do is prepare food when you have got time and put it in a covered container in the fridge – then cooking will be relatively quick when you do want to eat. Clean and chop some vegetables for your

Is organic produce really better for you?

The real answer is, frustratingly, "sort of". According to research carried out by the Food Standards Agency in the UK and similar organizations in France and Sweden, there is no solid scientific evidence to say that organic food is more nutritious than conventionally farmed food.But while there is no conclusive evidence that organic food will do you a massive amount more good than conventionally farmed food, it certainly won't do you any harm either.

The organic food movement can be said to have begun in the 1940s, when Walter James coined the term "organic farming" in his book *Look to the Land*, in which he put forward a model of "the farm as organism". But it was in the first decade of the twenty-first century that organic food really took off, becoming an industry worth billions in the US and UK. Organic certification for foodstuffs is tightly regulated: foods must be free of artificial additives and no synthetic pesticides may have been used during their cultivation.

The main big plus of organic fruit and vegetables is that it is kinder to the environment, because the soil is not over-farmed with the aid of chemical fertilizers, and pesticides are not sprayed into the air. Organic farms maintain biodiversity – populations of plants, insects and animals to a much better extent than conventional farms, and they also use less energy and produce less waste.

It is more likely that meat and poultry will have been raised more humanely on an organic farm: you know that the animals you're eating won't have been pumped up with growth hormones. Though you should really look to check if the words "free range" are on the packaging alongside "organic", to make sure that those chickens haven't been battery farmed. It should be mentioned that, in spite of Soil Association regulation, there is good and bad practice on organic farms as well as factory farms.

Agricultural activity	Conventional farming	Organic farming
Promoting plant growth	Chemical fertilizers	Natural fertilizers such as manure or compost
Keeping pests and disease down	Sprayed chemical insecticide	Birds, insects and traps
Killing weeds	Chemical herbicides to target specific plants	Remove by hand, and keep them down with mulch
Refreshing soil	Chemical fertilization	Rotation of fields
Feeding animals	Antibiotics, growth hormones, processed feed	Organic feed, grazing

evening meal while your morning cup of tea is brewing; or make enough soup for a couple of days and ladle it out of a pot in the fridge when you fancy some. Or, as it takes the same time to cook a big casserole as it does a smaller one, cook for more than one meal and freeze the rest – just make sure, if there are several meals' worth, you freeze it as individual meals, because thawing and re-freezing is likely to invite bacteria. Carrying out this batch cooking at times when you have little else to do will pay dividends during busy periods of the week. Also, it's worth noting that regulating your eating patterns will make it much easier to plan meals in advance.

T

Tip: If you are a grazer or like to snack while watching TV or at your desk, prepare yourself with boxes of healthy snacks such as carrots, celery sticks or dried fruit. Anticipate your snack attacks and have the healthy alternatives pre-prepared and ready to be grabbed, because if you have to peel a carrot or trim a piece of fruit when hungry, you'll probably reach past it for something instant such as a bag of crisps.

Three quick, delicious and nutritious dishes

Roast vegetables

Wash and peel (where necessary) a selection of vegetables – what you choose is up to you, but aubergines, courgettes, parsnips, garlic cloves and peppers are a good start. Chop them into five-centimetre pieces; sprinkle with salt and pepper; toss in olive oil and lemon juice; and roast in a hot oven for about thirty minutes, tossing three or

T

Tip: The ideal daily water consumption for a man (as recommended by the US Department of Agriculture) has gone up over the last decades, from between 1.5 and 2 to between 2 and 2.5 litres. This is because of the big increases in air conditioned environments and time spent in front of VDUs, both of which serve to dry out your body.

four times. Sprinkle with chopped flat-leaf parsley and serve.

Ratatouille

Chop up about 250g of tomatoes; slice a large onion; cut three courgettes into centimetre-thick slices; finely chop three cloves of garlic; and combine the ingredients in a saucepan that has a lid. Season with salt and pepper and add a splash of olive oil. Then put the lid on the pan and cook very slowly on a low heat for about twenty minutes, stirring frequently, until it looks like a stew. Serve.

(Either of the above is perfect by themselves or will make a very good-looking accompaniment to grilled meat or fish.)

Vegetable soup

Wash, peel (if necessary) and roughly chop whatever combination of veg takes your fancy – but it's usually a good idea to put some onion and garlic in there. Place in a saucepan that has a lid; season with salt and pepper; add enough water for about two centimetres on the bottom; fit the lid; then cook gently on a low heat for about fifteen

The healthiest shopping trolley & what it provides

Dairy

Low-fat or fat-free yoghurt Iodine, calcium, vitamins B2 and B12, phosphorus, protein.
Olive-oil spread As a substitute for butter, it will reduce the risks of heart disease, diabetes, obesity and colon cancer.
Skimmed milk Vitamins B2, D and K, calcium, iodine (protects the thyroid), potassium.
Low-fat feta cheese Vitamins B6 and B12 calcium, protein.
Eggs Protein, tryptophan (an essential amino acid), choline (a brain-boosting nutrient), vitamin B2.

Meat and poultry

Skinless chicken Vitamins B3 and B6, tryptophan, protein, selenium (an important metabolic catalyst).
Turkey pieces/slices Vitamins B3 and B6, tryptophan, protein, selenium.
Lean beef Tryptophan, protein, iron, zinc, selenium, phosphorus, vitamins B12, B6, B3 and B2.
Lean pork Vitamins B1, B2, B3 and B6, phosphorus, selenium, zinc.
Calves' liver Vitamins A, B2, B3, B5, B6, B12 and C, copper, folate, selenium, tryptophan, zinc, iron, protein, phosphorus.

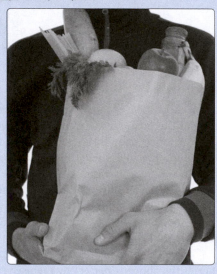

Fruit

Apricots Beta-carotene.
Avocados Cholesterol-lowering oleic acid.
Ruby grapefruit Vitamin C, soluble fibre, lycopene (an antioxidant), cancer-inhibiting limonene.
Kiwi fruit Vitamin C.
Pineapple Vitamins C and B1, bromelain (a digestive aid and an anti-inflammatory).
Figs Vitamin B6, potassium, fibre.
Blueberries Cell-protecting flavenoids, polyphenols (flush toxins and protect the heart).
Raisins Iron.
Raspberries Fibre, vitamin C, cancer-inhibiting ellagic acid.
Cantaloupe melon Potassium, vitamin C.
Bananas Potassium, carbohydrate.
Lemons and limes Vitamin C, cancer-inhibiting limonene.
Mangoes Alpha- and beta-carotene.

Pulses, nuts and grains

Lentils Fibre, protein, iron, folate, vitamin B1, manganese, iron, potassium, tryptophan.
Soy beans Protein, iron, omega-3 fatty acids, fibre, vitamins B2 and K, magnesium, potassium.
Kidney beans Protein, iron, tryptophan, fibre, vitamins B1 and K, magnesium, potassium, folate.
Whole oats Manganese, selenium, fibre, tryptophan, protein, vitamin B1.
Brown rice Manganese, selenium, magnesium, tryptophan.
Wholewheat pasta Complex carbohydrate, fibre, protein.
Walnuts Omega-3 fatty acids, manganese, copper, tryptophan.
Almonds Manganese, vitamins B2 and E, magnesium, tryptophan.
Peanuts Manganese, tryptophan, vitamin B3, protein, folate.
Sunflower seeds Vitamins E, B1 and B5, manganese, magnesium, tryptophan, selenium, magnesium.

Vegetables

Broccoli Vitamin C, beta-carotene, cancer-inhibiting sulphoraphane, immune system-boosting indoles.
Onions Flavenoids (a natural plant antioxidant).
Cabbage/spring greens Vitamins K and C, antioxidants.
Artichokes Fibre, silymarin (a powerful antioxidant).
Squash Vitamin C, beta-carotene.
Sweet potatoes Vitamins A and C, manganese, antioxidants.
Garlic Sulphur compounds that reduce LDL cholesterol, protect against cancer and lower blood-clotting risks.
Chinese cabbage Calcium.
Watercress Vitamins A and C, iron, folic acid, calcium, sulphoraphanes (anitoxidant and cancer-inhibiting).
Spinach Iron, carotenoid antioxidants (immune system boosters).
Tomatoes Lycopene (an antioxidant), coumarins (an anti-inflamatory, blood clot inhibitor).
Aubergines Fibre, chlorogenic acid (an antioxidant and LDL cholesterol inhibitor), nasunin (protects the brain cell membranes).
Green (or red or yellow) peppers Vitamins A, C and B6.

Fish and seafood

Salmon Omega-3 fatty acids, vitamins D, B3, B6 and B12, selenium, protein.
Crab Protein, phosphorous, vitamins B3, B12 and C, zinc and copper.
Sardines Calcium, iron, protein.
Mackerel Omega-3 fatty acids, protein, vitamin D.
Tuna Omega-3 fatty acids, vitamins B1, B3 and B6, selenium, protein, tryptophan.
Clams and mussels Vitamin B12, magnesium, potassium.

Drinks

Cranberry juice Vitamins C and K, fibre.
Green tea Flavenoids; regular green tea drinkers have lower rates of bacterial infection, heart disease, cancer and osteoporosis.
Don't buy orange or grapefruit juice: squeeze your own

Herbs and spices

Root ginger Magnesium, potassium, vitamin C, and is proven to aid digestion and circulation and to work as an anti-inflamatory.
Black pepper Vitamin K, iron, manganese, fibre, antioxidants, improves digestion.
Rosemary Fibre, iron, calcium, improves blood flow to the brain, boosts immune system, is an anti-inflamatory.
Thyme Flavenoids, vitamin K, boosts cell membranes of the heart, brain and kidneys.
Parsley Flavenoids, vitamins C and A, iron, polyacetylenes (inhibits cancer), freshens breath.
Cinnamon Manganese, fibre, cinnamaldehyde (prevents bacterial infection, inhibits blood clotting).

minutes, until the veg is soft. Tip it all into a blender, cover with water and liquidize; return the purée to the saucepan and add water to make it the consistency you prefer; bring to the boil and stir until smooth.

Eating out

There is no reason at all why you can't carry on enjoying restaurants and still eat healthily, provided you follow the same guidelines as you would when eating at home. Make the same informed choices from the menu as you would from the supermarket shelves, to pick a balanced meal. Even if the menu isn't exactly awash with healthy options, there are probably one or two options that aren't boiled beyond their nutritional life or swimming in fat – if there aren't you should consider eating somewhere else.

Don't be afraid to ask a waiter what's in a dish and if they are reluctant to tell you, find another restaurant. Also, if you want something cooked in a certain way, or served without dressing or sauce, most decent places should be happy to oblige. Even if you just want an unadorned salad or plain grilled skinless chicken they should treat it with the same culinary care and presentational flair as anything else. If they won't adapt their dishes on their menu it probably means their food isn't being cooked to order but simply reheated instead – another good reason not to give that establishment your money.

Fast food

You pretty much know what you're getting when you go to McDonald's or KFC or Subway, and you shouldn't be too shocked at the apparent imbalance between calorie and fat content and nutritional value. This doesn't mean abandoning burger or pizza joints for life. Just don't try to live on the stuff – you won't if you've seen Morgan Spurlock's movie *Super Size Me*. Try to follow these guidelines: stay away from anything breadcrumbed and fried – even if it is the healthier-sounding chicken or fish, it will still be a fat bomb. Ask yourself if you really need cheese and bacon; and avoid the sauces and dressings, as they will be minefields of salt and sugar. The good news is that many burger joints are now offering a choice as to how your sandwich is constructed, allowing you to avoid particular ingredients, which is far more relevant to your healthy-eating plan than supplementing a fatburger with a handful of McCarrots.

Sandwiches

Opting for wholemeal when it comes to the bread (or pitta or wrap), ditching the butter in favour of olive oil spread and going easy on the mayo – these are three things that ought to be second nature for anybody on a healthy eating plan. Your sandwich should be all about what's inside it; and that can be as nutritious as you want to make it. Homemade sandwiches are a great option for a healthy

Exactly what it says on the tin

What the label says	What it means
Organic	The food has come from a grower, farmer, processor or importer registered with a DEFRA-approved certification body. Pre-packed meals or dishes labelled organic must contain at least 95 percent organic ingredients. Organic ingredients are those grown or raised without the routine use of chemicals or hormones.
Free range	Only usually relevant to chickens, it means the hens have had continuous access to outside space. In the EU this has to be four square metres per hen; in the US there are no size restrictions.
Natural	This has no legal definition and therefore could mean anything, but the Food Standards Agency maintain it has to fulfil the basic requirements of the Trades Descriptions Act, therefore something calling itself "natural" is unlikely to have been knocked up in a laboratory.
Fat/sugar/cholesterol/sodium-free	The product contains less than 0.5g of fat or sugar per 100g/less than 2mg of cholesterol and below 2g of saturated fat per 100g/less than 5mg of sodium per 100g.
Low-fat/cholesterol/sodium	The product has no more than 3g of fat per 100g/less than 20mg of cholesterol and 2g of saturated fat/or less than 35mg of sodium.
No added sugar	This refers to regular refined sugar such as you'd put on the table; the product may still be sweetened with corn syrup or one of the other sugars such as dextrose, fructose or glucose.
Reduced-fat/sugar/sodium/cholesterol	This is a relative term, and can only be used to compare the item with its regular equivalent in the same range. Then it has to have at least fifty percent less of whatever ingredient it claims is reduced.

lunch if there is little choice locally or decent restaurants are prohibitively expensive. But you must remember to counter-balance the bread with a relative amount of mixed filling. Look upon building a butty in the same way as preparing a nutritionally balanced meal.

Of course, there is an almost impossible amount of choice on the sandwich shelves these days. The big chains selling pre-packed sandwiches usually offer some healthy options as part of their range, and give detailed nutritional information on the labels, allowing you to make your own informed choices. It is worth remembering

A

Expert advice: "Giving into your cravings isn't always a bad thing. Your body has a metabolic memory that tells you what you need by stimulating your desire for foods you've had in the past that contain the nutrients you're now short of."
Dr Sarah Schenker

The best of the web

food.gov.uk
The Food Standards Agency is an independent organization set up to represent the public's interests as regards food safety. They are the force in the UK promoting better labeling on food.

nutrition.gov
The official US government nutrition-dedicated site, packed with detailed, regularly updated information and healthy eating related reports and research.

nutrition.org.uk
The website of the British Nutrition Foundation, which although seeming to be aimed more at healthcare and nutrition professionals offers some very interesting reading. Those who already have a basic knowledge of food nutrition will get more out of it.

soilassociation.org
The body who certify organic producers and will tell you everything you need to know about organic farming, growing and eating.

healthyeating.net
A comprehensive and thoroughly enjoyable healthy eating site, with an emphasis on cooking and fantastic food.

nutritiondata.self.com
You need to register, but once you have this site will calculate the nutrition content of practically any food you care to name; it also offers dietary advice.

that the bread used for the majority of pre-packed sandwiches – whatever colour it might be – will not be nearly as nutritious as the bread you could buy to make your own sandwiches. So be aware that you probably won't be getting a great deal of fibre out of it.

Sandwich shops offer much greater scope for healthy eating than supermarkets, as you can choose exactly what goes in. But as with the pre-packed variety, don't expect to gain much other than carbohydrate from the bread, and always be wary of the pre-mixed fillings, as what is used to bind the tuna or the eggs or whatever together is liable to be inexpensive and bursting with fat, salt and sugar.

Tip: If you are going to eat sandwiches most days, invest in a breadmaker. They are remarkably cheap to buy and simple to use – you can put a loaf of bread on in less time than it takes to make a piece of toast. You choose which flour to use and then you can add fruit, walnuts, olives or practically anything else. The finished product usually works out as costing about twenty pence (forty cents) per loaf. As a bonus, home-baked bread is more substantial and requires more chewing – meaning you will eat less of it.

Ten top tips for healthy eating

▶ **Read food labels carefully**
You may be taking in far less nutrition than you realize.

▶ **Change your diet gradually**
Don't revamp your habits too radically as that will confuse your body and leave you resenting your diet, greatly reducing your chances of sticking to it.

▶ **Spread your nutrition across your whole diet**
Don't attempt to include half-a-dozen superfoods and not worry about the rest; look at getting some sort of benefit from every part of your diet, then vary it to incorporate as many different things as possible.

▶ **Treat restaurants much like you would your home**
Follow the same guidelines you would in your own kitchen and don't be afraid to ask questions or make off-menu requests. But don't take your trousers off, obviously.

▶ **A little bit of what you fancy does you good** Allow yourself a day off a week from your healthy eating plan – you've earned it.

▶ **Eat regular meals, especially breakfast** This will give you far more control over what you are eating as it will cut down the likelihood of your grazing during the day.

▶ **Keep healthy snacks ready**
If you are going to snack, keep a healthy alternative to hand – carrot sticks, dried fruit, satsumas and so on. Do this at home as well as at work.

▶ **A little change goes a long way** Small things like having that quarter pounder without the cheese or holding the mayo on a sandwich will add up to huge long-term benefits for your health.

▶ **Eat more raw food** It will not have lost the nutrients that get destroyed during cooking and the extra chewing involved will make you feel full, faster.

▶ **Keep the cookery simple**
Nothing is more likely to put you off eating fresh food than elaborate recipes and unusual ingredients – dishes such as grilled lean meat, roast vegetables and blended soups take just minutes to prepare and hit you with bags of unadulterated flavour.

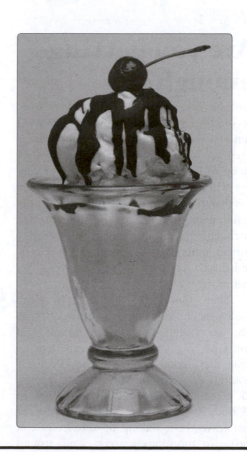

At night $\textcircled{2}$

Ideally you should go to sleep when you feel tired and wake up naturally when your physical and mental systems have completely refreshed themselves. At least that's how it used to work when we lived in an agricultural society and the only clock anybody needed was their body clock. But while this was clearly much better for us, it's unlikely that too many modern men are going to want to do anything as medieval as going to bed at sundown.

Are you getting enough?

Probably not. Sleep requirements vary from person to person, but most adult men need between seven and nine hours' good-quality sleep per night. A small percentage can get by on as little as five or six hours but very few will be able to function efficiently on less than that. However, although these sleep requirements are one of the fundamental, unchanging building blocks of being a human, some sixty percent of men in the UK and the US say they don't get anything like that much.

Then there's the question of sleep quality. A considerable proportion of those who are sleeping for the optimum eight hours per night clearly aren't experiencing sleep that's good enough to be effectively restorative. According to a recent survey, 75 percent of men between the ages of 25 and 50 experience difficulties sleeping that leave them waking up unrefreshed at least two mornings a week. And around half of that number felt so tired during the following days that they believed it affected their mental and physical performance.

These figures shouldn't come as a shock either, as modern society puts such pressures on men that the importance of a good night's sleep has been marginalized in a trade-off to wring more "productive" hours out of every day. Everybody works longer hours than ever before – in the UK people spend longer at work than any other nation in Europe, and in the US the average working week has increased by twenty percent in the last two decades. Men also have far more hands-on involvement in child-rearing and

F

Fact: Twelve percent of all serious road accidents in the UK are caused by tiredness; this figure rises to twenty percent for motorway accidents. That is far more than the amount caused by drink driving.

How it all works: sleep

The strangest thing about sleep is that, in spite of how vital it is to keeping us functioning, science doesn't actually know that much about it. What happens if you don't get enough is well known (see overleaf), as is the fact that sleep restores you to how you were before the day took its physical and mental toll. But how it actually achieves this is much less straightforward.

Growth hormones are secreted during sleep, which aid the repair and renewal of tissue. This is why babies, growing children and adolescents going through puberty need considerably more sleep as that is when their growth and bodily development happens. The notion of "beauty sleep" is because of the cell repair that sleep promotes. The immune system is recharged as we sleep, as the melatonin secreted acts as a strong antioxidant, and neurons within the cerebral cortex are regenerated, effectively refreshing the brain. Also, particularly during the Rapid Eye Movement (REM) periods of the sleep cycle, the brain reorganizes itself by sorting out what has made an impression that day through new connections between the synapses. These fresh pathways generate new, easily accessed memories, and it's believed that these apparently random thoughts being classified accounts for the often bizarre nature of our dreams.

Not all sleep is equally restful sleep, and during each undisturbed eight hours we will go through up to six sleep cycles consisting of four separate stages. Stage one, light sleep, is when the body gets itself into sleep mode by regulating and lowering cardiovascular rates and decreasing body temperature. Stage two is intermediate sleep, when blood pressure is lowered, allowing the body to totally relax, and it's during this period that the brain will be refreshed. Stage three, deep sleep, usually occurs after about twenty minutes and is the most difficult to wake up from. It's during this time that tissue growth and repair happens and our physical energy levels will be restored. Stage four, REM sleep, won't happen until you've been asleep for at least an hour. This is when you dream; the brain is more active and the eyes dart about behind the lids (hence the name). It's during these periods that the hormone cortisol is produced, which promotes alertness. As each REM stage gets longer as the night continues, if we get enough of them we wake up raring to go.

The natural sleep cycle

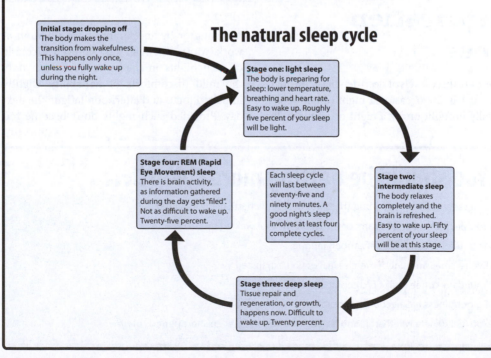

Initial stage: dropping off
The body makes the transition from wakefulness. This happens only once, unless you fully wake up during the night.

Stage one: light sleep
The body is preparing for sleep: lower temperature, breathing and heart rate. Easy to wake up. Roughly five percent of your sleep will be light.

Stage four: REM (Rapid Eye Movement) sleep
There is brain activity, as information gathered during the day gets "filed". Not as difficult to wake up. Twenty-five percent.

Each sleep cycle will last between seventy-five and ninety minutes. A good night's sleep involves at least four complete cycles.

Stage two: intermediate sleep
The body relaxes completely and the brain is refreshed. Easy to wake up. Fifty percent of your sleep will be at this stage.

Stage three: deep sleep
Tissue repair and regeneration, or growth, happens now. Difficult to wake up. Twenty percent.

domestic duties than their fathers did. Then, as members of the post-rock'n'roll generation, we're expected to continue with an exciting social life into middle age and beyond. It's a wonder we find time to get any sleep at all, and at the same time it's hardly surprising that, in some circles, not wasting your time sleeping is seen as some sort of macho badge of courage.

Although total sleep deprivation can, fairly quickly, have a devastating effect on the body (see box on p.42), of far greater concern are the creeping results of getting a couple of hours less than you need most nights of the week. It's this continual sacrificing of proper sleep that is one of the biggest contributors to the general stress levels and the low-grade maladies that are part of everyday life for so many twenty-first-century men.

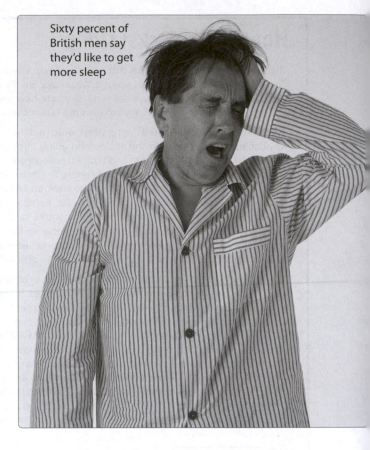
Sixty percent of British men say they'd like to get more sleep

What sleep deprivation does

There are three levels of sleep deficit to consider. The first is the occasional night of bad sleep, usually brought on by a night on the lash, by travelling or by an extraordinary situation at work. Most of us can survive even a couple of such nights in the same week with only the mild discomforts of irritability, slightly impaired focus and afternoon fatigue the next day. Provided such nights don't become too

You should be getting more sleep if…

You seem to catch every bug that's going around, particularly in winter.

You sleep through the alarm or turn it off without waking up.

You suffer crashing late-afternoon fatigue.

Even a small amount of exercise leaves you exhausted.

Your daily coffee intake is creeping up.

Forgetfulness has become noticeable.

You feel generally lethargic and lack concentration for even short periods of time.

regular, they'll do little lasting damage to your health as you can "catch up" the lost sleep by following it with a couple of early nights.

The next level is short-term sleep-deprivation, or acute insomnia. This is usually the result of something clearly identifiable, which can be isolated and ought to have a finite impact on your peace of mind and physical well-being. Among the most common causes are specific stresses such as a death in the family or a divorce, discomfort brought on by an injury or illness, or a problem that needs solving.

If you know you have a situation that may impair your sleeping patterns, make it as easy as you can for yourself by creating the ideal sleeping conditions, as detailed in the rest of this chapter, and try to go to bed earlier, preferably after a relaxing warm (but not too hot) bath. Only resort to medication under extreme circumstances, and then for as short a period of time as possible. If, as is common with this type of sleep disorder, you wake in the night and cannot get back to sleep, don't just lie there willing yourself into the land of nod. You will need to completely relax and this may mean getting out of bed (see box on p.44).

This level of sleep loss will be uncomfortable and will interfere to some

B

Best investment: pillows

A peaceful sleep is a restorative sleep, but that can only happen if your head and neck are properly supported, thus your pillow has to be on the case as well as merely in it. Yet where you lay your head is likely to be the most neglected aspect of your bed. The right pillow for you must offer sufficient support for your head, so that the top of the spine remains on the vertical axis, but the neck is allowed to droop forward slightly, as it would if you were standing up. Yet it should be soft enough to provide that psychological comfort factor. If you sleep on your side, a firmer pillow is recommended as your head will need the most support to stop it from sagging sideways, if you sleep on your back it should be medium-firm, while a front sleeper should go for the softest options so the head isn't pushed higher than the shoulders. The strain on neck muscles resulting from positioning your head too high or too low could be enough to disrupt your sleep without causing noticeable physical pain. Natural pillows mix different blends of down and feathers for, respectively, softness and firmness, while synthetic fillings offer a range of levels of support.

Choose your pillow in relation to your mattress, because the two will have to work in harmony with each other.

Your partner and you may want hugely different things out of a pillow, but as long as you match their cases, what's inside can suit your personal needs.

Don't wait until you renew your duvet or mattress to buy new pillows. Because they have to take the concentrated weight of your head they will wear out far more quickly – two to three years is what you can expect out of a good pillow.

Wash your pillow a couple of times a year – you'll be amazed at how it'll plump back up.

Buy pillows from a specialist bedding store or department, and don't be afraid to try out different types.

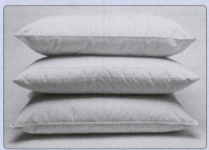

degree with your moods and abilities. Your powers of concentration and judgement will be greatly impaired and you will be far more susceptible to whatever bugs are going around as your immune system will start to suffer. But providing you are aware of your reduced capacities and are appropriately careful it shouldn't have too many long-term consequences. Also, as the causes of this type of impairment are finite, the effects on your sleep should be too.

Where real problems are occurring, especially among men, is with chronic insomnia. This is not always as dramatic as it might sound (i.e. not sleeping at all), as the term covers any form of sleep impairment

A week without sleep

Nights without sleep	What happens to you
One	Not much. The next day you'll be a bit grumpy and probably feel very tired from about four o'clock in the afternoon, but most of us can cope with missing one night's sleep.
Two	The early morning will be particularly difficult as, thanks to how your body clock is set, the urge to sleep will be strongest. You will be constantly irritable and concentration will be difficult. Physical fatigue becomes persistent.
Three	Mundane, automatic or repetitive tasks – driving, typing, operating machinery at work, etc – become very erratic, whereas anything that needs to be thought about actually "wakes the brain up" and gets done, albeit much more slowly than usual.
Four	Reasoning and rational reactions become less likely as the brain loses the ability to inhibit your emotions. Very short-term memory loss will occur – that is the inability to remember events since sleep deprivation began. Physical fatigue is, by now, acute and very uncomfortable.
Five	Speech is slurred, sentences don't flow and problem-solving abilities are falling apart as the brain's neurotransmitters become altered, meaning it is working harder and harder to accomplish less and less. Joints and muscles ache and your immune system will be severely compromised.
Six	The ability of neurotransmitters to function is now so reduced that dizziness and blurred vision will occur, while your sense of who you are – your personality – is becoming rapidly reduced.
Seven	The deterioration of your brain's ability to process thoughts will now be such that you will experience hallucinations and instances of paranoia and delusion.

that lasts for longer than a few weeks. The effects of this condition are similar to those of acute insomnia, but are indefinite and will become progressively worse over time. Then, because the fatigue, the lack of focus and the irritability become constants, they, and the insufficient levels of sleep that led to them, become accepted as a new norm which in turn is encroached upon when circumstance dictates. Long-term, chronic cases of insomnia will leave you with an increased risk of disease and infection as the immune system will be suffering. There is a much greater chance of your becoming obese; your long- and short-term memories stop working efficiently; and there is a much greater likelihood of depression.

While chronic insomnia is often brought on by an underlying physical or mental problem, these days it is as likely to be self-inflicted, with the ill-effects being all but ignored, to the degree that the sufferer believes nothing is actually wrong. If you feel you may be depriving yourself of sleep – that is, you regularly get less than seven hours, need an alarm to wake you and don't feel particularly refreshed in the morning – spend a week going to bed early every night (at least eight hours before you need to get up), not drinking in the evening and following our Ten Top Tips (see p.57).

If you feel much better after those seven nights, alter your sleeping habits accordingly; if it's made no difference then there may be something else wrong. Go and see your doctor, talk frankly and let him or her suggest a course of action.

Knock the nightcap on the head

Because alcohol is a sedative it will help you fall asleep quickly, but it will actively work

T

Tip: Apparently unexplained weight gain may be down to a lack of sleep. Sleep balances levels of the hormones ghrelin and leptin in our brains, which serve to regulate appetite by helping to control when we feel full or hungry.

against you staying that way for longer than a couple of hours. Once metabolized into your system, alcohol disrupts the deep sleep part of the cycle in a number of ways. This applies to more than just nightcaps, and is why, after a night on the booze, you may go out like a light but not feel at all refreshed in the morning.

Alcohol impedes the flow of tryptophan to the brain, which is the source of the neurotransmitter serotonin that is vital to maintaining deep sleep. It then triggers the release and production of adrenalin, which stimulates the brain towards wakefulness. Also – and this is particularly important for diabetics who enjoy a drink – it can lead to a drastic lowering of blood sugar known as night-time hypoglycemia. Under normal circumstances, when blood sugar levels drop, the liver converts carbohydrate reserves into glucose, which it releases

A

Expert advice: "Eating properly and at regular times will greatly help to stabilize sleep patterns and make sleep more restful, as the digestive system will not be working against the body as it tries to relax."
Dr Sarah Schenker

Getting back to sleep

Don't lie there trying too hard to get back to sleep. This conscious attempt to force yourself back to sleep will, in itself, wake you up, then the frustration of not actually managing it will start to stress you out, further contributing to your wakefulness. Get up and read, have a warm drink or do something relaxing until you start to nod off.

Whatever you do, don't have a smoke (in bed or anywhere else). Nicotine is a powerful stimulant, while the almost immediately ensuing withdrawal pangs will further serve to keep you awake.

into the bloodstream as replenishment. However, once the liver detects a quantity of alcohol in the bloodstream, it shuts down any glucose provision while it works to rid the body of this toxin, which can leave blood sugar levels plummeting. This in turn sparks the release of hormones that misguidedly attempt to address the situation by bringing on hunger, which stimulates the brain, disrupting deep sleep.

The drugs don't work either

Sleep medication – either prescription drugs or powerful over-the-counter pharmaceuticals – will never be a long-term answer to sleeping disorders. The majority of sleep medications on the market either go to work on the chemical balance of your brain

or slow down your central nervous system to bring on extreme drowsiness, but all any of them will do is relieve the symptoms of whatever type of insomnia is affecting you, rather than addressing the underlying causes. And their prolonged use – anything more than three or four weeks – can do you a considerable amount of harm.

It is relatively easy to get hooked on sleep medication, physiologically or psychologically (or both), meaning you will suffer withdrawal when you do give it up. Extended use can lead to a kind of hangover effect, in which a residue of the chemicals stays on in your system during the day, causing a continual feeling of drowsiness and a reduced ability to concentrate that feels not unlike chronic fatigue. Drug-induced sleep is never quite as restorative as natural sleep, becoming less so as medication use continues. Eventually the rhythms of your deep sleep become altered and REM sleep

Mythbuster: the older you are, the less sleep you need

The truth is the older you are the less sleep you'll *get*, which is very different. Once a man is fully grown – reached his twenties – he will need the same amount of sleep for the rest of his life. However, by the time he's reached his sixties he'll be getting less restorative sleep each night for a number

of reasons: the body produces less of the sleep hormone melatonin; he will be more likely to feel twinges of pain from joints or muscles; older people are more susceptible to changes in their sleeping environment; and calls of nature are liable to have an increasingly disruptive effect.

This is why so many older people get up so early, and may take naps during the day.

is disrupted, meaning that what you've been taking to help you sleep is, ironically, preventing you from sleeping properly.

That said, sleep medication can be effective in the short term, provided the causes of the sleeping problems are external and finite – such as jet lag, a job-shift change or a death in the family. However, if your sleeping problems are anything other than temporary, consult your doctor and make sure that together you concentrate on curing the insomnia rather than merely treating the symptoms with medication.

Power napping

When the phenomenon of "power napping" first came to public notice it was widely derided as nothing more than a cover for sleeping off a three-bottles-of-wine business lunch. The reality is, however, that taking a couple of short naps – and we do mean short – during the course of the day will go a long way towards reducing stress and keeping your creativity and cognitive powers sharp and focused. Power napping allows the brain to switch off for the duration, and to take advantage of the first two parts of the four-stage sleep cycle (see box on p.39) without sinking into deep sleep or REM sleep. As stage-two sleep re-powers electrical impulses in your nervous system, you will feel mentally regenerated, but without any of the sleep inertia and attendant wooziness on waking that comes with the later stages.

It's something that cats and old people have known for ages; now all you've got to do is get your boss to see it that way.

The secrets to productive power napping

Sleep for between ten and thirty minutes only – much more than that and you will tip over into deep sleep and awake groggy rather than refreshed.

Set the alarm.

Don't even attempt it if you have been drinking coffee all morning, as the caffeine will keep you awake.

Do it in the dark – either close the blinds or, if you've no sense of shame, wear a sleepmask.

Don't try to power nap after a high-fat/high-sugar meal: the energy involved in breaking that down will stop you dropping off.

Avoid power napping in the late afternoon, as you will be far more likely to drop into a deep sleep and not wake up for a while.

Don't get cold. As your body temperature drops when you are asleep and wrapping yourself in a blanket at your desk might be somewhat indiscreet, make sure the room remains warm enough.

Convince yourself, and your co-workers, that you're not just being lazy and that this will ultimately aid your productivity.

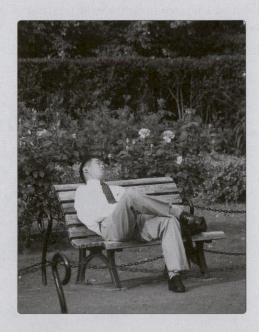

Types of sleep medication

Almost all the available over-the-counter brands contain antihistamine as their main active ingredient, and these products are in no way intended for prolonged use. Using them over an extended period can lead to constipation, forgetfulness, inability to concentrate and problems with your vision. The three most widely used types of prescription sleep medication are:

Benzodiazepines

These are tranquillizers, and work by slowing down the central nervous system. Side effects include continual drowsiness, reduced physical coordination and memory lapses.

Non-benzodiazepines

These increase the effects of gamma-aminobutyric acid (GABA), a brain chemical that inhibits the transmission of electrical impulses within the nervous system. They assist with creating restful sleep patterns rather than putting the user to sleep, and although safer than the benzodiazepines can become addictive. They are also used as antidepressants and as blood pressure regulators.

Melatonin receptor agonists

These hypnotics, such as ramelteon, increase the effects of the sleep chemical melatonin on the brain, thus bringing on drowsiness. Side effects can include nausea, headaches and dizzy spells; these are sleep onset drugs and have little effect on staying asleep.

Herbal helpers

There have been various herbal sleep potions in use since at least the days of the Ancient Egyptians, and many of them still prove popular today. They work by calming nerves and settling anxiety to ensure the taker is as relaxed as possible when trying to sleep. They should be used only as directed. The most effective and widely available are:

Valerian

A natural sedative that reduces cardiovascular rates to ease muscle tension and nervous stress, valerian is taken either in capsule form or brewed as tea. Because it slows the heart rate, you should be very careful not to take too much, and it can become psychologically addictive if you use it for too long.

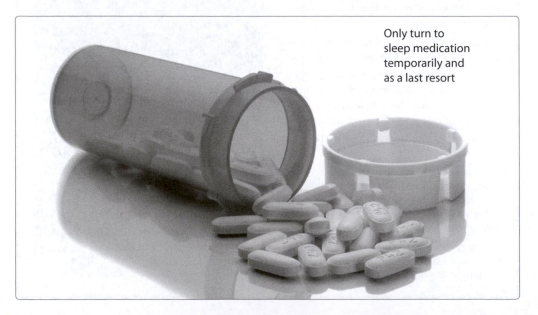

Only turn to sleep medication temporarily and as a last resort

How it all works: circadian rhythms

Better known as the body clock, circadian rhythms are the 24-hour sequences that human beings' lives operate on, evolved to coincide with the day/night cycle of the Earth's rotation. Circadian comes from the Latin words *circa* meaning "about" and *diem* meaning "day". The most basic of these cycles is the one that controls our feelings of sleepiness and wakefulness, coordinating them with it getting dark in the evening and light in the morning.

Although the body's circadian rhythms can be influenced by outside stimuli such as artificial light, noise or temperature, they are endogenously generated – that is, they originate inside the brain. They are triggered by the suprachiasmatic nucleus (SCN), which prompts the pineal and the adrenal glands to release the hormones that bring you in and out of the sleep cycle.

The SCN works on light-sensitive neurological signals originating in the optic nerve, and as the day starts to get dark it activates the pineal gland into production of melatonin, the hormone that promotes drowsiness. As the night progresses it will make sure that melatonin levels within the brain drop. Then when dawn breaks – the brain takes in a great deal of information about light levels through closed eyelids – production is stopped and cortisol is released from the adrenal glands. Also known as the "stress hormone", cortisol increases blood pressure and blood sugar levels and, thanks to the circadian rhythms, will be at its highest in your body early in the morning, when it serves to wake you up.

Signals from the SCN will have caused your heart rate and blood pressure to fall during the night. It will also control other aspects of the sleep/wake cycle, such as appetite suppression during the night, and dropping of body temperature.

It is the disruption of a person's circadian rhythms that brings on jet lag as, for instance, somebody travelling from the UK to New York will "lose" five hours on the real clock but their body clock is still set as it was, meaning an advanced circadian cycle. Thus they will feel tired early in the evening and wake up very early in the morning for two or three days, until the circadian rhythms reset themselves.

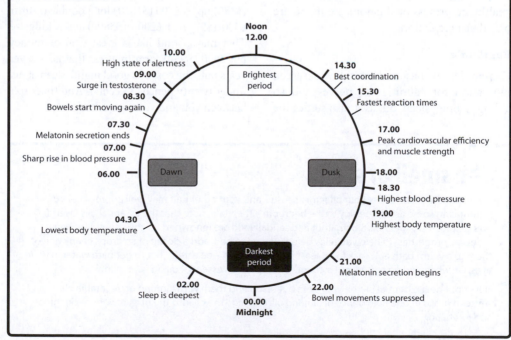

F

Fact: Over the last thirty years, the average height and weight of British men has increased significantly, yet the size of a standard bed hasn't. You may need a queen- or kingsize for you and your partner to get a decent night's sleep.

Passion flower

A very effective calming herb, passion flower is particularly useful if you suffer from periodic limb movement or restless leg syndrome (see p.54), as it will prevent muscle spasms. It is taken as tea.

St John's Wort

This herbal anti-depressant will improve the quality of your sleep rather than send you off, as it boosts the nervous system and calms anxiety. It is taken as tablets or capsules, but you should consult your healthcare professional before use if you are on other medication.

Camomile

Camomile tea has a thoroughly deserved reputation for calming the nerves and so aiding falling asleep, but as it also settles the

stomach it will ease any indigestion that may be keeping you awake.

Reishi mushroom

Often found in Chinese cooking, this wild-looking mushroom has been used in China to combat insomnia for centuries as it lowers blood pressure and has an all-round calming effect. Taken in capsules.

Getting the right mattresses

As you ought to be spending nearly one-third of your life asleep, your bed will be the best-used piece of furniture in your house. Thus paying attention to the mattress is a must.

The most important rule when buying a bed is to buy the biggest that is practical, but what type of mattress you choose (see box opposite) will be a matter of whatever feels best. A good mattress should last between seven and ten years, and will cost from around £200 ($380) up to £700 ($1350) for a double or from £300 ($575) to £2000 ($3800) for a kingsize. That may sound like a great deal of money, but £500 ($950) for a mattress that lasts seven years puts the cost of a good night's sleep at just under twenty pence (35 cents). And that's split between you and your other half.

The smell of sleep

If you want to make use of your olfactory sense – and your other half may well appreciate you introducing some aromatherapy to the bedroom – then take note that the essential oils lavender, orange blossom, spearmint, bergamot and sandalwood are renowned for their soothing, sleep-inducing properties. To help you relax before you go to bed, add a dozen or so drops of any one of them to a warm bath and soak for at least fifteen minutes – be careful not to get bath water in your eyes. Or, when you go to bed, put a couple of drops of an essential oil on your pillow.

Never put neat essential oils on your skin, but first blend them with almond or vegetable oil – fifteen drops in one fluid ounce of almond oil. Massage the oil into the back of your neck, throat and forehead.

At night ②

Type	Internal construction	Properties	Cost
Open-sprung	Rows of hourglass-style interconnected coil springs	The most commonly used mattress, it provides the least independent support as each spring's movement affects those adjoining, meaning couples tend to roll together.	Around £250 ($480) for a standard double
Pocket-sprung	Rows of hourglass-style coil springs, each self-contained in a fabric pocket	Encasing the springs allows them to move independently, meaning a sleeper's movement will have far less effect on their partner.	Around £500 ($950)
Latex	High-density latex foam	Moulds to the shape of the body as it moves, to provide pressure-relieving support; will also be hypoallergenic.	Around £650 ($1200)
Memory foam	NASA-developed viscoelastic	Softens in response to body heat and weight, moulding to your body shape and then holding that impression after you've shifted to allow you to settle back into it, minimizing disruption. This will provide total support while allowing natural movement. Will also be hypoallergenic.	Upwards of £750 ($1350)

However, more for the sake of your back than your wallet, make sure you and whoever else will be sleeping on it try out a mattress thoroughly and at the same time before you buy. Lie down on it together in all your regular sleeping positions, maintaining each one for several minutes. You should feel comfortable and supported and not roll towards each other, and there should be no noticeable sag as you move around or just continue to lie there.

Many mattress suppliers talk about "medium firm" as being the ideal degree of support. What that means is that the mattress holds your spine in the same position it would be in if you were standing up. The lack of support in too soft a mattress means the body bends and its weight forces the spine to sag and curve unnaturally. This leads to interrupted sleep as the body is not able to move or reposition itself so easily, as well

Turn it around

A mattress will last longer and provide better support if it is turned over or rotated every six months. This will stop it wearing unevenly, as it goes a long way to preventing any permanent internal contouring brought about by having the same shapes on it in essentially the same positions night after night. For sprung mattresses, alternate between rotating the mattress (spinning it so the foot becomes the head) and flipping it over (so the top face becomes the underneath). With latex and memory foam mattresses, do not flip over, merely rotate twice a year.

as backache upon getting up because the spine has been allowed to fall out of line, and fatigue in the muscles of the trunk because they will have been working to support you. Too hard a mattress means the only points supported are the heavier ones, and the resistance it gives to the body's weight puts too much pressure on the back as it will not be fully supported. This usually results in lower back pain and over time can lead to chronic backache.

Measurements of mattress support are given in spring gauge and spring count for open- and pocket-sprung mattresses. The lower the spring gauge figure the stronger the springs, thus offering greater support, and the higher the count the firmer the mattress will be. Latex mattresses should be at least nine inches thick; those with a sprung core offer more responsive support, though you will find them to be more expensive.

Sleep like a warthog

About one-third of all men habitually snore loudly enough to disturb their partner's sleep. This figure is much higher among older or

A

Expert advice: "Regular, restful sleep is a vital part of any fitness programme, especially as you get older. Sleep is when your body can repairs any damage done to the muscles by exercise." Gideon Remfry

overweight men, and it compares with about twelve percent of all women.

Snoring occurs at the back of the mouth, where the soft palate, the base of the tongue, the top of the throat and the uvula come together. When you are asleep, and the muscles in the jaw and mouth are fully relaxed, it is easy for this area to collapse to some extent, partially blocking the airway and causing the tissue to vibrate as air passes over it in either direction, creating the snoring sounds. The more the inside of the back of your mouth relaxes, the more it collapses, meaning an even smaller opening and considerably louder snoring.

Mouth anatomy is a major contributing factor to snoring, with a long uvula, a long or low soft palate and enlarged tonsils or

B

Best investment: mattress topper These have been very popular in the US for a long time, and are now starting to make headway in the UK. They are mattress-sized pads, quilted and down- or polyester-filled, that hook on to the top of the mattress, giving an extra layer underneath you. They will provide all-round extra support and, as you sink into it very slightly, give your bed an increased feeling of cosiness. A mattress topper will also extend the life of your mattress as they offer a degree of protection.

Don't buy a mattress topper online; go to a shop where you can physically handle or lie on one.

Wash or dry clean your mattress topper every time you turn your mattress.

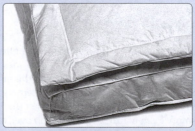

Drinking, smoking and snoring

The two most efficient causes of heavy snoring are alcohol and tobacco enjoyed that evening. The effect of a large amount of drink will be to relax the throat muscles, pretty much guaranteeing some obstruction to the airways. Smoking will greatly increase the likelihood of airway blockage as it causes both catarrh and a swelling of the inside of the throat. The chances of airway blockage will escalate in relation to the amount smoked and passive smokers will be similarly, if not quite so acutely, affected. To greatly reduce your chances of snoring, there should be a gap of at least four hours between your last alcoholic drink/smoke and going to sleep.

adenoids all working to narrow the airway and promote vibration. Boozing, smoking or taking drugs during the evening can have an adverse effect on the throat muscles (see box above), and the overweight are much more likely to snore loudly as layers of fat around the throat will push the sides of the airway in as the muscles relax. Nasal congestion can also cause snoring: partial obstruction will mean you have to pull harder to take in air, thus the tissues at the top of the throat are pulled closer together, increasing the likelihood of vibration. A complete blockage will mean you breathe with an open mouth,

a cause of snoring in itself. Nasal obstruction could be temporary, because of a cold, or a more permanent condition resulting from an inflamed or misaligned septum (the divide between your nostrils), in which case you should see your doctor.

Prevention, not cure

You can't really "cure" snoring, in the same way that you can, say, a sore throat, because it's caused by a set of circumstances creating a particular physical condition: your obstructed airway. All you can do is remove

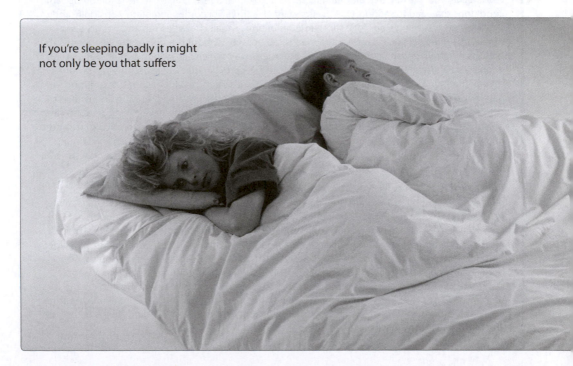

If you're sleeping badly it might not only be you that suffers

as many of the contributing circumstances as possible and work to keep the condition from occurring.

Many people snore simply because their mouth has come open as they sleep on their back, and a widespread remedy for this is to sew a tennis ball or golf ball into a pocket attached to the back of a T-shirt. The discomfort it causes when the snorer rolls onto his back makes it virtually impossible to settle, thus he will shift out of that position. Purpose-built chinstraps – or simply tying a headscarf around your chin with the knot on top of your head – will keep your mouth closed, while nasal strips are a popular option to keep the nose open.

Mandibular Advancement Devices (MADs) are gumshield-like plastic contraptions, worn at night, that fit over both sets of teeth to push the lower jaw and base of the tongue forward, creating a bigger airway opening and avoiding tissue vibration. These are softened in hot water then placed over the teeth and bitten down on to mould to a perfect fit. They are then left to harden on cooling. The upper and lower plates are hinged, and a screw adjustment is made to push the lower half up to 12 mm forward, holding the jaw in that position while you are asleep. These devices can cost between £50 and £100 ($95 to $190), and might not be necessary for every snorer, so seek professional advice before laying out for one.

A more drastic method is surgery, either with the knife or, as is becoming increasingly popular, with a laser. The traditional method involves a general anaesthetic and the soft palate

Obstructive sleep apnoea

Obstructive sleep apnoea (OSA) is the most common form of sleep disorder, affecting five percent of men over the age of thirty, although far fewer below that age. It is an extreme result of the same conditions that lead to snoring. OSA occurs when the airway becomes completely or significantly blocked and breathing stops for a short amount of time, usually between ten and twenty seconds (the word apnoea is Greek in origin and means temporarily without breath). As the sleeper misses breaths they will reposition themselves to open the airway, which can lead to stirring out of a deep sleep phase and into shallow sleep to start the sleep cycle again. Because this can occur several times an hour, it is extremely disruptive to a night's sleep, resulting in tiredness during the day. It also sees the possibility of dangerously raised blood pressure at night as the deprivation of oxygen to the bloodstream causes the heart to pump harder. It can also have a considerable effect on your partner, as the reopening of the airway is usually heralded by a loud explosive snort, and many claim that the person lying next to them regularly stopping breathing is such an alarming situation they are unable to relax enough to get a good night's sleep themselves. The OSA sufferer, of course, has no idea he's doing it.

The OSA sufferer is very likely to be a heavy snorer and, as with snoring, the likelihood increases relative to weight gain. Although the same methods of preventing snoring can be effective in the treatment of OSA, stopping your snoring may not prevent OSA. An increasingly common remedy, especially in the US, is the fitting of a Continuous Positive Airway Pressure (CPAP) device. This is a mask worn over the nose, or nose and mouth, through the night, which is connected to an oxygen cylinder that blows pressurized air into the airway with sufficient force to keep the soft tissue from collapsing and blocking the opening. The obvious drawback with this is that many people feel unable to sleep wearing the mask, but research has shown that those who do find it very successful. CPAPs should only be recommended for people with serious OSA – incidents occurring over twelve times an hour or lasting for more than twenty seconds – and should always be bought and fitted under the advice of a sleep disorder specialist.

Allergy alert

One of the most common causes of snoring is an allergy the snorer didn't know they had. The feathers in a pillow are a very likely candidate, as is the mattress filling or house dust mites in the bedroom.

Try different combinations of: a new foam-filled pillow; a mattress with a couple more sheets; and making your bedroom a dust-free zone by vaccuuming it on a daily basis and wiping all surfaces down with a damp cloth – not forgetting picture rails, door frames and skirting boards. Have your partner keep a snoring diary to find out what works.

and tissue surrounding the airway inlet being trimmed and tightened to prevent vibration. Laser surgery treatment is an outpatient procedure during which the soft palate and uvula are trimmed – this may require more than one session, as the doctor will go on shaving off tissue until the snoring stops.

A very straightforward prevention method, and one that might have an all-round beneficial effect, is a lifestyle change. Lose weight, as the more obese you are the more likely you are to snore; give up smoking, or at least cut down on the cigs; and don't go to bed half-cut.

Try to take it seriously

The thing about snoring is unless you have to sleep with a snorer, it's funny. Snoring has been a comedy staple since before movies had sound, and we seem to have been programmed from childhood to snigger at the sight and sound of somebody "sawing logs". Add to that the fact that most snorers – quite naturally – have no idea they're doing it, and it's often difficult to get them to fully appreciate how seriously disruptive it can be to domestic life. So if your partner tells you you've got a snoring problem, take their word for it and do something about it.

Sleepwalking guy

Somnambulism is another comedy failsafe, although in real life sleepwalking is seldom as widespread, consistent or as disruptive as snoring. Most is fairly trivial, a matter of getting up and walking around for a bit – often not leaving the room – then returning to bed. Occasionally, sleepwalkers will perform complex tasks or negotiate involved journeys – it's not unheard of for sleepwalkers to be found behind the wheel of a car. Although a sleepwalker's eyes will be open they will be unseeing, and this trance-

Mythbuster: waking a sleepwalker will give him a heart attack

Because sleepwalking usually occurs in the deepest phases of the sleep cycle, sleepwalkers will often start or jump quite violently (which is where this notion comes from) and be confused or disoriented. Should you wake one, be prepared for them not to know who you are or where they are. However, it isn't by any means necessary to wake a sleepwalker, as many will get back into bed and remain unaware of their night-time excursion. You may want to gently, but firmly, guide them back into bed.

like state is actually REM sleep. This is why sleepwalking is far more common among children, as their sleep-cycle involves a greater proportion of deep sleep than adults'. It has never been scientifically established that sleepwalkers are acting out dreams.

Much sleepwalking in adults is stress-related, which means you are possibly already having shallower, less restful sleep. Other major contributors are a chaotic sleep pattern or irregular sleep habits. Excessive alcohol can be a factor too, and a

Common sleep disorders

Disorder	Symptoms	Causes	Self-help
Restless leg syndrome	Uncomfortable twinges within the legs, creating the urge to move them; involuntary leg movement. RLS can occur before you fall asleep.	Stimulants before going to bed; smoking; very sedentary lifestyle.	Stretch or massage your leg muscles; take a warm (but not too hot) bath; take regular exercise such as walking, running or cycling.
Sleep paralysis	Inability to move experienced upon waking up or as you fall asleep; attacks usually last less than a minute. About fifty percent of all adults are believed to have been affected by it at some point.	A momentary disconnect between the brain and the body.	Although it can be frightening, sleep paralysis is harmless, but it cannot be prevented as it occurs randomly; nothing can be done about it other than to keep calm.
Narcolepsy	Drowsiness or even falling asleep during the day; disrupted and non-restful night-time sleep.	Science is unsure of what causes narcolepsy, but the most popular theory involves a chromosome disorder leading to a deficiency in sleep-controlling hormones.	Sufferers should seek professional help, and will most likely be prescribed a stimulant to keep them awake during the day, and thus promote deeper sleep at night.
Periodic limb movement	Cramping or rapid, involuntary movement of the limbs. (Not the same as restless leg syndrome, as PLM occurs only when the sufferer is asleep.)	There is primary or secondary PLM – the former occurs randomly, the latter is liable to be the result of an underlying condition – commonly diabetes or anaemia; it can also be a symptom of OSA or narcolepsy.	Most primary PLM sufferers require no treatment as it is widespread and harmless; if it is a symptom of another problem, that should be treated.

drunkard's disrupted sleep cycle can promote sleepwalking – a big problem with drunk sleepwalkers is urination in inappropriate locations.

Habitual sleepwalkers (more than once or twice within a couple of weeks) should make sure they are as relaxed as possible and totally prepared for a good night's sleep before going to bed (see box on p.57). Regular sleeping schedules and patterns will help to organize your sleep cycle more effectively. You should only need to seek medical help if, after bringing in these corrective measures, the night-time excursions persist.

Expert advice: "Men should take a more proactive approach towards sleep and make proper time for it. Sleeping well is as important as eating well, it's not something that happens when there is nothing else to do."
Dr Liliana Risi

Dream a scary dream

Nightmares occur only during REM stage sleep and will often invoke such a state of fear, panic or anxiety within the sleeper they will wake him or her up. Whether the sleeper remembers all or some of what scared them so much in the dream is as likely as it is not, but they will be aware of something wrong and therefore could wake in a state of panic. While nightmares are really little more than the brain rooting out some upsetting memories, as they are being dreamed they will feel very real, and should be addressed if they start to occur too often.

Nightmares are very prevalent among children, when they are considered a normal aspect of development, but in adults frequent – more than once a week – or recurring nightmares are a sign that all is not what it should be. Because you have no control over your dreams, the most immediate way to treat nightmares is to work out what is causing them and try and deal with that. The reasons behind them usually fall into one of two categories.

Mythbuster: cheese gives you nightmares

On the contrary, a small amount of cheese as a late-evening snack might actually help you sleep. As a dairy product, cheese is rich in calcium which will promote a feeling of calm. It is also a fairly good source of the amino acid tryptophan, which serves to calm the brain itself and so reduce stress levels to aid falling asleep.

The idea that eating cheese late at night causes nightmares is thought to date back to a 1950s health scare when it was believed – but never unequivocally proved – that the tyramine (another amino acid) in cheese was reacting with a popularly prescribed antidepressant to cause mild hallucinations, which manifested themselves as particularly vivid dreams.

Or perhaps it goes back even further, to the nineteenth century, when Dickens' Ebenezer Scrooge blamed his *A Christmas Carol* adventures on, among other things, "a crumb of cheese".

The best of the web

sleepfoundation.org
A US site discussing all aspects of sleep and with an e-newsletter and listings of specialist sleep centres and units within hospitals.

sleepnet.com
Another US site, with a lively sleep-related forum, and comprehensive links to sleep specialists both online and in person.

britishsnoring.co.uk
The website of the British Snoring & Sleep Apnoea Association, offering instant diagnosis and help, plus a wide range of anti-snoring products and personal consultation at their Surrey HQ.

sleepdisorders.about.com
A good starting point for investigating a wide range of sleep disorders in much more depth than most websites.

sleeping.org.uk
The membership website for the British Sleep Society, a registered charity aimed at healthcare professionals and dedicated to improving their understanding of sleep-related matters.

sleepcouncil.com
A British organization seeking to raise awareness of the importance of sleep. The website has many useful tips and a link to the Insomnia Helpline (020 8994 9874).

Inner stresses

The majority of nightmares occur around a stressful event in your life, and as that situation recedes in prominence so the dreams should stop. Such an event could be bereavement, or a problem at work, or the breakdown of a relationship, but reacting with the occasional nightmare is not a sign of any acute problems. Talking to friends and family about your anxieties will help, as will any of the methods for getting a good night's sleep described in this chapter.

More serious are the nightmares associated with post-traumatic stress, as the same situation can recur in a dream as the sleeper relives whatever awful events they were caught up in. This will need to be addressed with counselling and psychotherapy, therefore professional advice must be sought. Recurring nightmares can also be a result of undiagnosed depression, and if you think this might be the case, you should talk to your GP about it.

Extraneous influences

Regular heavy drinking is a prime suspect for causing frequent nightmares, as alcohol is a depressant and thus is very likely to have a negative effect on dreaming. An abrupt withdrawal from alcohol can lead to nightmares too, simply because that process results in anxiety, jumpiness, mood swings and poor sleep patterns. Suddenly giving up drugs – whether street drugs or prescription drugs – can have the same results, as it will throw the system in much the same way.

It could also be that the side-effects from drugs prescribed for another condition are behind your nightmares – beta blockers, antihistamines and appetite suppressants are often likely culprits. If your nightmares coincide with a course of prescription drugs, see your doctor immediately.

Ten top tips for sleeping better

▶ **Keep your bedroom exclusively for sleeping (and sex)** It contributes hugely to your sense of relaxation if in your mind your bedroom has no other associations than rest and sleep. And sex, obviously.

▶ **Sort out your bed** It's no wonder the most cited reason as to why a man prefers staying at his girlfriend's rather than her coming to his place is because "her bed smells so nice". Crisp, fresh bed linen, calming aromas and a general sense of sanctuary will let your body know you are serious about sleep.

▶ **Maintain your bedroom at a slightly lower temperature than the rest of the house** Ideally, you should aim for 15–18°C (60–65°F), as your body temperature will drop, and if the room is too warm it can work against you.

▶ **Make it as dark as possible** Your body is programmed to sleep when it's dark and be awake when it's light. As light can seep through the eyelids you should eliminate all light sources from the room – this includes LED clocks.

▶ **Don't watch TV in bed** If you do so until you fall asleep, your brain will be overstimulated, and this will delay your dropping off and make deep sleep harder to come by. Do something relaxing like reading or listening to soothing music instead.

▶ **Don't drink just before bedtime** Although alcohol's sedative powers will relax you, it will also disrupt your sleep a few hours later.

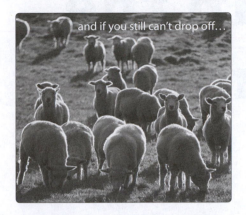

and if you still can't drop off…

▶ **Keep to as regular a routine as possible** It's recommended you go to bed and wake up at the same time every day, or as near as possible, because to drastically change those hours, even over the two days of the weekend, could be enough to reset your body clock.

▶ **Avoid a large or, worse still, spicy meal within two hours of bedtime** It will bring with it the likelihood of indigestion which will play havoc with your sleep patterns, and a full stomach is likely to increase pressure on the bladder.

▶ **Take regular exercise** Being physically tired at bedtime will always help you fall asleep, but don't exercise just before turning in as the increased blood flow will make you more alert, adrenalin will still be pumping around your system and your body temperature will be much higher than is conducive to dropping off.

▶ **Stay away from late-night stimulants** This isn't just cocaine and speed or tea and coffee; nicotine too is a powerful pick-me-up. Then don't forget that chocolate contains small amounts of theobromine, a stimulant in the same chemical family as caffeine.

In the mirror

Look good, feel good: it's always easier to be more confident about the world in general when you like what you see in the mirror. These days, not only is the world more hung up on what you look like but, thankfully, there has never been so much on offer to help you stay bright-eyed and bushy-tailed.

The skin you're in

A decade or two ago, the notion of a man with a skincare regime would've led to all manner of sniggering about his sexuality. These days, although it's still far from the norm for men to cleanse and moisturize with the same enthusiasm as their female partners, an increasing number are recognizing the benefits of skincare. Which isn't really surprising. Once you realize that flawlessly fresh-faced individual looking at you out of the mirror is the same man the rest of the world sees, it can be quite a boost to your self-esteem.

Healthy on the outside starts from the inside

The best thing you can do to achieve healthy, glowing skin is to drink at least two litres of water per day. It's as simple as that.

Sufficient water intake should be the basis of all good skincare routines, as it keeps your entire system hydrated. This allows nutrients to be absorbed, helps blood to circulate, flushes out toxins and prevents constipation. But most importantly, as human skin is around ninety percent water, it will make sure yours remains at its optimum, leaving it soft and radiant-looking.

Mythbuster: eating chocolate gives you acne

Diet has very little effect on acne, as its causes are mostly hormonal (see opposite) and its likelihood hereditary. Although eating huge amounts of oily or greasy food can manifest itself in extra oil on your skin and hair, even this isn't enough to cause acne, so a few bars of chocolate definitely won't make a difference.

How it all works: spots

Blackheads are not caused by dirt from outside getting under the skin, but a mixture of the naturally produced oil called sebum and the protein keratin getting trapped within a hair follicle to form a blockage. This will then get its colour from skin pigment (melanin) dissolved in the oil, which rises to the surface of the blocked opening. Whiteheads are the same accumulation of sebum and keratin without the dissolved melanin, and are formed at the surface of an already closed follicle.

Spots are a side effect of being run-down or constipated, as your system will not be functioning properly and toxins are not being shipped out. Although keeping your skin cleansed and exfoliated will help keep spots at bay by removing potential pore-plugging dirt and dead skin, the prime causes of pimples come from within.

Acne is an outbreak of blackheads, whiteheads or cysts caused by the excess of sebum produced in the hair follicles creating blockages and eruptions under the top layer of skin. It happens in adolescent boys as, during puberty, a surge in the male sex hormone androgen causes the production of sebum to go into overdrive, meaning the hair follicles can't get rid of it all via their usual natural processes. The problem usually clears up in your twenties, and the chances of full-blown acne lessen as we get older, but it can be triggered by high stress levels or continued use of anabolic steroids, as in each situation the adrenal gland will increase androgen production.

Although popping a zit is one of the most satisfying of cosmetic procedures known to man, it is also one of the worst for your overall complexion. Squeezing a spot will open up the follicle and push sebum and melanin out towards the mirror, but the same action will also push a percentage of it back into the adjacent tissue, resulting in a bigger, more painful spot. Instead, release blackheads and whiteheads by gently stretching and manipulating the skin around them to create an opening big enough for the oil to flow out.

An excess of oil can build up to form a blockage at the outer layer of skin

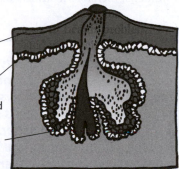

Outer layer of skin, mostly dead cells

Layer of new skin, where cells are formed

Sebum is produced in the hair follicle

Broadly speaking, the best diet for healthy skin is the same as it would be for overall health – cut out the junk food and excessive fat; maintain a good balance of vitamins, minerals and protein. To concentrate on healthy skin, however, vitamins C and E protect from sun damage, and thus inhibit premature ageing; vitamin A contributes particularly to keeping skin moist and also promotes quick healing; while the B vitamins

F

Fact: If you wash your face with soap, make sure it's a gentle soap recommended for the job rather than the same bar you'd wash your body with. General purpose soap is too strong for your face and will dry it out by stripping away its natural oils.

F *Fact: Constipation will show up on your face in the form of spotty or blotchy skin, as toxins usually removed through the digestive tract remain floating about in your body.*

T *Tip: When shopping for an exfoliating scrub go for those with the finest grains – the more expensive brands – as they will be the most gentle. The large grains in cheaper scrubs can damage lower layers of skin and leave it feeling raw.*

form the basis of skin cells and help with circulation. Iron will give you a healthy, even skin tone; omega-3 fatty acids, found in fish and some seeds, will help regulate your skin's moisture; and fibre transfers toxins – which would otherwise show up in your complexion – out through the digestive tract.

Real men exfoliate

Men's skin is about fifteen percent more oily than women's, therefore it attracts more dirt;

A *Expert advice: "Having plenty of sex can work as a bit of a beauty treatment, as it does wonders for your complexion in terms of keeping you looking younger. Because, during orgasm, you're in heightened sensitivity, there is a rush of blood, which means the blood vessels near the skin's surface are receiving more oxygen, which speeds up repairs to the cells in the skin. Research was carried out over time at the University of Caerphilly discovering that, among a thousand men and women, the ones that had sex at least three times a week looked ten years younger than those who didn't."*
Sarah Hedley

men also have bigger pores than women, so the dirt gets deeper into their skin more quickly. All of which conspires to mean that men have a far greater need to do a bit more than splash on the soap and water a couple of times a day. To keep your face looking fresh, the basic and most effective step is simply to expose the healthy skin by removing what is covering it up. This has to be done sympathetically, though.

Cleanse your face on a daily basis – last thing at night is ideal – with a cleanser recommended for your skin type. You may need to experiment before you find the right one – importantly, it should be formulated for men as that means it will be a little stronger. Soak a piece of cotton wool with the cleanser and rub gently over your face, then be amazed at the amount of dirt that comes off. Getting rid of this gunk removes the smaller particles that may clog your pores, and will take off the fine layer of grime that was dulling your complexion. In the morning, wash with warm water – not too hot or it may damage your capillaries – and facial soap.

Exfoliating needs to be done once a week, and it involves rubbing your face over with a mix of a grainy scrub and water, allowing the mild abrasion to lift off the layer of dead skin cells. This is an incredibly effective procedure, as to regularly remove this complexion-clouding layer will give your face an even, flawless appearance, probably knocking a few years off your age. After you have exfoliated there is no need to cleanse.

Following either cleansing or exfoliating, always moisturize your skin to replace natural oils removed by these processes. You will need to experiment to find which moisturizer is best for you, and how much you need to apply, but, like the cleanser, go for those formulated for male skin. Some moisturizers contain subtle bronzing agents, which is a safer way to get a suntan than lieing under a sunbed.

Smoker's skin and other self-inflictions

A sure-fire way for the skin on your face to look older than your years is a forty-a-day cigarette habit. Smoking activates the enzymes that break down collagen, the protein that provides elasticity to allow skin to remain taut as it moves. Without this it becomes loose and starts sagging, losing any natural glow to appear lifeless and prematurely aged.

Boozing won't help your complexion either, as the dehydrating effects of alcohol when drinking heavily will undermine the good work done by all that water you've been taking in. The result will be that your skin will dry out; it can also leave you with a permanently red face, as alcohol dilates the capillaries in the cheeks and nose to leave that angry-looking flush – a prime example being that sported by W.C. Fields. Excessive tiredness – another side effect of heavy drinking – can adversely affect your complexion, too. The skin cells repair themselves most efficiently while you sleep, and if you're not getting enough proper sleep then cell damage will start to show in the form of blotchiness and dry patches.

Ironically, although a decent tan is seen as a sign of good health, there's nothing particularly desirable about exposing your skin to intense sunlight. Ultraviolet radiation – UVA and UVB – is the main cause of premature ageing of the skin and skin cancer. It breaks down collagen to

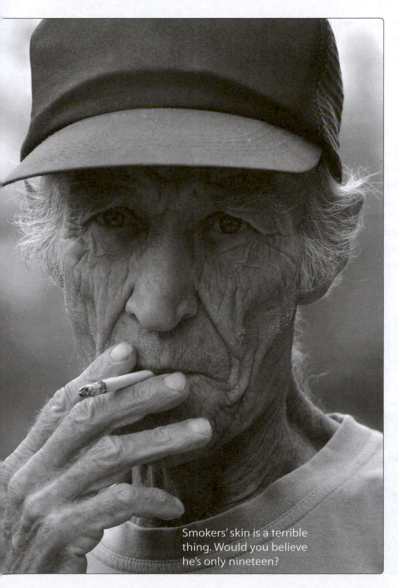
Smokers' skin is a terrible thing. Would you believe he's only nineteen?

Sunbeds: a safe option?

Now that the dangers of excessive exposure to ultraviolet rays have been widely acknowledged, responsible tanning salons limit the length of sessions to around five minutes. However, while it is claimed that sunbeds are much less risky for your skin than open-air sunbathing – because the doses of UV rays are regulated in terms of intensity and duration – a BBC report maintained that frequent sunbed users were 75 percent more liable to develop skin cancer and display signs of premature ageing. These findings support the view held by the majority of dermatologists: that any extra UVA and UVB radiation is an unnecessary risk, and that people who use sunbeds still go out in the sun. To this end, the only relatively safe tan will be the one you can buy in a bottle.

reduce elasticity and cause wrinkles, while promoting the formation of free radicals that can cause cancer by changing the genetic make-up of the skin's cells.

Shaving

Probably the most chore-like of our morning rituals, but also probably the most important. Looking unshaven is one of the few things we can't cover up and surveys have revealed it's the first thing job interviewers have noticed about a male candidate. It's also reckoned to be a turn-off for your partner in the bedroom and will be a cause of growing irritation throughout the day.

The closest shave

Use each razor blade or cartridge no more than four times and throw away disposables after one use, as they will no longer be sufficiently sharp. Rinse your face with hot water before lathering up, as this will soften your beard and make it easier to cut, but wash with cold water after shaving, as it will close your pores and move blood away from the skin surface to minimize any post-shave swelling or tenderness. Take your time, and leave the gel or cream on your face for at least a minute before starting in with the razor, as it will take that long to fully soften your beard.

Once you get the razor going, go over your face twice: the first time lightly and with the grain; the second time against it and slightly firmer, but don't press so hard it feels like it's dragging. Shave by feel rather than look, as your fingertips are the best judge of whether your face is smooth or not, and don't use a razor with a lubricating strip, as it will give a false impression of what your face feels like.

T

Tip: Shave after you've showered, as your beard will have been softened by the water and the steam in the bathroom. If the mirror is steamed up, there are products you can apply to it to keep it clear available at most pharmacies.

T

Tip: If your aftershave stings your skin with more than a mild tingling, it is too strong for you and is irritating your skin into tiny swellings. Switch to something without either alcohol, peppermint or citrus, or, better still, use a soothing, moisturizing cream.

To remove an ingrowing hair

Carefully release it from below the surface, using fine tweezers and a magnifying mirror. Then, once the end is free, do not pluck it out as it will grow back under the skin. Instead, leave it and shave as recommended in this chapter. Once a hair has been released, dab the area with witch hazel to treat any swelling or irritation.

Getting the bumps

Shaving or razor bumps occur when the shaved end of a hairshaft gets trapped inside a hair follicle and as it continues growing it presses up against the underside of the skin. This can cause painful "bumps" and a rash-like reddening of lighter skin. Men of African and African-Caribbean descent are far more prone to shaving bumps than Caucasians, as their hair will not grow straight, and therefore is more likely to turn inwards or sideways; also it is generally stronger, thus will push harder against the skin.

If you suffer from razor bumps, guard against them by taking the following steps:

Keep your skin in tip-top condition by exfoliating every day, using a soft facial brush rather than your fingers. A circular motion with the brush will remove dead skin cells, and clear away any dirt or grease blocking follicles, allowing hairs to grow beyond the skin's surface. Do not use a scrub that contains abrasive particles, though, as these can actually impede follicles. Opt for one with salicylic acid, a powerful exfoliant.

When shaving, use gel or cream with a large amount of moisturizer in it; avoid shaving foam as it tends to dry out the skin. Moisturize after shaving, and do not use post-shave products that contain alcohol, as these will close the follicles and dry the skin. Don't shave extra-close; if the hair is so short it momentarily pulls back beneath the skin after it has been cut, there is an

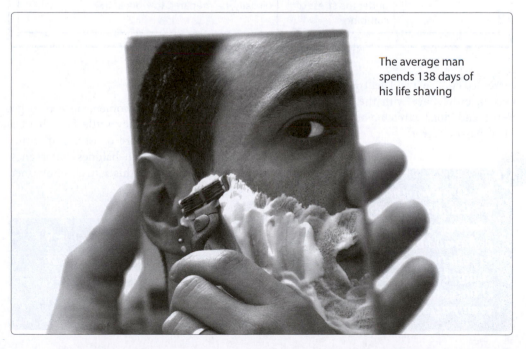

The average man spends 138 days of his life shaving

Get your hair right

Hair type	Particular problems	Remedies
Dry	Frequent breakage due to the lack of natural oils, making it brittle	Change hair care regime to use milder products and less frequently; avoid blow-drying or alcohol-based treatments; use products containing vitamin B; increase essential oils in diet.
Oily	Hair looks lank and wet; oil gets on clothes and skin	Wash daily with a mild shampoo; cut down on combing or brushing; reduce oil in diet; rinse with products that have lemon juice or vinegar bases.
Curly	Gets very dirty; becomes dry and brittle	Wash it daily; air dry, combing backwards with a large tooth comb; do not brush; apply a light oil daily.
Fine	Looks limp; is difficult to style	Use products with a protein or vitamin B base; wash and rinse in hot water to stimulate follicles; use a heavier gel for styling.
Thick	Tangles; has a hard feel to it; has a mind of its own	Wash three times a week, with a shampoo with no vitamin B or protein; pat semi-dry with towel, then apply low heat – from a distance – while brushing in the direction you want it to lie; avoid gels or mousse as they will increase its body.
African/African-Caribbean	Tendency to dryness; brittle and breaks under the stress of combing	Wash frequently; air dry, combing out gently; use products containing B vitamins; apply specialist oil daily; be prepared to work at it.

increased chance it will get trapped. For this reason, only shave with the grain of your beard and don't stretch your skin as the razor passes over it.

T *Tip: Once your hair is thoroughly wet, rub the dollop of shampoo in between your palms and then apply them to your head – if you whack it straight on to your hair, the chances are it won't distribute evenly across your scalp.*

Heads up

It's said that, unlike women, once men get past their twenties they settle on a haircut and stick with it, more or less, until either death or male pattern baldness intervenes. But whether or not this is true, most men

T *Tip: After swimming in a chlorinated pool, always wash your hair with shampoo and then rinse thoroughly before applying conditioner.*

T

Tip: Don't wash your hair while sitting in the bath because you will be rinsing it off in the dirt you've just washed out of it. This will make it very difficult to achieve any sort of shine.

T

Tip: If you have normal or oily hair and, during the summer, the sun is drying it out, treat it as dry hair for that period.

will feel more confident about life in general if what's going on above their eyebrows is the absolute best it can be.

Hair health

Healthy hair is, essentially, a contradiction in terms, as by the time a hair shaft has poked its way above your scalp it's already dead. What sort of shape it's in, however, represents a pretty accurate reflection of your general state of health. If you are in fine fettle, taking on a good balance of vitamins and minerals and drinking the requisite two litres of water each day, your hair will display this fact to the world; but if you are run-down or deficient in nutrients, you locks will bear witness to that too.

Of course, what you do to your hair will have a huge effect on what it looks like and

how long it lasts, but it will always have a much better chance if you are healthy to start off with.

Hair dos and hair don'ts

A simple approach to hair care will always be the best. Adding gel or styling mousse will be a matter of choice, but one that should only be taken once the hair itself is in tip-top condition.

How often you should wash your hair depends on your daily routine, your environment and how much styling product you use. It may need washing every day – if you work out daily, get filthy at work, or use a lot of styling products – or it may not warrant it more than once a week. But the more it gets washed the milder the shampoo you should be using. Stronger shampoos will strip the hair of its natural proteins and oils; if this is happening too regularly the hair

Making a stink

Sweat doesn't actually smell. Body odour comes about when sweat hangs around on the skin allowing bacteria to feed on it, causing it to break down into the aromatic fatty acids which produce that unpleasant odour. The groin and armpits will be the main culprits, as the glands in those areas produce the oils and proteins the bacteria thrive on, as opposed to the rest of the body which will, largely, sweat salty water. Your feet will have their own unique ripeness because as well as producing the bacteria-friendly oils and proteins, being shut away in warm, dark, unventilated socks and shoes breeds fungus that will add to the stench.

Stopping the stink is a matter of inhibiting sweat production in those areas so that the bacteria has less to feed on and regularly washing with antibacterial soap – this will not be the same soap you should be using on your face – to remove old sweat and any developing cultures. Dirty clothes are a breeding ground for bacteria, which feed on the sweat that has dried into the fabric. Feet should be dried thoroughly after washing and dusted with antifungal powder; take your socks and shoes off as often as is politely possible, to allow them to air.

F *Fact: The life of the average male hair is between three and five years, growing between one and two centimetres per month. It grows faster at night than during the day and accelerates when the weather gets warm.*

T *Tip: Always keep the hairdryer moving as it is very easy to damage your hair or burn your scalp without realizing – a burnt scalp may not hurt but the hair follicles will be damaged and dried out, thus more oil will be released in that patch to compensate.*

won't regenerate these elements and will become lacklustre and brittle. Conditioning after each wash – or using a shampoo with a built-in conditioner – replaces these natural oils, and will form a protective barrier against the hair drying out or getting damaged by its environment.

When washing, pay particular attention to the hairline at the front of your head, the nape of your neck and the area just above your ears, as these areas tend to attract the most dirt yet get the least attention during shampooing. Work the shampoo in gently with your fingertips, remembering that your

hair is most vulnerable when it's wet, leave it for a minute or two, then rinse under clean, warm (not hot) running water. After this, rinse once more and rinse again – the most common reason for people having lifeless-looking hair is that all the shampoo, and thus all the dirt, hasn't rinsed away.

If you are only washing your hair once or twice a week, it's probably best to repeat the shampooing stage.

If you are applying conditioner, dilute it in a cup instead of putting it directly on

M

Mythbusters: baldness balderdash

Hanging upside down cures it This theory assumes that increasing the blood flow to the scalp and the hair follicles will stimulate hair growth. But there is no scientific evidence whatsoever that you will experience anything other than dizziness.

Stress makes your hair fall out It won't, but it may make it vanish faster if you were going that way anyway. This is because of the general low physical condition you'll be in because you are stressed.

Baldness skips a generation This is based on the disproved idea that you inherit the

baldness gene solely from your mother, who can only have got it from her father.

Masturbation as a boy will cause baldness as a man It won't make you go blind, either.

Bald men are more intelligent A myth perpetuated by the film and TV industry which, for a long time, has used the image of a balding, bespectacled "egghead" as visual shorthand for intellectual.

Bald men are more virile This idea is due to the baldness gene being linked to the male sex hormone, but there is no proof of this whatsoever. However, if it's what women believe then it's little wonder slapheads aren't arguing with it.

Eat your hair healthy

Complaint	Dietary cause	Remedy
Dry hair	Lack of essential fatty acids	Oily fish; seeds – particularly flaxseeds and pumpkin seeds; olives; nuts; avocados
Greasy lank hair	Lack of vitamin B; much too much oily food	Wholegrain products; dairy; eggs; leafy green vegetables; cut down on fried food
Thinning hair	Iron deficiency; low protein levels	Red meat; liver; leafy green vegetables; wholegrain products; beans; eggs; dairy; soya products; fish
Weak, easily broken hair or split ends	Lack of silica (it promotes hair strength); low protein levels; deficiency in vitamins A, B, C, E, K	Silica is found in strawberries, rice, leafy green vegetables, onions, cucumber, celery and cabbage; protein is in dairy, milk, eggs and fish; vitamin A in carrots and broccoli; B in green vegetables and seeds; C in citrus fruits; E in avocados, whole grains and green vegetables; K in seafood, dairy, green vegetables and yoghurt

your hair, as this will allow for a more even application and make complete rinsing out much easier. Make sure the conditioner is massaged into the ends of your hair, as that is where it will be needed most. Leave it on for four or five minutes before rinsing off with the same thoroughness as for the shampoo.

The best way to dry your hair is to allow it to air dry without you touching it but, as that is not always practical, towel dry by patting and blotting rather than rubbing. If you have to use a hairdryer, make sure you keep it moving, keep the heat setting down as low as possible and don't use it every day.

The bald truth

Approximately 37 percent of all men will suffer male pattern baldness (MPB) of varying degrees – 95 percent of male hair loss is due to MPB rather than any secondary cause. It can start happening at any point beyond puberty, but the most common age range for it to kick in is between thirty and forty-five. Although it appears to be random in how it causes hair loss, it will almost always start at the crown and/or the temples and progress from there, hence the term "pattern".

Wiggy wiggy wiggy

Unless you've got the finance and the 24-hour maintenance crew to be able to sport a syrup as completely convincing as Sean Connery's in *The Hunt For Red October*, don't even think about the hairpiece as a viable option. A cheapie toupee, which means anything costing less than four figures – and you'll need two of them for when one's being cleaned – will fool nobody, and may even get you pointed at in the street. Just because nobody actually talks about your dodgy-looking wig, doesn't mean nobody's noticed it.

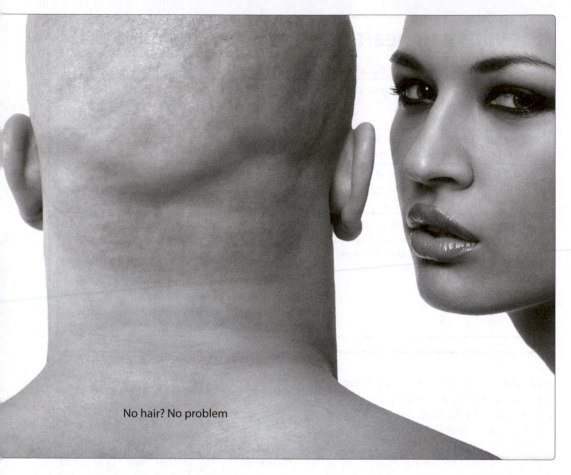

No hair? No problem

Will you go bald?

As seemingly arbitrary as how it affects you, is who it will affect. Every day, thanks to combing, washing and other frictions, we lose between seventy and two hundred hairs from our scalps – a fraction of the 120,000 that will be on a healthy head of hair – and baldness occurs because the hairs we lose are not being replaced. This will be due to the effects of the hormone dihydrotestosterone (DHT), a by-product of the male sex hormone testosterone. DHT attacks groups of hair follicles, leaving them alive but shrinking them, causing the production of weaker and finer hair until they become so narrow they can no longer produce hair at all.

Because MPB is hormonal you will be genetically predisposed to it, but, as yet, science has not found a way of determining who will go bald and to what degree. It was long believed that because MPB is linked to genes that are part of the X chromosome, which is handed down from your mother, baldness on your mother's father's side is a

T *Tip: The best time for that initial headshave – or even a new hair cut – is Friday evening, because you'll have at least two days to get used to what you look like before you have to turn up at work with it. This will hugely help your confidence.*

reliable indicator. However, recent research has shown there are more genes involved, some of which come from your father, meaning you could inherit it from anywhere in your family tree.

Miracle cures

Google "cures for baldness" and you'll come up with more potential – and potentially expensive – miracle cures than you could shake a stick at. For years there has been a largely unscrupulous quasi-scientific industry circling around men with receding hairlines and deep pockets, who are desperate to recapture their former glories. And the combination of Internet opportunities and today's obsession with youth and looks has made this considerably more lucrative. The truth is, because it is genetic there is no real "cure" for male pattern baldness, although there are a couple of options to slow it down a little by promoting vigorous hair growth.

Minoxidil was originally used as an oral medication to lower high blood pressure, but when a hair-growth side effect was discovered it was developed into a scalp application – it is the principal ingredient of Regaine (Rogaine in the US) hair treatments. Quite why it encourages hair growth is not known, but it is believed that as it dilates blood vessels so it stimulates the hair follicles. It works most effectively on the hairline at the front of your head, but any added hair growth will cease when you stop the treatment.

Finasteride is a drug that was developed as a treatment for prostate problems, and has been marketed as a remedy for hair loss under the brand name Propecia for

A *Expert advice: "If you want to look your best for your partner, be malleable – allow your woman to style your clothes and hair. It will leave you looking better in a way that women will appreciate – guaranteed – as so many men, even the stylish ones, dress for their mates rather than for women. Also, if you are going shopping, and you ask her to come with you and give you a bit of advice, then follow that advice. It will let her know you are really confident and comfortable in your own skin. There are few things that are more impressive about a man than his being comfortable in his own skin. You'll make her feel better about you; it will save you a lot of shopping headaches; and at the end of it you'll be dressed, according to her, the sexiest you can be. A win win win situation." Sarah Hedley*

about ten years. It works by inhibiting production of the enzyme that creates DHT from testosterone, therefore slowing down the damage to hair follicles and preventing further hair loss rather than initiating new growth. Once again, the effects only last as long as the treatment continues.

Traction alopecia… pull the other one!

Traction alopecia is the process by which hair follicles are killed off by having their hairs pulled at so hard that they come out with the root. It's common among those of African or African-Caribbean descent with cane row or braided hairstyles, or men with tightly stretched ponytails.

If Wayne Rooney can do it...

Hair transplanting involves tiny pieces of hair-growing scalp being removed from a "donor site" at the back or the sides of the head, and relocated into openings cut into the bald or thinning areas. The number of hairs in each "plug" varies from ten to fifteen, down to one or two, and most transplant operations will involve a mixture of different-sized pieces. To achieve the most pleasing – and convincing – results, multiple surgery sessions will be required, with several weeks' healing between each, meaning it might take a year before you are able to appreciate the end result.

While hair transplanting has been shown to work, it has also left as many transplantees with weeping scalps, scars and mad-looking tufts of hair sprouting apparently randomly from their heads. The starting point for anybody considering a hair transplant should be personal recommendation, or, because the skill of the surgeon is paramount, you should at least be able to see an example of their work in the flesh rather than in a photograph. After that, the rule of thumb is that you get what you pay for. It's hard to say how much the treatment will cost because the number of sessions can vary, as can the number of plugs transplanted.

It's not for everybody, though. Those with fine or thin hair should not consider

B

Best investments: specifically designed headshaver

There are many razors and electric shavers on the market with specially shaped blades, ergonomically designed to be used on the head. These will save you time, discomfort and the potentially humiliating experience of having to go to work with squares of tissue stuck to the cuts on your otherwise gleaming pate.
The Gillette Fusion Power Stealth (right) was designed with headshaving in mind and has blades that flex to fit the contours of your skull as you apply light pressure.

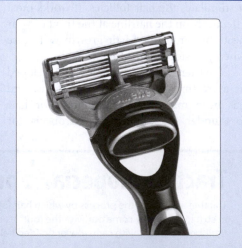

Is your hair loss illness-related?

Hair loss can happen as a result of an underlying condition or a course of treatment you are taking for something. In these cases it will be more immediately noticeable as large amounts of hair will come out when you wash it or comb it, or will be appearing on your pillow or clothes' collars. If it is related to another complaint it will be accompanied by other symptoms, and the primary cause should be treated on advice from your doctor. As a rule, once the primary problem clears up so will the hair loss. If it appears to have come about as a side effect of a treatment you are undergoing, once again, consult your doctor.

Conditions that might cause hair loss

Thyroid and pituitary conditions
Lupus
Diabetes
Radiotherapy or chemotherapy
Anything that brings on fever and high temperatures, such as flu or viral infections
Steroid treatments
Fungal infections of the scalp
Post-surgical trauma
Iron or protein deficiency

it as an option, and you should wait until your male pattern baldness has reached its conclusion – a hairline that continues to recede after bald bits have been filled in will leave some very odd-looking gaps.

Headshaving

The huge advantage of approaching a rapidly receding hairline by shaving the rest of it off is that you will no longer be "that bloke who's losing his hair" but "that fella with the shaved head". The crucial difference being

that it now looks like your idea: you could have a luxuriant head of hair and be merely following a fashion.

Be warned, though: much as a clean pate will always look more dynamic than well-established male pattern baldness or – horror of horrors – a comb-over, it's not a look that will suit everybody. Small round heads are best suited to this style, while pointy heads, uneven skulls or big bulges at the back are less so. However it's worth remembering your head will look enormous the first time you see it without hair – everybody's does.

Strong features can be both a blessing

Go grey gracefully

Grey hair is the result of a lack of melanin in the hair follicle, meaning there is no pigmentation in the new growth of hair and it will be white – grey hairs are actually white, it's simply that mixed in with coloured ones the effect is grey. Forty percent of men will have some grey hair by the time they reach their fortieth birthday, with many of them getting it well before then.

There is nothing you can do about it. No food supplements or dietary changes will reverse this process or stop it happening, so just go with it. And if you decide on a dye job then get it done professionally. DIY results are seldom very subtle.

and a curse, as while a clean head will accentuate a firm jawline or the sort of eyes that women find irresistible, a big nose or ears will look even bigger. Also, if you have

Ten top tips for looking better

▶ **If it's going, don't even think about a comb-over**
The only way you'll get away with it is if you have the same size bank account as Donald Trump. And even that won't stop people sniggering behind their hands.

▶ **Drink more water** Your skin is ninety percent water, thus keeping well hydrated will keep it looking fresh.

▶ **When towel-drying your hair pat and blot only** It is very fragile when it's wet and rubbing it will cause breakage.

▶ **Go easy on the smoking and drinking and whatever**
People who burn the candle at both ends tend to look the part, because it dries your skin out. Seen Keith Richards lately?

▶ **Invest in an ergonomically designed razor** If you are going to shave your head, it will save a great deal of general grief.

▶ **Don't wash your face with regular soap** It will dry out your skin's natural oils. Use specially formulated facial soap or face wash.

▶ **Never clean your teeth with lemon juice** It may get them white, but it will also strip them of their enamel.

▶ **After every dip in a chlorinated swimming pool** you should shampoo your hair and rinse off thoroughly, as lingering pool chemicals will dry out your hair.

▶ **Never squeeze a spot** This could push the excess oil back into your skin. Stretch and manipulate the skin around it to release the oil.

▶ **Buy your own skincare products** Men's brands will be specially formulated for male skin and the chances are hers won't be strong enough for you.

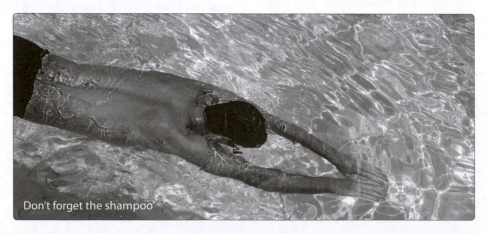
Don't forget the shampoo

the shape of face that can't wear hats, or you simply feel uncomfortable in them, it's probably not a good idea to shave your head as you will need to go hat shopping fairly quickly – in summer the sun will scorch your scalp, and in winter you will lose a huge amount of heat through your head.

Smoothing it off

It is advisable to get your first headshave done professionally. This is because people will put your freshly shaved scalp under enormous scrutiny during those first few days and the last thing you want is any nicks or cuts or patches of stubble spoiling that vista of gleaming, oiled scalp. Besides, you're about to shave all your hair off, so you've got enough to worry about at this point. Any old-school barber who does wet shaves will do it, as will the more modern practitioners who have the required electric equipment. After that, you'll need to start flying solo because you'll need to redo it every few days. Although the DIY approach isn't particularly difficult, the skin on your scalp is far more sensitive than on your face, thus shaving it requires more care and patience.

First-timers, whatever the method of shaving used, should cut hair down to a Number One or, at most, 3mm (an eighth of an inch). Then, and each time after that you shave it, take a hot shower first, as that will soften the hair, relax the scalp and open the hair follicles as much as possible. After that, while the hair is still damp, gently massage diluted tea tree oil into your scalp with your fingertips and follow these simple steps:

If wet shaving:

1. Apply a well-lubricated shaving gel or cream – not foam – massage in well, and allow to stand for at least five minutes.
2. Using a new blade each time, shave with light, long strokes – there will be no obvious grain to follow as, unlike your face, the hair on your head grows in many different directions.
3. Don't go over shaved patches again, as this will only irritate the scalp.
4. Change the blade immediately if you feel it's no longer cutting smoothly.
5. With a hand-held mirror go over any bits still lathered up, then check by feel that the shave is clean.
6. When attending to any still-stubbly spots, be careful not to redo any shaved bits.
7. Rinse off head with cold water.

Dress to impress

Suits are sexy, according to our resident sex and relationships expert Sarah Hedley. To wear a suit in a situation in which you didn't have to wear one, and to wear it in such a way that it is immediately obvious that you are dressed that way through choice and not because you've been told to, can repay enormously when it comes to impressing women. It makes you look like a) you're making a bit of effort; b) you're self-assured enough to be dressing how you want to; and c) which is the clincher, you've given careful consideration to what other people might like to look at on you.

According to Sarah, "Women have been dressing for men for years and know exactly how to get attention and exactly how much attention they are going to get by showing a particular amount of cleavage or a certain length of skirt. Guys, however, don't seem to be aware of it and, single guys especially, are more likely just to dress for themselves or so as not to stand out from their mates. That's why when a guy wears a suit in a situation where others might not, it looks like he is dressing because he understands how it's going to work for him and that's pretty impressive. That said, it's got to be the right suit, not one that says 'I work in a bank so my mum bought me this'. And it has to fit properly because that will mean you'll be much more relaxed in it."

8. Pat dry with a towel, as rubbing your freshly shaved head will scrape your scalp.

9. Gently dab over with witch hazel to close pores and treat any tiny nicks.

10. Massage scalp with a tea tree oil-based moisturizer to prevent infection and bring up a healthy sheen – a moisturizer should be applied to the scalp every morning, whether you have shaved it or not.

If electric shaving:

1. Gently and lightly pass the shaver over the head in long orderly strokes – don't use the rotary rubbing technique as this will greatly aggravate or even cut your scalp.

2. Using the mirror and fingertips, check for missed patches and go over them carefully.

3. Be patient! Because you have to be more careful, electric shaving your head will take proportionately longer than electric shaving your face, and, even including the lathering up, longer than wet shaving it.

4. Gently dab with witch hazel to close pores and treat any nicks.

5. Massage scalp with a tea tree oil-based moisturizer to prevent infection and bring up a healthy sheen – tea tree moisturizer should be applied to the scalp every morning, whether you have shaved it or not.

As part of your routine

In each case, you'll need to shave your head at least once every three days – the best practice is to fall into the same routine as shaving your face – but make sure you follow a daily scalp care routine. It should be cleansed with cotton wool and facial cleanser every day, as without hair to cover it up it will be a magnet for airborne dirt. But never exfoliate, as that will dry it out and leave it sore.

After cleansing, apply a moisturizer and in the summer be careful to use sunscreen. Moisturizing the scalp is particularly important for those of African or African-Caribbean descent as black skin tends to be naturally drier, and the sunscreen element should not be ignored. It is also recommended that you shampoo your scalp a couple of times a week, with a product containing tea tree or another scalp conditioner.

Going dental

British men have, on average, almost seven fewer teeth than they ought to – 25.3, instead of the full 32. It's a level of toothlessness approaching pre-NHS days, the result of over half of us having some sort of untreated tooth decay and thirty percent having untreated gum disease, about a quarter of which is serious.

As visits to the dentist by adults in the UK are becoming fewer and further between, it's unlikely this is going to improve any time soon. Therefore we need to do everything we can for ourselves to hang on to our pearly whites.

Plaque attack

The natural bacteria in the mouth combine with food particles and saliva to form plaque, an acidic, sticky build up on your teeth. If allowed to remain there, plaque will eat through the enamel to the tooth's dentine layer, then through the pulp, exposing the nerves. Toothache is the first sign this is happening, and once plaque gets inside an un-filled hole in the tooth the process speeds up and eventually the tooth will fall out.

Bacterial plaque also causes gum disease (gingivitis), which if untreated leads to

T *Tip: The most reliable natural tooth whitener is a mixture of baking soda and salt, which will also kill the bacteria that causes plaque.*

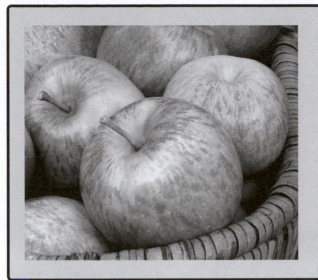

The not-so healthy options

Not only is the amount of hidden sugar in the Western diet contributing to galloping rates of tooth decay, but some apparently dental-friendly food is working against us.

Fruit in particular is being bred to be sweeter, therefore increasing sugar content – some varieties of apple, notably Pink Lady and Braeburn, contain as much sugar as a can of fizzy drink.

periodontitis, a condition that loosens the tooth from the surrounding gum, meaning it will eventually fall out – gum disease is responsible for more tooth loss than actual tooth decay. The first symptoms of gum disease are noticeably red and swollen gums, if it progresses to periodontitis, the gums will bleed during tooth brushing and often during the night.

The bacteria at the basis of plaque formation thrive on foods such as cakes, soft drinks, sweets and some fruits, as these are rich in sugars and starches that cause acid production to boom. Gum disease will also be advanced by smoking, poor nutrition – particularly vitamin C deficiency – stress and diabetes.

Dental defences

Looking after your teeth and gums is more a matter of dedication than any particular science, keeping them clean and avoiding massive amounts of damaging foods should form the basis of any dental care regime. Follow these guidelines to maintain maximum dental health:

Brush twice a day with a fluoride toothpaste

Fluoride, which is added to the water in the UK, strengthens the tooth's enamel and reduces the amount of acid produced by the mouth's bacteria, thus cutting down plaque.

Floss each time you brush

Or use intra-dental brushes, as the gaps between the teeth, especially at the gumline, are notorious for plaque build up.

Use an electric toothbrush

They are so much more efficient in plaque removal and general teeth cleaning.

T

Tip: If you get a tooth knocked clean out, wrap it in plastic to keep it as hygienic as possible and take it immediately to an emergency dental hospital. It may be possible to put it back in.

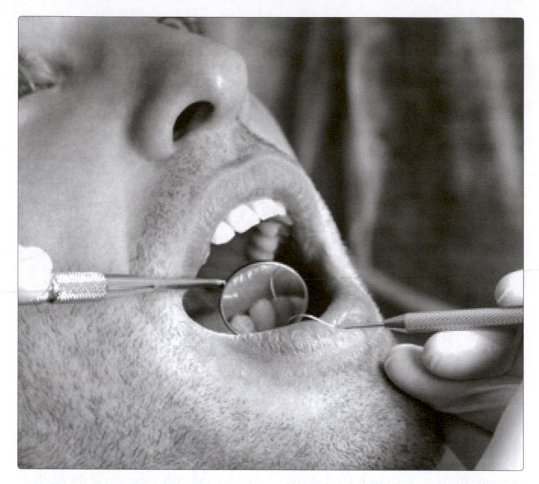

Change your toothbrush (or its head) more often

At least four times a year, and don't wait until it looks knackered.

Use less toothpaste

A pea-sized blob is ample, anything more than that is a waste.

Invest in a tongue scraper

Proper tongue scraping is vital to remove the large amount of bacteria that will be living on the tongue's soft surface; merely going over it with a toothbrush isn't good enough.

Cut down on sugar

Less sweets and sugary drinks will reduce plaque production, and a well balanced diet contributes enormously to all-round oral health.

Don't forget nature's toothbrushes

Eating crunchy vegetables like carrot or celery sticks after a meal will help remove any plaque that might be forming.

That gleaming smile

Everybody's teeth are different, and they can vary in shade quite dramatically from person to person – fewer than fifty percent of us have perfectly white teeth. Add to this the degree of staining that can occur from smoking or black coffee, red wine and tea, and the reality is that our teeth get more discoloured with age. It's no wonder keeping them pearly white requires effort beyond brushing twice a day.

Whitening or smokers' toothpastes can be effective, and there are two main types: abrasives and bleaches. The former contain tiny abrasive particles that will destain your teeth by friction, and are not recommended for older men as this action will also wear away tooth enamel that will be naturally thinner. Toothpastes containing peroxide are reliable tooth whiteners, but to be effective the active ingredient needs to be in contact with the surface of the tooth for an extended period, thus at least five minutes' brushing each session is required. Even then it will take

several weeks of daily brushing for either type of toothpaste to show significant results.

Professional bleaching is probably the best way to remove stains from your teeth, and most dentists will carry it out. The gums and soft tissue will be protected by gel or a rubber shield, and hydrogen peroxide will be applied to the teeth by encasing them in a custom-fitted, gumshield-like device that is filled with the chemical. Your dentist will fit the mouth pieces, and conduct the first couple of sessions – the teeth need to stay in the solution for between thirty minutes and an hour – then you will carry on at home for two or three sessions a week for about a month. There are several home tooth-bleaching kits on the market, but it is always advisable to get it started by a dentist.

Anatomy of a tooth

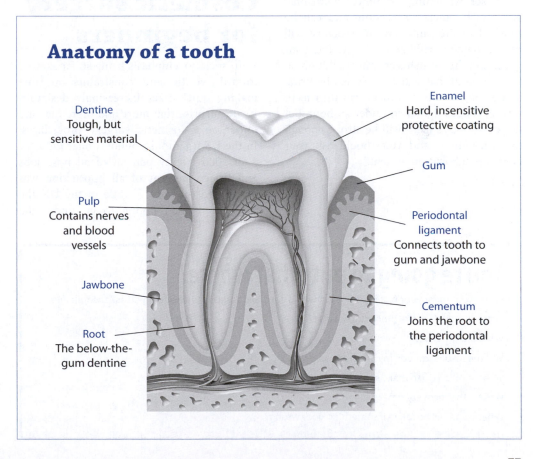

Dentine
Tough, but sensitive material

Enamel
Hard, insensitive protective coating

Gum

Pulp
Contains nerves and blood vessels

Periodontal ligament
Connects tooth to gum and jawbone

Jawbone

Cementum
Joins the root to the periodontal ligament

Root
The below-the-gum dentine

The best of the web

dentalhealth.org (UK)
The British Dental Health Foundation, offering advice about all things dental, including tooth whitening.

naaf.org
The website for the National Alopecia Areata Foundation, which offers support and practical advice as it seeks to raise awareness about this hair-loss condition.

grooming-health.com
A comprehensive male grooming site, offering tips, advice, a question-answering service, and up-to-the-minute product reviews.

dh.gov.uk/en/Publichealth/CosmeticSurgery/index
The Department of Health's website has the most comprehensive advice and information section for those considering cosmetic surgery.

headshave.baldlygo.com
Virtual headshaving online. Check out what several celebrities might look like with clean heads, then post your own picture and try it out for yourself.

Laser whitening, or power whitening, is a much quicker procedure and can be finished in the same day. Your dentist will fit a protective rubber shield around your gums and then brush a chemical solution on to your teeth that will be activated by firing a laser on it. This treatment can turn teeth several shades lighter in under an hour, but not everybody's teeth will be strong enough to withstand it and you should ask your dentist to advise you on that.

Cosmetic surgery for beginners

With society's emphasis being so far skewed towards youth, and constraints on time making quick fixes increasingly desirable, it's no surprise that more and more men are undergoing cosmetic surgery procedures. In the US it's a multi-billion-dollar industry – in 2006 twenty percent of all nose jobs and fifteen percent of all liposuction was performed on men – while in the UK the number of men opting to go under the

You're going to put what *where?*

When you go for your first consultation with a cosmetic surgeon, make sure you ask the following:

What *exactly* does the procedure involve?

What are the risks?

Will the results impede my life in any way?

What should I do to make sure everything goes as smoothly as possible?

What is the recovery time?

What steps will be taken if something goes wrong?

Don't get tucked up for a nip and a tuck

How much it will cost will vary enormously from surgeon to surgeon, and even the same procedure can cost different amounts for different people, as each will involve a unique amount of work. However, ball park figures for the more popular operations are:

Rhinoplasty (nose job) £2000 (In the US $4000)

Liposuction £1500 ($3000)

Ear surgery £2000 ($4000)

Botox £170 ($340)

Facelift £4000 ($8000)

Pectoral implants £2000 ($4000)

knife has risen by three hundred percent over the last five years. And as techniques get ever more sophisticated, so the range of procedures on offer gets ever wider. As well as the long-established nose jobs and botox injections, popular ops now include pectoral and buttock implants to become instantly ripped, cheekbone augmentation and jawline reshaping for that full-on chiselled look, and penis enlargement for obvious reasons. Should you be one of the millions of men apparently thinking about getting a nip or a tuck or a bit put in, there are certain aspects you should first consider.

Before you take even the first step towards the scalpel, think long and hard about why you want this particular operation. It's very dangerous to assume that instantly altering your appearance will solve your problems or improve your life just as quickly. Difficulties you had in life pre-surgery will still be there post-op. After you've thought that one through, choose a surgeon that is registered either with (in the UK) the General Medical Council's Specialist Register of Plastic Surgeons, or (in the US) the American Society of Plastic Surgeons, and even then it's best to go on personal recommendation, from somebody whose results you can inspect.

Once you meet your surgeon, he or she should be able to use digital technology to show you what you will look like after the procedure. They should also never try to talk you into anything you're not sure about. Don't commit yourself to anything too hastily, as there's plenty out there to choose from.

In the middle

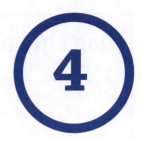

The old spare tyre ... a bit of a pot ... the beer gut ... love handles ... all coy euphemisms that give the impression men have an almost affectionate relationship with the activity of putting on weight. Or maybe it's a grimly ironic acceptance of what seems to be something of a default setting these days, as huge portions of bad food and less day-to-day exercise (as discussed elsewhere) conspire to pile on the pounds. However, in order to do something permanent about putting it on – or keeping it off – you'll need to understand exactly what fat is and how much damage it can do to you.

Apples and pears

You won't just get up one morning, look down and not be able to see your feet – it's a far more insidious process than that. Due to the decreasing speed of their metabolism, if men carried on eating and exercising at exactly the same levels from their twenties into their fifties, they would gain, on average, nearly two kilograms of fat a year.

Of course, genetic differences mean this is far from an exact science, and there is no way of predicting who would put on how much weight. What is pretty much a certainty is that you will put it on around your waist in the form of a big belly.

Belly belly bad

As a man, you will be naturally predisposed to putting centimetres on the waistline as the years roll by. This contrasts with the situation for women, whose accumulation of later-life fat will pad out the hips, buttocks and thighs before it starts to settle on the belly.

Science is baffled as to why you will be apple-shaped whereas she will be pear-shaped, but one thing doctors are sure about is that your belly fat will be very bad news. If left to its own devices, there's a good chance your belly will turn round and kill you.

Surrendering to a "middle-aged spread" is one of the worst things you can do. Belly fat is the most unabashedly toxic type of fat there is, and piling on the pounds around your waist will threaten your coronary health to a far greater degree than a big backside. Also, by virtue of where you're carrying this heavy weight, your belly can affect several other aspects of your physical well-being such as your energy levels and the state of your back.

F

Fact: The vast majority of young male gym goers see a "ripped" six-pack as the foremost reason they are there, with big biceps coming a pretty close second.

How it all works: putting on and shedding fat

Body fat is excess muscle fuel – fat or carbohydrate – stored in fat cells, also known as adipose cells, to make sure we have a reserve of energy if times get hard. An adult man will have between seventy million and two hundred million fat cells, which expand in size rather than increase in number to accommodate extra fat, and are located either just below the skin (subcutaneous fat) or within the abdominal cavity (visceral fat). A certain degree of fat is vital to our systems, with up to sixteen percent of the body's weight being healthy for men, and around twenty percent for women.

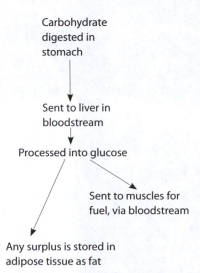

Carbohydrate digested in stomach

↓

Sent to liver in bloodstream

↓

Processed into glucose

Sent to muscles for fuel, via bloodstream

Any surplus is stored in adipose tissue as fat

Our bodies move when fat, glucose or glycogen are delivered to the muscles through the bloodstream, where it is combined with oxygen, also arriving via the bloodstream, to form adenosine triphosphate, or ATP, the energy that powers the muscle cells.

Inevitably, taking on board more fuel than is being used causes an excess, which the body puts into storage as fat. When a large number of calories have been consumed, the fat cells produce enzymes that capture any unburned fatty acids and glucose, drawing them into the cells where they will be converted to fat and kept as a fuel reserve. Hence an inactive overeater puts on weight. However, increased activity or a low-calorie eating plan causes a loss of fat because, as more energy is required than has been consumed, the body draws on these loaded cells and breaks the stored fat down into glycerol and fatty acid – the same components the digestive system reduces the fat we eat to – which allows it to be released into the bloodstream. Once there, the fatty acid goes directly to the muscles to be turned into ATP, while the glycerol is taken to the liver to be stored and converted into glycogen for future fuel.

Unsurprisingly, the quickest way to accumulate fat is to eat a great deal of food that is high in fat. This is because glucose burns far more efficiently in the muscles than fat, and is thus the body's fuel of choice, while the fat cells can process fatty acids into fat almost ten times as easily – it takes 23 calories of internal energy to convert 100 calories of glucose into fat for storage, but only 2.5 to convert the same amount of fat.

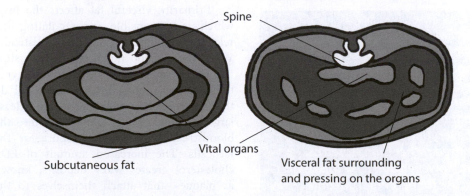

Spine

Vital organs

Subcutaneous fat

Visceral fat surrounding and pressing on the organs

The fat going on your waist will have a high concentration of visceral (or intra-abdominal) fat, whereas fat being accumulated elsewhere will be subcutaneous (it sits on the surface just below the skin or within the muscles). Although you need a degree of visceral fat to surround and protect your organs, it shouldn't be so much that it starts to show in the form of a belly. It will pack tightly around the vital organs – it is far denser than subcutaneous fat – and attack your heart by playing havoc with your insulin control mechanisms, thus sending your cholesterol levels soaring. This is why, historically, men are more susceptible to heart disease than women, and anybody with a higher than thirty percent concentration of visceral fat is a prime candidate for type 2 diabetes, stroke, heart disease and high blood pressure. They will be much more at risk than the unfit or those with all-over fat.

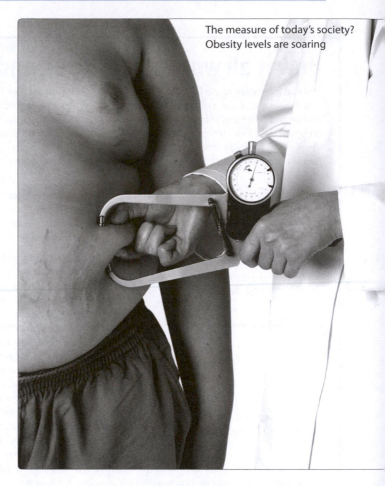

The measure of today's society? Obesity levels are soaring

Metabolic mayhem

There are so many adverse conditions occurring in the body as a result of excess belly fat that they have been given the collective name Metabolic Syndrome – or Insulin Resistance Syndrome. At the centre of these conditions is the system's inability to efficiently metabolize visceral fat.

Primarily, visceral fat affects the liver, which is responsible for regulating the release of cholesterol into the bloodstream. When there is too much fat in the system the liver goes into overdrive trying to process it, and a healthy liver will do this *too* efficiently, meaning it will release large amounts of LDL cholesterol into the bloodstream to act as transport for the fat cells. The increased amount of LDL cholesterol creates waxy deposits, known as plaques, that attach themselves to the artery walls to narrow and eventually block

T

Tip: Eat less more often as, ideally, your digestive system should be given five smaller meals a day to deal with rather than three large ones. If you can do that, you increase the chances of everything you've eaten being utilized rather than stored as fat. However, don't use this as an excuse for perpetual grazing.

them. There will also be too much glycerol being taken into the liver for processing into glucose.

Eventually, the liver becomes overworked and functions far less efficiently. When that happens the fat starts to build up in it, swelling the organ and causing a condition known as non-alcoholic fatty liver disease. This, in extreme forms, can be a precursor to cirrhosis.

Visceral fat also releases a chemical known as angiotensinogen, which combines with renin, by itself a harmless secretion from the kidneys, to cause the narrowing of blood vessels. The fatty acids produced by the belly fat also release molecules that adhere to and roughen the interior artery

F

Fact: Visceral fat causes so many problems within the body and has such a proactive effect on the vital organs it surrounds that scientists are starting to view it as an organ in its own right, rather than a digestive by-product.

walls, making it easier for the plaques to take hold. All of this conspires to vastly increase your chances of high blood pressure, stroke or cardiovascular disease.

Seven habits of highly overweight people

Food shopping when hungry
You are guaranteed to buy more than you need, then will be obliged to eat it. Incidentally, the same rules apply if you've had a couple of drinks before heading towards the supermarket.

Being bored in proximity to convenience food
Hanging about at airports, waiting for colleagues in coffee shops, watching mindless television, stopping at a motorway service station on a long drive… all these are situations that will drive you to reach for the snacks or sandwiches, whether you're hungry or not. Keep a healthy alternative to hand.

Not eating breakfast
After eight hours' sleep you need to fuel up almost as soon as you get up, and to skip breakfast will trick your body into starvation mode, meaning it hoards reserve calories as body fat, plus late morning hunger will find you snacking before lunch.

Drinking too much
This isn't just beer or wine, but giant fizzy drinks or orange juice or tea and coffee with sugar. Opt for cold water.

Not getting enough sleep
Sleep deprivation means a reduction in cortisol secretion, the hormone that controls your appetite, and that can end up with you experiencing increased fat storage.

Not planning meals in advance
Too often this results in grabbing whatever is to hand and easy to prepare, which usually means fast food or convenience food. Spend some time at the weekend sorting out what you're going to eat during the days ahead.

I've started so I'll finish
It is deeply ingrained in so many of us to finish what is on our plates – the problem is it's liable to be a great deal more than it used to be. Too much, in fact. Leave some behind.

Body Mass Index

A widely used method of determining how fit or fat you are is the Body Mass Index, or BMI. It is a 150-year-old calculation designed to assess how overweight a person might be relative to their height, and display the result as a single figure.

To calculate your BMI divide your weight in kilograms by the square of your height, as measured in metres, then apply the resultant figure to the chart below. But do so with a healthy-sized pinch of salt: the Body Mass Index may be the definition of choice when it comes to formalizing the current obesity crisis but it is a notoriously rudimentary system and doesn't make any allowances for race, gender, age or muscle mass.

Body Mass Index	Weight status
Below 17	Possible malnutrition
17.1–18.5	Underweight
18.6–25	Normal
25.1–30	Overweight
30.1–40	Obese
Over 40	Morbidly obese

BMI Calculator
$$\frac{\text{Weight (kg)}}{\text{Height (m) x Height (m)}}$$

Alternatively, click on **nhlbisupport.com/bmi**, feed your figures in and let the online calculator do the hard work.

Expert advice: "Keeping your weight down is a whole lifestyle approach, so you can't eat what you like and then come down to the gym and assume a good workout every once in a while is going to take care of it. To get fit and stay fit and make sure your body's operating at full capacity you have to have a combined exercise and diet programme. The two go hand in hand."
Gideon Remfry

A big, hard belly will raise the likelihood of type 2 diabetes as well. The presence of visceral fat will create a condition in the system known as insulin resistance, in which the body's cells no longer respond to insulin as a regulator of blood sugar levels. With glucose levels running unchecked in the bloodstream the pancreas ramps up insulin production to try to clear things out and that serves to make things worse as the body's metabolic balance is further tilted off centre. Such a state of affairs is a fairly certain precursor to diabetes.

Likely lads

Genetics plays a huge role in how you will accumulate fat, but there are several environmental causes that are entirely

Mythbuster: the ladies love the love handles

In a survey of women carried out by an American dating website, in the "He should have..." checklist a flat stomach was the third most important factor when it came to first impressions of a man – after well-cared-for hair and good teeth, but slightly ahead of clean shoes. However, a big belly also came second in the "Instant turn-off" category, just behind being badly dressed. With the men in the same survey, "Lose some weight" was far and away the top answer to "How would you want to change your appearance?"

within your realm to control. Saturated fats are a major contributor to visceral fat, so men with diets high in animal fats or dairy should change their ways. Excessive alcohol consumption is another trigger – hence the "beer belly" notion – and will damage the liver and further contribute to its malfunctioning. Interestingly, though, there has been some recent research to suggest that moderate drinking – a glass of wine a night, say – will actually work to prevent visceral fat. Smokers, too, have a much higher chance of developing a big belly – a recent study in Japan showed men who smoked accumulated visceral fat at a much higher rate than non-smokers, although scientists have yet to fully understand why.

The other prime candidates are the perpetually stressed. Although it's frequently assumed that stressed people burn off fat with nervous energy, belly fat actually occurs as the direct result of stress. When you are under strain a hormone called cortisol is produced by the adrenal gland and released into the system to raise blood pressure and

T *Tip: Be careful with sauces and dressings, especially mayonnaise-based concoctions, as they can contain massive amounts of fat and sugar.*

You should be worried about the killer in front of you if…

You have a waist measurement of more than 100cm or 39 inches Measure your waist by standing up straight, lifting your clothes and running the tape around your body halfway between your hip bone and lowest rib; keep the tape level all the way around and don't let it cut into your flesh.

Your belly is hard Because visceral fat accumulates so densely within the abdominal cavity, many big bellies will feel hard when other fat areas on the same body are wobbly. To assess what sort of fat you are carrying in front of you try to shake your belly to see if it flops about; if it stays still you have a high proportion of visceral fat.

You get more than thirty percent of your calorific intake from saturated fats (dairy, meat, eggs) or trans fats (hydrogenated fats found in processed foods, commercial fried food, hard margarine). These fats are far more likely to manifest themselves in the body as visceral fat than the unsaturated varieties are.

Fat sex probably isn't the best sex

That extra poundage could seriously affect your sexual performance. The obese are twice as likely to suffer from erectile dysfunction because the blood supply needed to inflate the spongy tissue in the penis is impeded by narrower arteries and blood vessels, plus there's the fact that the blood has further to travel.

blood sugar. Research at Yale University has shown that sustained high levels of cortisol in men of all ages and older women promote the accumulation of fat around the belly. And the test subjects' girths went up in direct relation – the greater the stress, the more cortisol produced, the more visceral fat, the bigger the belly.

Don't think this doesn't apply to you

It is possible to be of slim build, with no visible signs of a belly, but still have a dangerous level of visceral fat in your body, because it's all about percentages. Between ten and fifteen percent of visceral fat (as a percentage of your total body fat) is fine and normal; if it is approaching thirty percent you are heading for trouble, and if it is over that, do something about it right now.

On the other hand, it's possible to be vastly overweight but with pretty healthy visceral/subcutaneous fat ratios – recently in Japan, a team of Sumo wrestlers were tested for fat make-up and were found, in spite of their size, to have lower levels of visceral fat and blood cholesterol than apparently healthy non-athletes. This endorses the theory that exercise keeps visceral levels low.

Or are you just fat?

The type of fat that most of us have, and quite a few of us have too much of, is subcutaneous fat, the soft, loose, expandable layer of connective tissue – known as adipose tissue – that exists just below the skin. For men it is far more likely to be on their upper body, whereas women tend to accumulate it lower down.

Fact: An average-sized and averagely active man with 25 percent body fat is storing approximately enough energy to last him a month.

Doctor, doctor…

Any of the warning signs described in this chapter ought to be enough to convince you to do something about your belly; however an accurate measurement of how much visceral fat you have in your belly can only be done with a CAT scan. To get one of these you will have to visit your doctor, but it is highly unlikely he or she will send you for a test as pricey as that. What they are certain to do, though, is measure your waist, then your blood sugar, blood pressure and blood cholesterol and talk to you about your lifestyle, to ascertain how much of a risk you are running.

Fat planet

The percentage of adults who are obese in the following countries:

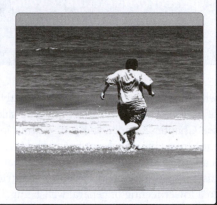

United States: 36 percent

Australia: 28 percent

United Kingdom: 25 percent

Germany: 16 percent

France: 11 percent

Japan: 3 percent

Source: World Health Organization

Subcutaneous fat forms a protective layer that exists to cushion and insulate the body, and is where excess nutrients are stored to provide energy in lean times. The reason the body converts excess carbohydrate to fat is because it represents a far more compact way of storing it, as fat contains very little water, and in terms of providing energy per gram, it takes up less than half the space of carbohydrate or protein. However, the problem lies with the fat that isn't being burned and is fuelling little other than the present obesity crisis.

This is the kind of low level, casual fat that has crept up on such a large percentage of the population, and although it isn't necessarily the stone killer visceral fat might be, at worst it will contribute to all of the same problems and at best it's not a particularly good look. Then there are the difficulties its sheer physical volume can cause. Every extra 10kg (22lb) of body fat a man puts on will require an added 29km (18 miles) of blood vessels to serve the extra tissue, yet he will only have the same-sized heart to pump blood through them. This puts a considerable strain on your ticker.

Also, when you do anything in the upright position, the extra weight will have to be supported by your hips, knees and ankles, creating a great deal of cumulative wear and tear on your joints. Carrying all that unnecessary poundage also increases the amount of effort you'll have to put in to perform just about any regular task, which is

A

Expert advice: "There has to be a happy medium, and the rule of thumb is eighty/twenty: if you have good food going into your body eighty percent of the time then you'll be able to handle twenty percent of your diet being not so healthy with very few ill effects."
Gideon Remfry

why overweight people are so frequently out of breath. Then it will affect how you sleep – see Chapter 2. Once you start getting jowly, the airway in your throat becomes restricted, leading to the snoring and apnoea that will disrupt your sleep patterns and so contribute to a lower feeling of general well-being.

The runaway weight train

One of the biggest reasons for doing whatever it takes to avoid piling on the pounds is that the weight you're starting to accumulate will very quickly assume a momentum that will become progressively harder to stop. This is why it's such a relatively short step from overweight to obese, and the causes of this unhealthy spiral can be psychological as well as physiological.

Top of the list is a vicious circle of inertia. Although an overweight person will use more energy performing exactly the same action as a less-heavy individual, the chances are the former will perform far fewer movements. This can be as a result of the physical problems resulting from weight gain – stressed joints, breathlessness, tiredness and so on – restricting movement, or simply because the brain is subconsciously aware of the extra effort involved and so will demand as little movement as possible. Either way, it means less exercise of any kind, thus fewer calories burned off, and this state of affairs will spiral as your weight goes up.

Society's attitude towards the overweight doesn't help either. Many in the UK feel it is the unseen "ism" that doesn't get the acknowledgement given to, say, racism or sexism. It can lead to widespread discrimination and such psychological problems as low self-esteem, anxiety and even depression. This in turn ramps up a weight gain cycle by precipitating such fat-friendly situations as increased alcohol intake, comfort eating, binge eating and reduced physical activity.

Calories counted

A calorie is the unit of measurement for the energy needed to raise the temperature of one gram of water by ten degrees Celsius. A kilo calorie (kcal or C) is equivalent to 1000 calories. This is what's used on packaging to denote the amount of energy provided by a particular food.

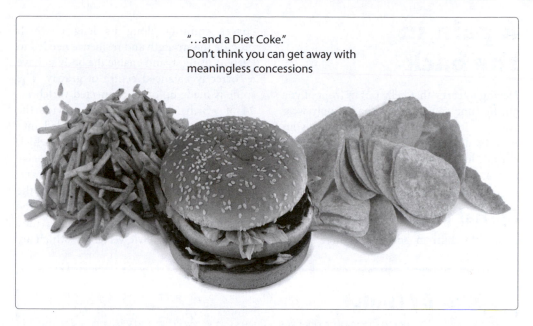

"…and a Diet Coke."
Don't think you can get away with
meaningless concessions

Then there's the possibility that dieting itself will contribute to continuing weight gain. Many weight-loss eating plans are simply too drastic, and the system's reaction to a sudden and sustained fall in calorific intake is one of metabolic panic – assuming starvation is imminent, the body starts storing fat to cope with this and so weight actually goes up. This can prompt the "diets just don't work for me" syndrome, which won't do any dieter's motivation much good and can set off the psychological problems discussed above.

"Yo-yo" dieting, periodic crash dieting alternated with unhealthy or binge eating, can be a problem too, as the reaction to the confusion caused within the metabolism is one of playing it safe, which means storing fat. In this case, the dieting often becomes more extreme to achieve the same results, which can lead to health problems beyond those associated with weight gain.

T

Tip: Taking the skin off a piece of chicken before you cook it will reduce the fat content by over 75 percent. Even if your chosen method of cooking is frying.

Check your calorie intake

It's very easy to take on far more calories than you need without actually realizing it. An averagely active man will need about 2800 kcal per day, compared with a woman's 2000 or a pre-adolescent child's 1750. Now consider that the average slice of pizza contains around 300 calories, a pint of lager around 200, a quarter pounder with cheese 500, a tuna baguette with mayo 530, a bag of crisps 175 and a 100g bar of Cadbury's Dairy Milk chocolate 530. There are many interactive calorie-counter websites or apps that will allow you to calculate what it is you're taking on board and how you might need to address it.

A pain in the back

Having to carry that belly out in front of you all the time can do more than simply wear you out. It can affect your spine, alter your posture and become the major factor in the chronic lower back pain that affects so many men as they approach middle age.

Spinal trap

A healthy human spine has three gentle curves running along its length, which provide the strength and resilience needed to keep us upright, and enable the body to have a correctly balanced centre of gravity. The spine is made up of 33 connected vertebrae, 24 of which are moveable, to provide the necessary flexibility. They are divided into three groups: cervical, the top seven, which support the head; thoracic, the next twelve down, to which the ribs are connected; and the lumbar, the five largest and lowest of the flexible vertebrae, which bear most of the weight of the trunk. The remaining nine vertebrae are the pelvic vertebrae, which are

Spoilt by choice

As a society, we've got to a point that what's on offer has evolved way beyond what's necessary for survival. And faced with such a selection, we are far too often choosing beyond our needs.

"In the twenty-first century, we've got greater spending power, there's greater availability of foods and we have greater choice," Dr Sarah Schenker explains. "But it's far more multifactoral than that. There's the way society is now: we're eating on the run, we're eating alone, we're substituting different meals for different times in order to fit them in with our lives, and how much time people spend out of the home eating their meals is important – younger people, especially young men, are probably eating the majority of their meals away from the home, except at weekends.

All of this has led to the breakdown of the traditional three meals a day, and that is a very big change in how we eat because of the choices it puts in front of people. Before, when there was much less choice, we ate fairly instinctively. Now with anything you like on offer, faced with the choice of an apple or a bag of crisps or a bar of chocolate, most people will go for the crisps or chocolate because they're much more available and they taste nicer.

When there was only a limited choice of local produce, or food that was in season, which you had to assemble, prepare and cook yourself, there was a far greater chance you would go for something like fish or chicken or something nutritious. Largely because that was what was there, and there wasn't any particular convenience factor to be considered because you were going to have to cook it yourself anyway. You simply made time in your day. Now, although those choices are still available, you're also faced with the choice that means you have everything done for you and you can eat anything at any time, anywhere. While it's not necessarily human nature to choose what's bad for you, it becomes very difficult to avoid what is convenient and being presented to you so attractively. Immediate gratification is very hard to fight.

Also, the move away from previous traditional meal times has meant nobody is hungry any more – or not hungry in the traditional sense. Just slightly unsatisfied. When people were sitting down to three meals a day, they hadn't eaten for maybe six hours, so they were ready for a nutritious meal – a large meal. Their bodies wanted it and would be letting them know, because that's what hunger is: your body telling you it's low on nutrients. People graze all day long now, so they're seldom hungry enough to want a proper meal. And to make it worse, they're not grazing on particularly nutritious food, because the choice of grazing food these days is immense and very attractively presented. You could eat cakes all day long."

T

Tip: Eat more slowly and you'll eat less. It takes the brain about twenty minutes from when you started eating to register if your stomach is full, and because these days we tend to eat much faster often we pass the point of being full without realizing it and continue, eating too much.

fused together into two groups – the sacrum, the five directly below the lumbar, and the coccyx, the four at the base of the spine.

The lumbar section of the spine is absolutely crucial to maintaining your comfort as it effectively holds up everything above the hips, distributing the load while you are either active or resting. This lower segment of the spine will be principally supported by the core muscles of the abdomen and the lower back, in combination with those around the hips, buttocks and pelvic area. It's in this area that lower back pain occurs, and because a large belly can radically affect its delicate balance, any man carrying that sort of load will greatly increase his chances of persistent lower back pain.

It's why fat guys waddle

Gaining a large, solid belly will alter your posture, which will contribute to more than just lower back pain. Having to support that excess weight just in front of your lumbar vertebrae will start to pull them forward, extending the natural curve of the spine which, in turn, will cause the pelvis to tilt too far forward. This means the legs have to move out from under the hips as you walk, kicking forward and spending a much greater part of the stride cycle in front of the body than is natural. Hence the waddle, which will add to the strain on the knees, which are already supporting excess poundage.

In this situation, the chances are that the muscles around the pelvis, buttocks and lower back are not well developed – likely a result of a lack of exercise – and therefore cannot provide extra support. This altered posture means the head has to adjust itself to stay level, and the pulling forward involved will put extra strain on the neck and the shoulders.

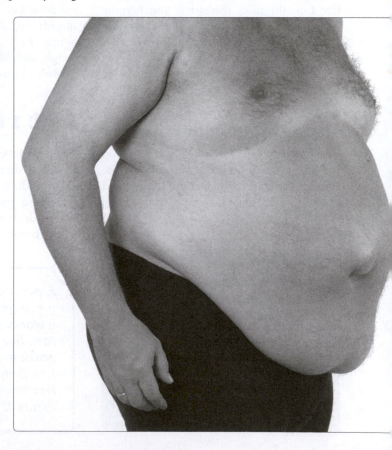

How many sugars?

Added sugar in the modern diet is one of the most dangerous sources of empty calories, as they often lurk under confusing pseudonyms, and are far more prevalent than you might imagine and will play merry hell with your blood glucose levels.

The most popular aliases for added sugar are...
dextrose, fructose, glucose, corn syrup, lactose, maltose, sucrose, high-fructose corn syrup, molasses, fruit juice concentrate, malt syrup and corn sweetener.

You are most likely to find the highest proportion of added sugar in...
soft drinks (not diet soft drinks), cakes, biscuits, commercial fruit juice, fruit squash, dairy-based desserts including some yoghurts, bread and other baked goods.

Within the lower back itself, the distortion of the vertebrae puts enormous strain on the discs – these are the spongy slices of tissue that allow the vertebrae to move against each other in comfort. Once the spine starts to be pulled out of line like this, the discs themselves can become damaged. These discs, and the out-of-position spine, can also create pressure on nerves leading from the spinal column. Any of these situations will lead to sharp lower back pains or even sciatica.

Dragging you down

The extra weight also puts added stress on the ligaments and tendons surrounding the spine – this can result in painful tears and strains, which may cause the surrounding

muscle to spasm, producing powerful pain waves. This occurs because the core muscles that surround the spine have a duty to protect it, and when a joint or ligament is stressed the brain instructs the muscle to contract tightly around it to provide a solid defence. These muscles themselves will already be subject to added strain through simply having to support the belly's extra weight and, like those mentioned above, will probably be underdeveloped to start off with.

Get rid of it

Losing that belly might not be rocket science – eat less, do more, is pretty much all it takes – but to do it efficiently, effectively and with minimum risk to your health, there are a few guidelines that should be followed. Your ideal combination of exercise and diet will

T

Tip: Don't feel obliged to finish what's on your plate – in spite of what your mum taught you! Over the last decade the size of portions in restaurants and takeaways has risen dramatically, meaning it's very easy to overeat without being aware of it.

Expert advice: "The fruit and veg message is a strong one because it works. People who are eating their five fruit and vegetables portions a day are healthier, are less likely to be obese and have less illness: that is well documented." Dr Sarah Schenker

be a matter of taking elements from both the food and fitness sections of this book, then applying them to a weight loss conclusion – one that rebalances your calories in/calories out equation.

No need to give up everything

Crash diets might work in the short term and mean you drop a few kilograms during the first few weeks, but in the long term they will not be sustainable without damaging your health. Likewise, such extreme diets as the Grapefruit Plan, or the Cabbage Soup Diet, or the Beyonce-endorsed maple-syrup-and-cayenne-pepper diet, are not recommended for any length of time. Low carb, or worse still no carb, diets are not a good idea either, as they tend to involve compensations in other areas – specifically loading up the meat and dairy – which can seriously bump up your cholesterol levels.

The basis of any sensible weight loss eating plan is simply to cut out fats, refined sugar and simple carbohydrates, but retain sufficient protein, nutrients, natural sugars and complex carbohydrates. Although cutting the carbs on plans like Atkins or South Beach will show spectacular early results, complex carbs, as found in whole grains, are vital to give you the energy to start the exercise programme that will form the other side of your weight loss schedule.

Put some effort in

Exercise is vital to healthily managed long-term weight loss, if for no other reason than that raising your calorific expenditure will allow you to offset some of your intake, meaning you can enjoy the odd pizza or a couple of beers without feeling guilty. Also, while it improves your cardiovascular levels and generally makes you feel better, exercise will stimulate your metabolism into burning

calories far more efficiently. Then, every kilogram of muscle you put on will require more calories burned to maintain the same weight in fat.

Perhaps as importantly, exercise will give you something positive to be doing rather than simply feeling like you are giving things up, and help you focus on becoming fitter and healthier, rather than merely thinner. Men who adopt an exercise programme to go along with their eating plan are more than twice as likely to keep the weight off than those who don't. This is believed to be because keeping fit becomes a habit.

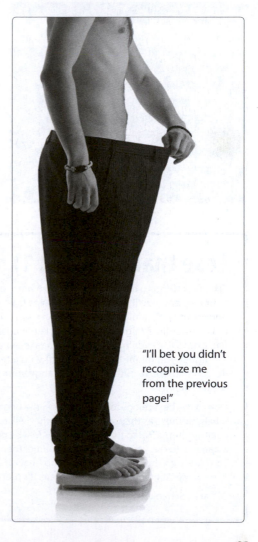

"I'll bet you didn't recognize me from the previous page!"

Keep a food diary

Before you start a new eating plan, keep a food diary for a couple of weeks, logging everything you eat, an estimation of its calorific content, at what time and with whom you ate, and leave space for comments. That way you can accurately address what needs to be changed on your personal menu – nutrition-wise as well as from the weight loss point of view – and look at the situations and the company in which you are eating what, as that can have a serious impact on your weight management.

F

Fact: Over the past 25 years the number of calories Americans consume through drinks – soda, fruit juice, alcohol, milk – has more than doubled. The average daily intake coming purely from beverages has gone up from 260 to 560 calories with no corresponding reduction on the food side.

Beware of diet pills

Thanks to Internet shopping, the slimming pill business has boomed during the last few years, and the sort of weight-loss drugs that would need a prescription in the UK or the US are being bought as "diet supplements" in unregulated overseas marketplaces. Although these pills will usually prove successful for a quick weight loss fix, they should never be contemplated on a long-term basis, as they are powerful, dangerous and potentially addictive drugs. Which is why they are so tightly monitored in the first place.

Slimming pills mostly fall into three categories: appetite suppressants, metabolism accelerants and fat blockers, or combinations thereof, and each has its own set of potential dangers. The first type boost the levels of the hormones such as serotonin in the brain, to bring about feelings of fullness or satisfaction. They can quickly become addictive, as when the body stops getting the nourishment it needs because you're simply

---

Lose that gut (Part 1)

"The first thing to do is look at how the high fat and high added sugar foods are getting into your diet and you'll probably find that at least one is cropping up in each meal or each eating opportunity. You might have a Danish pastry for breakfast; then at break time pick up a can of Coke; lunchtime might involve a packet of crisps; then mid-afternoon you have a chocolate bar. Come the evening, perhaps it's a takeaway. Or perhaps if you've eaten something healthy for dinner you might then finish it off with a few cans of lager. Then what do you cut first? How do you take those initial steps to change your eating habits, because they're going to be the most difficult?

One of the best things to think about in the beginning is what you have in between the main meals, because as they are secondary they will be easier to change. Think what would be the healthy alternative to that can of Coke? Maybe pick out something from another food group, like a banana, to get you through to lunchtime. Then in the afternoon, instead of the chocolate try a yoghurt from the calcium-based group. That's how you can start changing the balance of things. Then carry on going forward from there. It's pretty simple."

Dr Sarah Schenker

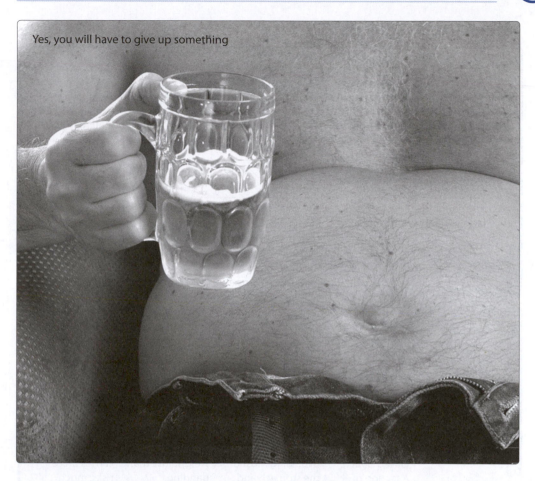

Yes, you will have to give up something

not eating enough, it starts to bypass the boosted hormones and put other hunger-recognition systems in place. This often leads to increased dosages, because the feelings of satisfaction the drugs bring on represent something of a high, so psychological addiction isn't far behind. And with it comes all the personality changes and anxieties associated with mood-altering drugs. Recent US studies have also shown prolonged use

T

Tip: Chew each mouthful for longer and you'll feel full sooner, because chewing is the action the brain associates with eating. Therefore doing it for longer is far more likely to satisfy your hunger pangs.

T

Tip: Too many diets don't last because they focus too much on what you shouldn't be eating, thus you end up thinking about those "bad foods" all the time. Rather than be negative, concentrate on what you should be eating and how much good it's doing you.

Bypass, banding or balloons?

Of course not every weight loss method involves working hard to change your lifestyle, and the alternative is to go under the knife. The three most common procedures are gastric banding, gastric bypassing and the insertion of a gastric balloon, and none of them should be entered into until you've talked it over with your doctor.

Type of operation	What it involves	How it works	Pros	Cons
Gastric banding (or lap banding)	A restrictive band is placed around the stomach, to divide off a small pouch at the top and leave a small opening into the main chamber.	The small pouch fills up quickly, food then passes slowly through the opening to be digested as normal. It leaves you feeling full almost immediately, and greatly limits the amount of food that can be eaten.	Recovery time of around two weeks; a less complicated operation than bypass, therefore a shorter stay in hospital; less expensive (by around 30 percent); reversible.	Lower, slower weight loss than gastric bypass; not suitable for the hugely obese (BMI over 45).
Gastric bypass	The stomach is stapled across near the top, to create a small closed pouch; a section of small intestine is run from this directly into the lower intestine.	Food passes straight from the pouch into the lower intestine, bypassing most of the stomach and small intestine. It also hugely reduces the number of calories that can be absorbed.	Suitable for the very obese; results in greater, quicker weight loss than banding.	It is a major procedure, therefore expensive; carries more risks; much longer recovery time; difficult to reverse.
Gastric balloon	A 500cc balloon is inserted into your stomach through your mouth.	The balloon is inflated by filling it with a sterile saline solution, meaning your stomach is partially full before you even start eating, thus you eat less.	Relatively inexpensive; performed under local anaesthetic; can be done as an outpatient.	Weight loss is slow; the balloon can leave you feeling constantly bloated.

of appetite suppressants damages the heart valves as well.

The metabolic accelerants contain amphetamine-like substances – ephedra or ephedrine is the most common – which can cause all the psychological problems of speed drugs, such as aggression, mood swings, paranoia, plus such physiological troubles as raised blood pressure, strain on the heart and an increased likelihood of heart attack and stroke.

F Fact: In the US, the average daily calorific intake for grown men is 3600 per day, almost 33 percent more than they actually need. The average for the UK is not much better, at 3400.

T Tip: If you're a regular light drinker take a couple of nights off each week. A 125ml glass of wine contains around 88 calories, while a half-litre of beer can contain between 180 and 220 (depending on what type of beer), so taking three glasses of wine or pints of beer out of your intake, twice a week, could save you between five hundred and twelve hundred calories per week. And help you sleep better on those two nights.

Fat blockers inhibit the actions of the enzymes that break fat down in the intestines in order for it to be absorbed through the intestine wall, thus they prevent the actual digestion of around forty percent of all fat consumed. These drugs have to be administered and taken in precise amounts, as their major side effect is that even a small amount of variation from the correct dosage can result in a total loss of bowel control.

Change your habits

Do you always have a burger when you meet the guys on the way to the game? Will you usually pick up a bag of chips when you get off the bus late at night? Is there a beer-and-pizza ritual that is involved every time you watch a DVD at home? Losing weight

Suck it up

Liposuction, or lipoplasty, is a body-sculpting procedure that targets specific areas of fat build-up, and is becoming increasingly popular among men. It's relatively simple – a hollow stainless steel needle is inserted into the area concerned and the offending fat, quite literally, sucked out. This technique is only effective on subcutaneous fat – the neck and face or buttocks and "love handles" are prime candidates – and cannot be applied to visceral fat, so you're still going to have to put in a bit of effort to lose that gut.

Before you sign up for it though, it is worth bearing in mind that over fifty percent of liposuction recipients put that fat back on within five years. This is either because those particular accumulations were genetic, or because the individuals never paid any attention to the science or theories of weight loss and so never addressed the bad habits that put the fat there in the first place.

Lose that gut (Part 2)

"To get rid of that gut you've got to look at food first. Especially for younger men, the first thing to do is cut out the rubbish from the diet. This has to be done straight away, because you can't begin to address it while you're still eating badly. Then you've got to look at resistance training on a regular scale, and that means three times a week, because the more lean muscle tissue you have the more efficient you will be at burning body fat. You can do cardiovascular training; it's great and should be a part of your routine. You burn body fat while you're doing it; when you stop, the burn stops and there's no after-effects. But as it takes more energy for the body to support lean muscle tissue than it does fat, you continue to burn calories while you are at rest. Thus if you create as much lean muscle as possible, you maximize your efficiency at burning body fat."

Gideon Remfry

is as much about altering what you do as it is about changing what you actually eat. Focusing on this very often reveals that it's your circumstances dictating your diet rather than the other way around.

As you start planning your new eating regime, look for patterns, places and associations in your life that may lead you into eating badly as a habit – keeping a daily food diary will help to make things clearer.

If you can identify such regular situations, the best thing you can do, rather than avoid them completely and possibly feel resentful, is to adapt your approach to them. Get off the bus at a different stop so you avoid passing your favourite chip shop; turn up to meet the others a bit later so there's less time to eat or sink that extra pint; eat (healthily) before you settle down to watch a film and you'll be less likely to stuff yourself with pizza.

Don't eat that, eat this!

High calorie	Lower calorie
Mozzarella cheese	Feta cheese
Chicken	Skinless chicken
Draught Guinness	Bottled Guinness
Sandwiches	Wraps
Cream	Plain yoghurt
Waffles	Pancakes
Deep pan pizza	Thin crust pizza
BK Big Fish	BK Whopper
Streaky bacon	Back bacon
Ice cream	Sorbet
White chocolate	Plain chocolate
Bagel	Croissant
Rack of lamb	Rib of beef
Spaghetti Bolognaise	Fettuccini Alfredo
Apple crumble	Apple pie
Hamburger	Hot dog
Lager	Bitter
Sirloin steak	Pork chop
Waldorf salad	Caesar salad

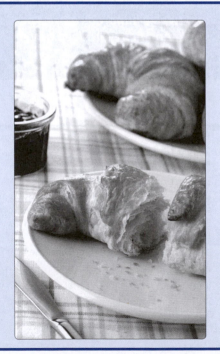

Calories burned

These are the calories burned per hour by a 76kg (168lb) man; the sports' figures err on the side of the casual participant rather than the fiercely competitive. Ideally, your exercise plan should involve burning at least 1500 calories per week, falling to 1200 once you get over the age of sixty.

Activity	Calories burned per hour
Boxing	850
Squash	850
Running (ten-minute miles)	710
Martial arts	710
Rugby	700
Cycling (on the road)	620
Rowing	600
Swimming (freestyle)	600
Circuit training	570
Tennis (singles)	570
Football (US)	560
Basketball	550
Football (soccer)	550
Raquetball	500
Rollerblading	500
Skiing (general)	450
Badminton	350
Walking (moderate-to-brisk pace)	300
Golf (walking and carrying your clubs)	290
Weight training	220

You'll be amazed at how many calories you'll be missing out on just by paying attention to what you are doing.

Slowly does it

Weight lost quickly is weight that's liable to be put back on almost as speedily. Any seemingly miraculous plan that promises ten kilograms lost in as many days is in fact going to be ridding your body of retained water and muscle mass rather than fat, and this will soon reappear as your system restabilizes. Fat falls off relatively slowly, and you should be aiming for a weight loss of between one and two pounds per week as a result of small

F *Fact: One single gram of fat contains three times the calories of a single gram of protein or carbohydrate.*

Fatherhood makes you fat

It's not just new mums that put on "baby weight". Recent research in Australia found that first-time fathers gained an average of three kilograms during their baby's first year. This weight gain was repeated with every subsequent child. It's believed that this is due to a combination of life being thrown into chaos – sleep patterns and meal times severely disrupted – increased stress and an abandonment of previous activities such as playing football or going to the gym. And the most worrying part of the report was that once gained this weight was never lost.

The best thing for expectant fathers to do is prepare for this in advance. Read your partner's baby books, as they will be crammed with dietary information that looks at healthy eating with one eye on weight control. Also, once your baby is a bit older (five months is generally recommended), you might consider buying a "running buggy": a way of getting in some power walking while pushing the pram.

changes in your lifestyle and eating habits. Also, the longer a weight loss plan lasts, the more likely it is to become an integral part of your life rather than something to be endured for a specific amount of time, which means you will have a much better chance of sticking to it.

Half a kilogram of body fat is worth about 3500 calories, so to lose a kilogram in a week you'll need to rebalance your personal equation by an average of 1000

F

Fact: Restaurant portions in the US are, on average, twice the size they are in France.

T

Tip: So many foods that are high in fat are low in fibre too, meaning a double whammy of accumulating fat on our bodies while not clearing out harmful deposits.

The best of the web

weightlossforall.com
A US site dedicated to helping you lose weight, and among the eating tips and programmes it offers a comprehensive chart of the calorific content of food.

myfooddiary.com
A membership website offering a vast manner of dietary advice and assistance, including a service that will analyse your food diary and provide suggestions as to how you can get the best out of your eating plan.

thedietchannel.com
Tips to help you diet and tests to establish what sort of diet you need; plus health-oriented eating plans and regularly changing diet-related features.

menshealth.com/bellyoff
Pretty much what it says on the tin, a very successful weight loss scheme for men, detailing diets and workouts, and keeping a running total of the pounds lost by Belly Off Club members.

calories every day. Taking 600 or 700 hundred calories a day out of the average Western diet isn't overly difficult – change a lunchtime sandwich to a salad, but pass on the mayonnaise; skip those two or three pints after work; or switch from deep pan to crispy base pizza. Then you can see off a further 1500 to 2000 calories simply with an hour's running or playing football three times a week. As long as you build on each week's achievements it won't be long before you can see the results.

Ten top tips for losing weight

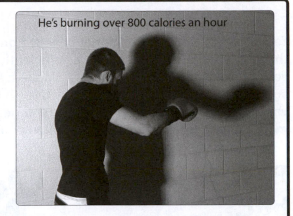
He's burning over 800 calories an hour

▶ **Take on enough carbohydrate to exercise**
Any sensible weight loss programme will involve an exercise regime as well as an eating plan, so make sure you are eating enough of what you need to work out.

▶ **Don't listen to other people**
Everybody is different, so what is right for somebody else's weight loss plan may be completely wrong for you.

▶ **Listen to other people** Equally, the experiences of people around you may be relevant as you consider what your weight loss options might be. But only as a guideline. Also, talking to your friends and family about how you are getting on will help keep you motivated.

▶ **Only eat when you're hungry**
This may sound very obvious but one of the driving factors behind the West's obesity problem is people eating out of habit, or boredom, and not because they need to.

▶ **Drink more water** Often, when you think you are hungry, you are in fact thirsty. Water will also fill your stomach with no calorific intake whatsoever.

▶ **Drink colder water** It will cool you down internally and your body will burn a few calories, bringing itself back to its normal temperature.

▶ **Don't make your regime too spartan** Otherwise you simply won't stick to it. Or you'll be unhappy. Or, most probably, both.

▶ **Look at all your habits** There will be patterns of behaviour attached to your piling on the pounds and if you look at changing them it will be a great deal easier to eat and exercise correctly.

▶ **Give in to your cravings** As long as you do so with restraint. If you fancy a bar of chocolate or some other off-plan treat, buy it – but only eat half of it.

▶ **Sub-size me** Go for the regular instead of large (or small instead of regular) option; have the starter-size portion as a main course. Or simply leave something on your plate other than the pattern.

In the guts

To get the maximum nutritional benefit from the food you eat, it has to pass through your digestive system as efficiently as possible. Too often, though, your body has its work cut out for it. Modern lifestyle and diet conspire to work against its natural – and most effective – ways of processing food, causing various levels of discomfort. And as you get older, it becomes progressively more difficult to keep things moving along quite as they should.

Easy to swallow, but…

Your digestive system gets ready to swing into action well before you start eating. In fact, you don't need to be sitting at the table or even seeing or smelling food – merely thinking about food will make your mouth water. The production of saliva is the first stage of the gastric process; saliva contains the digestive enzyme amylase, which works in conjunction with chewing to break the food down into something that can be easily swallowed.

Once our food has been broken down, reflex actions, instinct and the digestive process take over – see box opposite – and

F

Fact: There are more nerve cells in the stomach and intestines than in the spinal column.

we no longer have too much control. What we can do, though, is make sure all these automatic processes function as well as is possible.

Problem is, we don't seem to be doing that very well, as far and away the number-one reason for men visiting the doctor, both in the UK and the US, is gastrointestinal.

Stress

Just as relaxation promotes good digestion, stress has the opposite effect. Indeed, the ties between your stomach and your brain are so significant that the expression "gut feeling" is far from figurative. Excitement, stress and fear can all manifest themselves in your digestive system.

When the brain is put under pressure in stressful situations, and the fight or flight condition kicks in, one of the first things it does is to shut down the digestive system.

Mythbuster: Stress gives you stomach ulcers

Though stress is not the initial cause of gastric ulcers, it can definitely aggravate them – the release of extra cortisol during a "fight or flight" moment will cause a surge in stomach acid.

How it all works: digestion

Once the teeth, tongue and the introduction of saliva have mashed the food down into a swallowable mass, it passes through the throat into the oesophagus, a tube lined with muscles that push it towards the stomach with an action known as peristalsis. This involves rippling contractions and relaxations of the intestine itself, pushing the broken-down food along the tube – movements that would look like a snake swallowing its prey. As a rhythmic action – the peristalsis wave – it happens along the entire length of the digestive tract, from the oesophagus, through the small intestine and along the large intestine to the colon.

At the base of the oesophagus is a sphincter, a ring-shaped muscle that acts as a valve to permit food to pass into the stomach but not back up the other way. Once in the stomach, food will be broken down further into smaller, easily digestible particles as it mixes with the acids and enzymes produced there. Food leaves the stomach as a sludgy, semi-liquid substance called chyme; it then passes into the small intestine, where it will be further deconstructed, allowing nutrients to be transferred into the system. An adult's small intestine will be five metres (seventeen feet) from end to end; as the chyme passes through the three sections of its length – the duodenum, jejunum and ileum – the nutrient-extraction process continues and the chyme is broken down even further as a series of different chemicals go to work on it.

Once through the small intestine the chyme is moved to the large intestine, a wider tube, about one and a half metres in length and divided into three parts: the caecum, colon and rectum. It passes quickly through the caecum into the colon, where the water content is drawn off and re-absorbed into the system; the dried-out chyme is packed into solid faeces which are collected in the rectum. These will then be excreted through the anus.

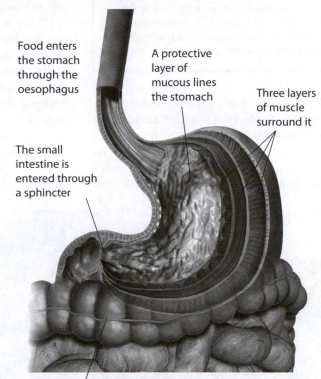

Food enters the stomach through the oesophagus

A protective layer of mucous lines the stomach

Three layers of muscle surround it

The small intestine is entered through a sphincter

The colon collects waste before releasing it through the anus

The time it takes

In the mouth: one to two minutes

In the oesophagus: ten seconds

In the stomach: two to four hours

In the small intestine: one to six hours

In the large intestine: could be as long as several days

M

Mythbuster: Drinking milk cures stomach acid problems

While milk will immediately soothe the painful effects of excess acid, it will go on to contribute to the problem. Milk is rich in calcium; this promotes the production of the hormone gastrin, which triggers the release of stomach acid.

The brain does this so that no further energy is used to break down food and blood can be diverted from the stomach to muscles and other organs vital to an action scenario. We have been hard-wired this way, more with a view to taking on a sabre-toothed tiger than to making a presentation at a sales conference. This is what causes the sensation of butterflies in the stomach, as such speedy internal activity produces the fluttering feelings to a degree related to the level of stress. In extreme cases of fear, the bowels and bladder may empty themselves without warning, simply to relieve you of any surplus weight.

This is how it works in extreme and unexpected circumstances, but serious problems occur when your default setting is feeling under pressure. When suffering from such chronic stress, your body's protective systems become overburdened, with the digestion system being the autonomic nervous function (involuntary vital function) most prominently affected.

The body loses nourishment as digestion is perpetually impaired, while

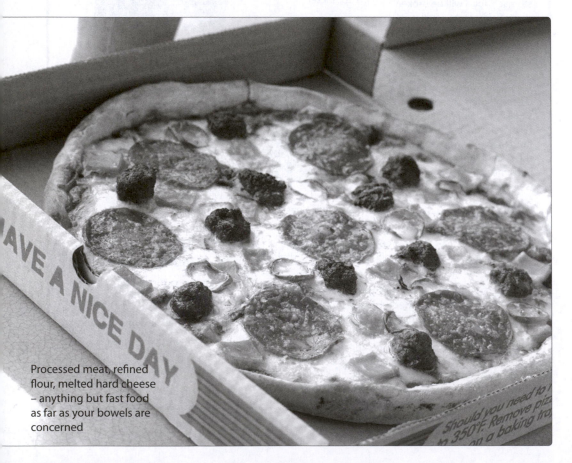

Processed meat, refined flour, melted hard cheese – anything but fast food as far as your bowels are concerned

the problems caused by undigested food in the gut multiply (see box on p.111). Constant high levels of cortisol – the stress hormone – are produced, overstimulating gastric acid production, one of the most common causes of gastritis as the excess acid attacks the linings of the stomach or the small intestine to cause inflammation. Although excess stomach acid can be countered with chewable or liquid antacids – Milk of Magnesia (also known as Pepto-Bismol) is the best known – this should only be a temporary measure. Over time, prolonged use of antacids will reduce the necessary levels of gastric acid, and that will seriously impede the digestive system, in turn blocking the absorption of iron and B vitamins.

Bellyachin' at a glance

Condition	Symptoms	Causes	Cure
Acid reflux, a.k.a. heartburn	Burning sensation behind the breastbone	Digestive juices passing up from the stomach into the oesophagus	Avoid peppermint, coffee, fruit juice and chocolate; cut down on the drinking; stop smoking
Indigestion	Nausea, excess gas, pain deep within the abdominal cavity, churning in the stomach, acid reflux	Eating too quickly, excess stomach acid, overeating, spicy food, activity straight after eating, stress	Antacid; avoid spicy food; eat slower and relax afterwards; chew your food more
Peptic ulcers	Sharp burning pain in the stomach, nausea, bloating	Breach in the mucous lining of the intestinal tract, allowing acid to attack sensitive tissue	Acid-lowering medicine; avoid caffeine, spicy food and smoking until it is healed
Food poisoning (see box on p.109)	Vomiting, dizziness, sweating, diarrhoea, weakness	Contaminated food, unwashed hands	No solid food and plenty of water until it passes
Wind	Burping, farting	Eating too quickly, gassy carbonated drinks	Chew your food more thoroughly and don't gulp it down; avoid fizzy drinks
Trapped wind	Stabbing pain deep within abdominal cavity	As above, but the air is caught inside the intestine	A warm drink will expand the intestine and dislodge it
Gastroenteritis a.k.a. Delhi Belly or Montezuma's revenge	An extreme form of food poisoning (dysentery, cholera and typhoid are all serious forms); symptoms as for food poisoning above	Bacterial or viral infection from food or untreated water; poor hygiene	Drink plenty of water; eat bland food; rest

F

Fact: The more overweight you are the more likely you are to suffer from frequent acid reflux.

Acid overload

Gastritis is the inflammation of the protective layer of mucous that lines the stomach and intestines, and is the most common of intestinal-related complaints among adult men. It can manifest itself in a number of different ways, and has about as many causes.

Quite apart from the stress factor and the overproduction of stomach acid, this film of mucous is prone to attack from bacterial, fungal or parasitic infection, the last most commonly transferred to your gut by undercooked shellfish. Prolonged use of anti-inflammatory painkillers (NSAIDs) such as aspirin, ibuprofen and naproxen will inhibit the production of substances that protect and sustain the mucous layer. Excessive alcohol or coffee drinking or overly spicy food will attack the mucous, while cigarette smoking contributes to gastritis as nicotine increases the production of stomach acid. Old age is another factor, as the older a man gets, the thinner the mucous lining in his stomach becomes.

Gastritis can be acute, manifesting itself in sudden burning sensations in the abdomen, indigestion or nausea; or it can be chronic, building up slowly over time with a continual dull ache, general loss of appetite and a constantly bloated feeling, with the side effect of plentiful gas. The latter condition is also given to sharp twinges of pain, if the intestinal tract is further irritated by something like a boost of cortisol or a particularly lively curry. Both acute and chronic gastritis can cause vomiting, and in extreme cases the stomach lining will actually bleed, with the blood showing up in vomit or faeces.

To treat gastritis, taking antacid will counter the painful effect of the stomach's acid, but then the underlying cause needs to be addressed. Often that's a process of elimination. Your immediate action should be to cut out any of the potential irritants listed above, and if that makes no difference then you probably have an infection. If you believe this to be the case, visit your doctor, who, if you test positive, will prescribe a course of antibiotics. As these infections can be stubborn, be sure to complete the course and then visit your doctor to make sure you are in the clear.

You could have a gut flora problem

The chances are, given today's diets and lifestyles, that keeping your gut flora in a healthy balance will not be happening by itself and you will need to introduce pro- or prebiotics. Any of the following could mean an imbalance of bacteria in your gut:

You suddenly become allergic to things and develop food sensitivities.
Unexplained weight gain, often accompanied by cravings for sweet foods.
Frequent constipation or bouts of diarrhoea.
Night sweats and disrupted sleep patterns.
Bad breath or bleeding gums.
Colds or low-level infections refuse to clear up.

If any of these is the case, introduce a course of pro- and prebiotics to your diet. If, after a couple of weeks, the symptoms persist, visit your doctor.

Biotics decoded

Antibiotics While these clear up all manner of diseases, they will also wipe out the good bacteria in your gut as they can't tell the difference. Following a course of antibiotics, reintroduce the probiotics to your system.

Probiotics The good bacteria that reside in your gut to protect against damaging bacteria – the good guys are stronger – forming the basis of your immune system. Found naturally in yoghurt or can be taken as supplements.

Prebiotics The food that the gut's probiotics need to thrive and which occurs naturally in whey as well as some fruit, vegetables and whole grains.

Understanding ulcers

A gastric ulcer is a kind of premier league gastritis, and it occurs when the layer of mucous is completely eaten away on a small patch of the intestinal or stomach wall, a couple of centimetres in diameter. The sensitive lining will then be exposed to the ravages of stomach acid, leading to jolts of very sharp pain if acid levels surge. Around ten percent of the population of the UK will suffer from gastric ulcers at some point in their lives, with men being twice as susceptible as women, and most sufferers aged between thirty and fifty.

Although the accepted term is "stomach ulcer", it is unlikely to actually be in the stomach. The correct term is peptic ulcer, as it can occur in the oesophagus, the stomach or the duodenum section of the small intestine. The first is very rare because food is not digested in the oesophagus and doesn't stay there for very long; instead it's usually caused by frequent regurgitation of acid. The second, the stomach ulcer, is far more common in women than men.

Ulcers among men take root mostly in the duodenal section of the small intestine, and the usual cause is food's liquid content arriving, while the solid parts remain in the stomach. The arrival of the liquid triggers the release of acid in anticipation of digestion, but when no solids turn up there is nothing to absorb that acid and it attacks the inner walls. Food not chewed properly promotes this situation, as does a diet with a high proportion of hard-to-break-down food – red meat, hard cheese and processed foods. It should be noted that all externally introduced causes of gastritis also contribute to the formation of ulcers.

The good news is that peptic ulcers are relatively easy to treat. Initially, acid will be

A

Expert advice: "Men in the UK and the US are not achieving nearly the target for fibre. They should be getting at least eighteen grams of fibre per day, but, in Britain, among men, the average is less than twelve. It means there is very poor bowel health out there, which is affecting everything else to do with our digestion and well-being. Men have to eat more fibre." Dr Sarah Schenker

F

Fact: Around fifteen percent of men will develop a peptic ulcer at some time in their life, probably between the ages of thirty and fifty.

T

Tip: Too much coffee or alcohol can stop your bowel movements, as they are both diuretics and therefore will greatly reduce the amount of water in your system.

countered with an antacid or acid blocker (also known as an H2 Blocker), then medicines containing either sucralfate or misoprostol will be prescribed. These will form a protective coating over the sore to promote swift healing. A natural way to protect against ulcers is by taking zinc, as it strengthens the epithelial cells in the layer of stomach lining below the mucous and reduces the release of acid-producing histamine.

Gut level

One of the biggest contributors to continued good health is what's going on among the bacteria in residence in your small and large intestines – your gut flora. It's in here that "friendly" bacteria – probiotics – produce B vitamins, vitamin K and amino acids,

regulate digestive acid levels in the intestines and help keep your digestive system moving so your bowels remain regular. These bacteria – lactobacilli and bifidobacteria in particular – also fight off such harmful bacteria as "C. diff" (Clostridium difficile), "A. Strep" (A. streptococcus) and some strains of "E. coli" (Escherichia coli) by protecting against toxins and pathogens being introduced to your system.

This is an important aspect of your immune system, as it guards against allergies, colds and flu. It is also believed that it will prevent irritable bowel syndrome, and that a healthy balance of gut flora is a reliable first line of defence against cancer of the colon.

Maintaining the balance of good/bad bacteria in the gut can easily be overlooked, and not drinking enough water, eating too much junk food, a chaotic meal pattern or a course of antibiotics can tip the scales away from good intestinal health. Live yoghurt or the fermented milk drink kefir contain a good supply of both lactobacilli and bifidobacteria or, outside of these dairy products, probiotics can be taken in the form of liquid or capsule supplements.

However, once the friendly bacteria have been introduced to the system they need to be fed, and you'll need to be taking a

B

Best investment: pineapples As well as being an excellent source of vitamins C and B1, pineapple is one of the most effective digestive aids there is. The fruit is rich in powerful enzymes that break down protein (proteolytic enzyme bromelain) and thus are a huge asset when it comes to digesting such stubborn foods as meat or hard cheese.

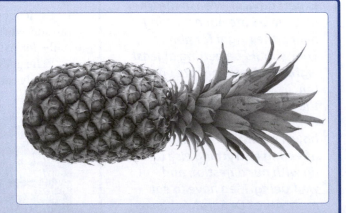

What's your poison?

Type	Causes	Effects	Prevention
Salmonella	Under-cooked meat or poultry; cross-contamination of raw and cooked meat or poultry; unpasteurized dairy products; raw eggs; cream or milk "on the turn" and the sauces or fillings it may be used in.	Cramps, diarrhoea, vomiting, fever	Cook meat and poultry thoroughly; keep raw and cooked apart; wash utensils, hands and surfaces well after contact with raw meat or poultry – no matter how fleeting; avoid unpasteurized dairy; cook uninspected eggs; and keep milk and cream – and any dishes they are used in – in the fridge.
Listeria	Undercooked meat or poultry; cross-contamination of raw and cooked meat or poultry; unpasteurized dairy products; under-cooked or raw seafood; unwashed fruit and vegetables.	Cramps, diarrhoea, vomiting, fever, skin lesions, chills	Cook meat and poultry thoroughly; keep raw and cooked apart; wash utensils, hands and surfaces well after any contact with raw meat or poultry; avoid unpasteurized dairy; and thoroughly wash any fruit and vegetables you don't peel.
Staphlococcus	Pre-prepared salads in which the mayonnaise may be off; cream or milk "on the turn" and sauces or fillings it may be used in.	Cramps, diarrhoea, vomiting, fever, headaches, general weakness	Keep salads, milk and cream – and anything they are used in – in the fridge.
E. coli	Unwashed fruit and vegetables; under-cooked meat or poultry; cross-contamination of raw and cooked meat or poultry.	Cramps, diarrhoea, gas, vomiting, fever	Thoroughly wash any fruit and vegetables you don't peel; cook meat and poultry thoroughly; keep raw and cooked apart; and wash utensils, hands and surfaces well after contact with raw meat or poultry – no matter how fleeting.

How it all works: the kidneys

The kidneys are situated near the small of your back, on either side of the spinal column: they collect waste – the unwanted by-products of internal chemical reactions – from the bloodstream; then they get rid of it. They do this by filtering around 150 litres (317 US pints) of blood per day as it flows into them, via the renal artery, which branches off the aorta that runs directly from the heart. The kidneys remove waste by passing the blood through tiny filtering units known as nephrons, then mixing it with water to become urine and depositing this into cavities called calyces. From there it is carried away by the ureter to the bladder, where it is stored before being passed out of the body through the penis via the urethra. The kidneys will get rid of about two litres of water and waste per day from a grown man.

As well as simply disposing of waste through urine, the kidneys also control the level of water within our bodies, passing more into the bladder if there is too much, or prompting feelings of thirst if there is too little. This is why you are left still feeling thirsty after some drinks, because the kidneys are still crying out for water. Another important function of the kidneys is to regulate the levels of chemicals like salt, potassium and phosphorus in the system, and remove any harmful excesses.

Each kidney contains over a million nephrons, which act as filtration units

Renal artery carries blood to the kidneys

Renal vein carries filtered blood away from the kidneys

The ureter carries waste to the bladder via urine

Each nephron contains an intricate network of tiny tubes and channels to remove all waste products

Kidney stones occur when chemicals aren't passed out through urine and build up sufficiently to form solid chunks of matter within any part of your urinary tract. These can be incredibly painful, and are either removed surgically or treated with drugs to break them down into pieces small enough to be passed through the urethra. This can be quite an experience in itself, given that a piece can be several millimetres across and far from smooth on the outside.

Kidney stones are almost three times as common among men as women, affecting men in their twenties and thirties in particular, and Caucasians are the most susceptible racial group. Symptoms of a kidney stone include: stabbing pains in your lower back; blood in your urine; painful urination; a constant desire to go; and flu-like fever and vomiting.

Irritable bowel syndrome

This is a collective term for functional bowel disorders that do not fall into any other category. The most common symptoms of irritable bowel syndrome (IBS) are: chronic constipation and/ or persistent diarrhoea; and prolonged cramps and/or bloating in the lower intestine. Medical science is unsure of the internal causes of IBS, but it is believed the main culprits are oversensitive nerves that cause peristalsis to happen too often and too fiercely while eating, or nerves that may be aggravated when the bowel is full and expanded.

If you think you have IBS, visit your doctor who will conduct a physical examination and give you a blood test. They will also discuss your lifestyle with you, as stress has been linked to the condition, inasmuch as it has an adverse effect on the digestive system. What your doctor won't do, however, is cure IBS, as at the time of writing there is no cure for it, merely changes that can help relieve it.

The principal culprits will be dietary: fatty foods, fried foods, alcohol, caffeinated drinks, fizzy drinks, chocolate and milk products have all been proved to exacerbate IBS symptoms. But as everybody's condition is unique, it will be necessary for a sufferer to work out what it is that causes their IBS to flare up and cut that out – this is best done by keeping a food diary over a month or so to implement a process of elimination. Adding fibre to your diet can help – though not if one of your symptoms is diarrhoea – and eating smaller meals more often will help your digestive system cope more efficiently, reducing the scope for irritation.

regular supply of prebiotics on board. These can be found in whey (what's left of milk when the curd has been removed to make cheese) or, for the lactose intolerant, in the carbohydrate fibre oligosaccharides, found in fruit, vegetables and whole grains.

Garlic, onions, tomatoes, Jerusalem artichokes and bananas are all rich in prebiotics, but the amounts contained are still tiny – it takes twenty bananas to yield a gram of oligosaccharide, around half the RDA – so taking prebiotics in the form of supplements is recommended.

F

Fact: Although the kidneys are one of the hardest working organs in your body, they are seldom stretched. Many people live healthy and active lives with just one functioning kidney.

Waste management

Getting rid of the stuff we don't want is every bit as important as making the most of what we need.

How often is regular?

How often you should move your bowels depends entirely on who you are – everybody's different and their body's digestive timetable will vary accordingly. A 24-hour cycle of solid waste disposal is the most common, but it's by no means universal – only sixty percent of us go every day – and that will be due to habit formed out of convenience and comfort as much as anything gastric. Anything between three times a day and three times a week is considered perfectly healthy, and these figures will start to decrease with age.

The physical act of getting up in the morning will trigger an urge to defecate

A

Expert advice: "Laxatives are not a good idea in anything other than the very short term. They don't add anything to your system, and you will be missing out on all the other nutrients you get if you keep your bowels healthy with whole food."
Dr Sarah Schenker

Take it easy

Bowel movements should happen easily and almost by gravity, with no need for squeezing or straining, and the easiest will involve soft, bulky stools that hold themselves together. This will be achieved by a diet high in fibre and with plenty of water. The indigestible fibre will hold onto water to create a stool of a soft consistency, and without the fibre, what is passed into the rectum will be low on water content and therefore can be uncomfortably hard. Somewhat obviously, the more water there is to start off with, the more the fibre will have to retain – a healthy stool should be around 75 percent water.

as the movement itself will shift the large intestine, triggering the rectum to send signals that it wants rid of the waste it's been storing up during the night. Also it is not unusual to want to go fairly soon after a big meal; this is called "gastrocolic reflex" and is triggered by an expanded stomach, the goal being to make more room further along the digestive tract. This reflex is strongest in children, and gets weaker as you pass into adulthood.

T

Tip: Regular exercise will go a long way to keeping the rest of you regular, as it stimulates movement in the large intestine.

Your mum knew what she was talking about

Don't eat too fast. Otherwise you'll swallow too much air with your food, leading to wind or indigestion.

Chew every mouthful properly. The enzymes that extract the nutrients from food work on the particles' surface area only, and the smaller the pieces of food, the greater the surface area for them to react with.

Don't eat standing up. It will cause you to eat faster than if you were properly relaxed at the table, thus the points mentioned above come into play.

Don't start running around immediately after you've eaten. Apart from feeling uncomfortable, it is harder for your body to digest food properly if you are exercising right after a meal.

Don't put too much food in your mouth. Smaller mouthfuls encourage you to chew your food more thoroughly – besides, cheeks bulging out like a hamster is never a good look.

Don't talk with your mouth full. Quite apart from turning the stomach of whoever is sitting opposite you, you will take in a great deal of air, meaning gas attacks will surely follow.

Drink a glass of water during your meal and after you've finished eating. Water aids the production of digestive juices, eases the flow of food along the digestive tract and keeps faeces soft.

Faeces are the colour they are because of pigmentation formed by the bacteria in the gut reacting with bile that travels the gastric tract, and the smell is from sulphur compounds produced by the bacteria in the colon. Sulphur-rich foods such as cabbage, broccoli, brussel sprouts and beans tend to make this more acute.

Keep it moving

Constipation is second only to gastritis as the most common intestinal complaint in the US, but as Americans spend more than $700 million each year on over-the-counter laxatives – that's over two dollars for every man, woman and child – it's safe to assume there's a great deal more that doesn't get as far as the doctor. As well as infrequency or lack of bowel movements, the term also covers difficult movements, hard or uncomfortable stools and the feeling the bowels are not yet emptied after a movement.

The truth is everybody will get constipated to some degree at some point in their lives, and around two percent of us are bunged up at any one time. The good news is, as far as you're concerned, women are twice as likely to be affected as men.

Constipation occurs in the large intestine, when the stool is unable to pass through the colon or the rectum and out through the anus, and is usually because the waste matter is too hard and dry or collecting in too large a mass. Functional (or mild) constipation is pretty much an expected by-product of today's diet and lifestyle; it will be temporary and usually clears up by itself, or with a bit of help by switching to a fibre-rich diet and drinking plenty of water.

The older you are, the more attention you need to pay to this, as your digestion will be naturally slowing down, thus waste will spend longer in the colon, meaning more water will be extracted from it. Deal with constipation by adjusting your eating/drinking habits rather than resorting to laxatives, which should only be taken on advice from your doctor.

Chronic constipation is any of the above symptoms that continue for more than two weeks after you have addressed the issue with diet and exercise. You should consult your doctor if that is the case, because there may be a more serious underlying problem – chronic constipation is an early symptom of cancer of the colon, and can also be a side effect of irritable bowel syndrome, diabetes or Parkinson's disease.

The enema within

Although the medical profession has yet to acknowledge there is any value in enemas or colonic irrigation – they are not covered by Britain's NHS – they are a popular recommendation among the alternative health community. They have been used by

> **T** Tip: When you gotta go – go. Providing it is convenient and appropriate, that is. Holding on to a bowel movement too long, too often, will harden the stool and increase the likelihood of constipation.

> **F** Fact: Most constipation isn't constipation at all, merely digestive sluggishness, as to be classified as constipation it must involve fewer than three bowel movements during the course of a week.

mankind for thousands of years, and it's easy to understand why.

Each involves the cleansing of the colon and lower intestine by introducing a liquid – saline solution or very weak coffee are the most effective – to dislodge the build-up of faecal waste on the intestinal walls. In both cases, a tube is inserted into the anus and the liquid flowed in either by gravity or gentle pressure. An enema will involve the fluid being held in the intestine for ten minutes or so while the abdomen is gently massaged; colonic irrigation is a continuous flow through an "in" and "out" tube. As dislodging years' worth of intestinal crud build-up will be a progressive process, both will involve several sessions, with the liquid penetrating a bit further along the intestine and stripping it closer to the actual wall each time.

The effects of colonic cleansing on a man who has, for years, been eating an indiscriminate diet of modern food can be quite astonishing. Once the liquid penetrates properly what comes out is solid, rubbery and intestine-shaped, both in continuous length

F

Fact: Horses get hiccups more frequently than humans do; they just don't make any sound.

21st-century blockages

The most common causes of constipation in modern times are:

- Lack of water
- Diet low in fibre
- Too much processed food
- Side effect of taking iron or calcium supplements
- Too much hard-to-digest food such as hard cheese or red meat

and outside patterning, and often black in colour. There will be a feeling of lightness and flexibility around the midsection, and a boost to general well-being as nutrients get absorbed far quicker and more efficiently through the newly exposed intestinal walls. A side effect of this last point is it won't take much to get you tipsy.

An important point to remember after either an enema or colonic irrigation is to replace the good bacteria in the gut, as the cleanse will have removed them along with all the harmful stuff.

The best of the web

alternative-healthzine.com
A site rich in tips and techniques to do with alternative health and healing. It has a huge section on digestion, the liver and colon.

Eufic.org
The European Food Information Council is packed with internal healthcare articles and diet-related tips – the section on a healthy gut is excellent.

Colonhealth.net
The Colon Therapists Network's website welcomes civilians and will supply all the information you need about colonic health.

Ten top tips for digestive health

▶ **Take zinc if you are stressed**
It will strengthen the stomach lining against any excess stomach acid.

▶ **Don't drink milk to soothe a stomach ulcer** It will ultimately make it worse – opt instead for a specially formulated antacid.

▶ **Reintroduce the good bacteria to your gut** Do this after a course of antibiotics, as the antibiotics will have killed them off as well.

▶ **Don't eat standing up**
It will cause you to eat faster, chew less thoroughly and swallow more air, all of which are overtures for indigestion.

▶ **Dislodge trapped wind with a warm drink** It will expand the intestine and shift the trapped air pocket.

▶ **Don't worry if you don't "go" every day** Just sixty percent of the population have a daily bowel movement. Only if you're going fewer than three a week should you be alarmed.

▶ **Chew your food thoroughly**
It will stand a much better chance of being efficiently digested.

▶ **To avoid constipation drink plenty of water** Stools should be 75 percent water and lack of it in the system is the most common cause of constipation.

▶ **Get a colonic irrigation**
It should be compulsory for any man over the age of thirty, as it will shift the layers of crud lining his digestive tract and allow it to function properly again.

▶ **Eat live yoghurt regularly**
It will maintain the necessary levels of friendly bacteria in your gut.

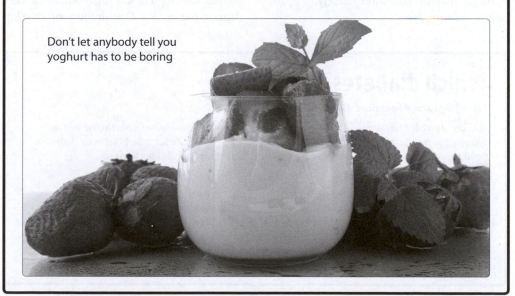
Don't let anybody tell you yoghurt has to be boring

Diabetes

Until relatively recently, diabetes had nowhere near the high profile of heart disease or lung cancer in terms of public awareness. But during the last twenty years it has become one of the world's major health issues. There are over 150,000 new cases diagnosed in the UK every year, where the number of diabetics is expected to reach the four million mark by 2025. It is rising four times as fast among men over thirty than among women of the same age. It is a chronic, progressive condition, for which there is no cure. But it can be managed with lifestyle changes and medication.

What is diabetes?

In order to metabolize carbohydrates into energy, the body breaks it down into glucose, a simple sugar, which is delivered to the muscles. Insulin, a hormone produced in the pancreas, enables this to be absorbed into cells. Diabetics with type 1 diabetes are unable to naturally metabolize glucose, as they do not produce insulin; while those suffering from type 2 do not produce enough insulin (or, alternatively, cannot utilise it properly).

Because the glucose cannot be turned into energy, it can build up in the bloodstream to dangerous levels – a condition known as hyperglycemia – which causes dizziness, extreme thirst and general feelings of weakness. In extreme cases, prolonged high blood-sugar levels can result in ketoacidosis, when, without glucose to fuel the muscles, the body starts to burn off fat and the waste from this process, known as ketones, combines with the unused glucose to turn the blood acidic. Without immediate treatment, ketoacidosis can cause a diabetic coma.

What are the symptoms?

As a condition related to the bloodstream, diabetes affects both the large and small arteries, so will have an impact on many different parts of the body. A type 2 diabetic is three times more likely to suffer heart disease than a non-diabetic – that's the same rate as a non-diabetic who has already had a heart attack. Their risk of having a stroke is also three times higher than non-diabetics, although whether or not the subject is overweight is a strong determining factor.

Kidney disease is common among diabetics, as high blood sugar will eventually damage the organs. One in four will develop

Which diabetes?

Type 1 (insulin-dependent diabetes)

This occurs when the pancreas does not produce any insulin due to a malfunction in the immune system, and results in increased blood glucose levels. There is no cure for type 1 diabetes: diabetics need to monitor their blood sugar levels and administer regular insulin injections.

Type 2 (adult-onset diabetes)

Type 2 diabetes sufferers are able to produce insulin. But they fall into two categories: they are either only capable doing so in an insufficient quantity, or they have a metabolism that is unable to utilize insulin efficiently, meaning blood sugar levels will not be correctly regulated. Around 90 percent of all diabetics have type 2. It occurs most commonly in overweight people and is often the result of a sedentary, unhealthy lifestyle. Glucose can build up in the blood due to a poor diet, or when the amount of exercise taken is insufficient to burn it off.

nephropathy (kidney disease); while forty per cent of dialysis patients are diabetics. One of the symptoms of diabetes is a blurring of vision, because changes in blood sugar effect the eye's lens; while untreated diabetes will damage the tiny blood vessels in the eye's retina, making it a common cause of blindness.

Diabetic neuropathy is a diabetes-induced condition that damages the nerves in the feet (and sometimes the hands) leading to increasing loss of feeling, which can be made worse by problems with circulation. In the UK and the US, foot problems are the most likely reason for a diabetic to be admitted to hospital, while type 2 diabetes is the leading cause of foot or lower limb amputations.

Who is most likely to get it?

Anybody can develop type 1 diabetes at any point in life, but it is considerably more likely if either parent has it. Type 2 diabetes is far more related to lifestyle: it can appear to run in families but this is often because some of the conditions that increase the likelihood are hereditary, or because of a similar way of life. Men are more likely to get type 2 than women, and if you are of Asian, African or African-Caribbean descent the risk is up to ten times higher. Those with high blood pressure or high cholesterol – particularly a high ratio of LDL (low-density lipoprotein) cholesterol to HDL (high-density lipoprotein) cholesterol – are more likely to develop the condition, as are the overweight and the sedentary.

Excessive weight greatly increases the risks of type 2 diabetes. The obese have much higher blood sugar levels, thus need to produce more insulin to manage it. Furthermore, a body that persistently overeats will not use its insulin as efficiently, because of the condition known as insulin resistance: if there is a rise in blood sugar, the body produces extra insulin in order to cope with it, which then triggers a temporary shutdown of the cells' insulin receptors. It does this to discourage further overeating,

Am I a diabetic?

You may have diabetes if you are experiencing a combination of these symptoms:

Perpetual tiredness
Frequent urination – especially during the night
Blurred vision
Perpetual and often extreme thirst
Genital itching
Unexplained weight loss
Dry skin
Cuts and grazes taking a long time to heal
Increased hunger

In the case of type 1 diabetes, these symptoms will come on quickly. But for type 2, the condition may build up slowly, and symptoms may get passed off as something else – stress, a virus, getting old and so on – with diabetes only being identified via a medical examination. If you suspect you might have diabetes, keep a written record of any of the above symptoms that occur over a two-week period, then take your findings to your doctor.

but when this insulin is not absorbed, the pancreas produces even more, thus more receptors are closed and the bloodstream is flooded with glucose.

What to do about diabetes

Type 1 diabetes can only be managed by regular and careful monitoring of blood-sugar levels with special equipment, and injections of insulin to compensate for the lack of production. Because type 2 is lifestyle-related, it can be managed by changing that damaging way of life and adopting healthy eating and regulated exercise programmes.

Diabetes fact and fiction

"If you are fat you will get diabetes"

Fiction Type 1 diabetes can affect anybody, and although obesity is a major factor in type 2, so are family history, ethnicity and lifestyle. The vast majority of overweight people are not diabetic, just as not all diabetics are not overweight.

"Diabetics can't eat cakes or sweets"

Fiction Provided the sugar is part of a healthy meal plan in which other carbohydrates have been balanced out to compensate, you can take full advantage of the dessert menu. But avoid sugar taken on its own: i.e. fizzy drinks or oversweetened coffee.

"You can still have a drink"

Fact In moderation, that is. Alcohol contains dangerous amounts of sugar for a diabetic, and large amounts can interfere with the liver as it tries to deal with low blood glucose levels.

"Diabetes is hereditary"

Faction It's true in a sense. Although the majority of diabetics have another family member who is, there will be many more relatives of diabetics that will not develop the condition.

"Diabetics can't do sports"

Fiction For type 2 diabetics, exercise should quickly become an important part of their lifestyle, but they will need to make sure their carbohydrate intake is increased and blood sugar is monitored before, during and after competing in any sport.

"You will never 'get better' from diabetes"

Fact Unfortunately diabetes can't be cured, though it can be successfully managed, and there's no reason why it should dominate your life.

Diabetes by the numbers

An estimated 7 percent of the world's population is diabetic.

By 2030 the worldwide percentage is expected to have risen to nearly 10 percent.

1.8 percent of the UK's population (2.9 million people) are diabetic.

There are an estimated 850,000 undiagnosed sufferers of type 2 diabetes in the UK.

Diabetes effects an estimated 10 percent of Americans: 28.8 million people, of whom an estimated 7 million are undiagnosed.

Per capita, the United Arab Emirates has the highest ratio of diabetics – 18.7 percent.

(*Sources: Diabetes UK/Department of Health & Human Services USA/World Health Organization*)

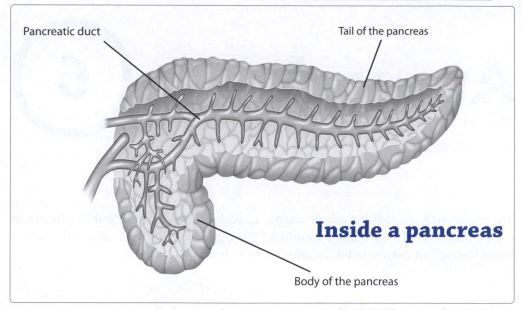

Pancreatic duct

Tail of the pancreas

Inside a pancreas

Body of the pancreas

I've just been diagnosed diabetic!

It's not the end of the world. These simple steps will put you in control, allowing you to make the changes you'll need with a minimum of stress.

• Look on the bright side: at least you now know what all that tiredness and thirstiness was about.

• Tell your partner, as she or he is going to have to work with you on this.

• Get a thorough physical examination, including an eye test, so you'll know if there are any added complications.

• If you feel you left the surgery before the information properly sank in, make an appointment to go back and have a proper conversation about it.

• Read up about diabetes: the more you understand the condition, the better you'll be able to cope with it.

• Positively plan your new lifestyle, so it seems like an improvement rather than a penance: investigate interesting healthy eating and take up a sport as exercise.

The best of the Web

diabetes.org.uk
A UK charity that provides information, advice and assistance for those affected by diabetes, while campaigning to halt the increase of the condition.

diabetes.co.uk
A global diabetes community, with a very lively forum among the advice and information pages.

diabetes.com
A US website with no-frills information about type 2 diabetes.

At work

Anybody with a full-time job probably spends more of their waking hours at work than they do with their families. What goes on there is going to have a huge impact on their overall happiness, health and well-being.

Why we want to work

That we need to work in order to be able to live well is pretty much a given – making benefit fraud really work for you would probably take a huge amount of effort these days. The better paid your job is, the better you can afford to live.

However, perhaps more significant than work's monetary worth is its massive psychological importance, especially among men for whom the hunter-gatherer gene remains a dominant part of their make-up. The reason so many retired people take on part-time work, often far below the status of what they used to do, is less about the pay packet and more about the simple act of doing a job. It allows a man to maintain his sense of self-worth.

And what do you do?

As human beings we are genetically programmed to make some sort of contribution to the advancement of the species and to the world around us. Perhaps it's because men can't have children that this need is often expressed through work.

Beyond any differences it might make to our environment, work has two important bearings on our lives.

What we do is frequently what defines who we are, as far as other people are concerned. In many cases this can serve to frustrate, especially when you're introduced to somebody and your job is the factor that decides what they think of you.

Equally, however, it can provide a flattering platform for prestige and recognition as you chat your way across the dinner parties of the world. Indeed, as a method of keeping score with your peers, what you do is generally taken more seriously than how much money you might seem to have.

Ultimately, there is so much that is vital to the well-being of our psyche that is maintained by having the right job. As well as the basic, and very powerful, need to feel useful, a man's work can satisfy creative urges. This can be crucial, as unfulfilled ambitions are a massive cause of frustration among men as they approach middle age.

Then there is the problem-solving side of any level of work. This can produce immense inner satisfaction as it brings with it a feeling of being in control. Completing the series of finite tasks that comprise most jobs fulfils our subconscious desire for closure – closures that might not be as forthcoming in other areas of life. Also, progression at work will be as gratifying as advancement in your personal or family life and probably more easily quantifiable.

Is your job the right job for you?

Although simply having a job is important, anybody who has ever been in a job that is genuinely making them miserable – as opposed to simply not liking it very much – will appreciate that having the right

---

How to get ahead at work
(without your nose turning noticeably brown)

Take a public speaking course
It will do wonders for your confidence and presentational skills.

Don't ask questions you could have answered yourself
Most bosses would rather you solved your own problems than bothered them.

Don't get distracted
Facebook, YouTube and the like are for lunchbreaks and after hours.

An apparently emotionally unstable worker will not get promoted
Stop and calm down, and leave that furious email in your draft folder for a few hours, then read it again.

Go beyond the call of duty (but within reason)
Don't slope off home every time everyone else in the office has to stay late, and take responsibility for things that need attention but might not be in your area. (While this may appear to contradict some of this book's other good health advice, it is merely a once-in-a-while suggestion – it should never be allowed to become the norm.)

Let yourself be noticed rather than clamour for attention
Most company creeps are earmarked as such early on and toadying will only get them so far.

Work smart not hard
There's a commonly held notion among many bosses that if an employee is having to stay late every night they are doing something wrong – having a life outside will stand you in much better stead than burning the midnight oil.

Take a training course or two
If your firm runs courses then take them: that's what they're there for; the people who organize them will appreciate your interest. Besides, you'll be learning a new skill at somebody else's expense.

Keep up to date with your field
If you want to do well in it you'll need to know what is happening outside your firm as well as in it. This will put you across as a Big Picture kinda guy.

Appear to want to progress
If you turn down two opportunities for promotion, don't expect to be given a third, as you will be marked as "lacking in ambition". (But, equally, pay attention to the point above about not creeping.)

Be yourself
It will serve you well in the long run.

job is vital. As you go through life your requirements and expectations will evolve; so what the best job for you is will alter. One thing that won't change, however, is that wrong jobs rarely turn into right jobs over the course of time.

Anecdotal evidence has long suggested that being in the wrong job is a far from unusual situation, and this was backed up in 2008 by a survey from the British government's Skills Commission. It showed that over forty percent of the British workforce believed they had been in the wrong job at some time; twenty percent said they were currently in such a situation; and it is estimated that, of the average working life,

nearly five years is spent doing something unsuitable.

This is a state of affairs that, according to the Chartered Management Institute, is on the increase. In its 2010 survey of recruitment companies, it concluded there had been a ten percent increase in staff turnovers across the board since 2008. While the majority of reasons given for employees changing jobs were positive – promotion, more money, better environments and so on – the upsurge was being fuelled by people moving because they were dissatisfied with what they were doing.

Being in the wrong job, often without fully realizing it, can cause a huge amount of

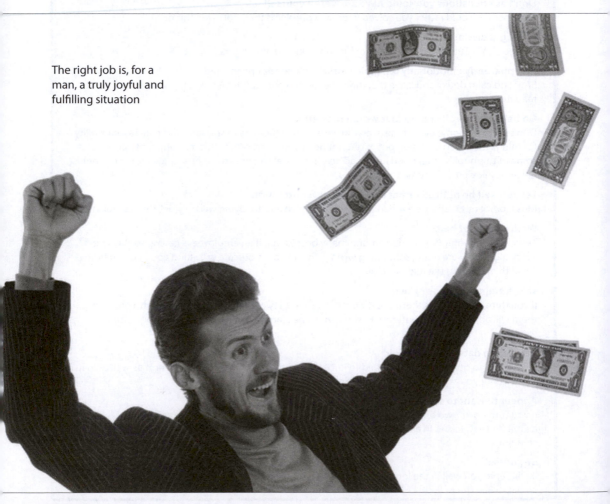

The right job is, for a man, a truly joyful and fulfilling situation

Is it worth it?

When clinically assessing your job's suitability, divide a blank sheet of paper into "For" and "Against" columns, and weigh it up. These are some of the points everybody should consider:

You dread Monday morning
You might not even realize you do, but if you are continually more tired than you should be on Monday mornings, it may be because subtly increased stress levels mean you're not sleeping well on Sunday night.

Your firm's ambitions no longer measure up to your own
It can be damagingly frustrating to be stuck in a situation you believe will not allow you to progress to the level you aspire to.

You don't get along with your colleagues
Whether this is due to a different outlook on how the firm functions or you simply don't like each other, a lack of pleasant personal interplay at work can be wretched.

You don't feel as if you are being listened to
Everybody has ideas and some of them are good, so the people above you ought to hear you out. If your suggestions aren't being taken seriously it implies you aren't either.

"Decompression" when you leave for the day seems to be taking longer and longer
This can often lead to drinking too much, or can have an adverse effect on your domestic life if it means work-related problems come home with you.

You've hit the Glass Ceiling
They are very real, and if it seems like you've suddenly stopped progressing for no apparent reason you're probably squashed up against one.

stress, because underutilization of your skills can only lead to frustration, as can being expected to perform tasks that are beyond you. And because you'll spend so much time at work, having to do something you simply don't have any feel for or interest in is going to make your career path seem more like a prison sentence.

Signs can be apparent even before you start a new job: if you don't hit it off with your prospective boss at interview stage, the chances are you never will; and a lengthy commute that eats into your evenings won't get any shorter; whilst taking a job for the money, as a means to an end, is only a good idea so long as you realize the money's all you'll ever get out of it.

Feeling the pressure

Work-related stress accounts for around 14 million lost working days in the UK per year, once the depression and anxiety brought on by it is taken into account. This costs the British economy some £4 billion annually. In the US, it is estimated that occupational stress costs employers around $200 billion per annum in terms of absenteeism, reduced productivity, compensation payments, higher staff turnovers, and costlier health insurance. The United Nations International Labor Organization is calling stress at work a "global epidemic".

This is a situation that is unlikely to change, given the pressures in the workplace towards longer hours. We are expected to do more in less time, we are provided with

How it all works: stress

When confronted with danger or entering a stressful situation, our exteroceptors (eyes, ears, nose et al) send sensory nerve impulses along the spinal cord and the brain stem, alerting the brain to what is happening. Once these signals have been processed within the brain stem, commands called autonomic nerve responses are sent back down the spinal cord (the central nervous system). Autonomic nerve fibres are part of the peripheral nerve system that connects the brain, via the spinal cord, to the body's internal organs and glands. The signals that run along them serve to regulate the body's internal environment. Autonomic nerve responses are not under our conscious control but operate purely on internal impulse, and fall into two categories, sympathetic and parasympathetic; the former prepares the body for action and the latter is a calming influence.

The sympathetic responses to stress cause the pupils to dilate to let in the maximum amount of light and promote clear vision, the bronchial tubes to open to allow the most air into the lungs, the stomach lining stops producing digestive enzymes and the liver releases extra glucose into the bloodstream for energy. None of this we have any control over, and is an instantaneous natural reaction. Most importantly, the sympathetic nerve impulses stimulate the adrenal gland, and its reactions form the driving force of our reaction to stress.

The adrenal gland sits on a cushion of fat on top of the kidneys, and under normal conditions plays a role in the production and deployment of energy, but in times of stress it is pushed into overdrive. Its outer layer, the cortex, starts producing extra amounts of the corticosteroid hormones, one of which is cortisol, also known as the "stress hormone". In normal circumstances our cortisol levels are highest in the early morning, as it helps us wake up, but now, in preparation for fight or flight, this amount will greatly raise the blood pressure, allow blood sugar levels to rise by increasing the breaking down of glycogen; it also has anti-inflammatory properties. The inner part of the gland, the medulla, releases the hormone epinephrine – adrenalin – which increases the heart rate and stroke volume, and boosts the supplies of oxygen and glucose to the brain and the muscles by constricting the blood vessels in the skin but dilating those in the muscles. It raises the levels of glycogen production in the liver and has a suppressive effect on the immune system, so no internal energy is being wasted.

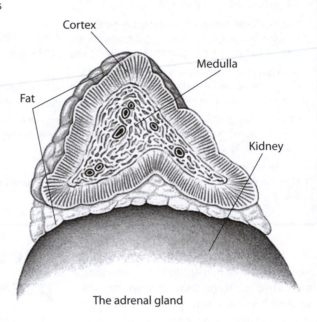

Cortex

Medulla

Fat

Kidney

The adrenal gland

The adrenal gland will keep these levels up as long as the brain continues to feel under threat, which is why chronic stress can be so physically damaging, but if the situation is resolved the parasympathetic responses kick in. They will constrict the pupils, contract the bronchial tubes, resume the production of stomach enzymes, reduce glucose levels and normalize activity in the adrenal gland.

less training and we have lower levels of job security. Work-related stress tends to have a far greater psychological effect on men than domestic- or relationship-based pressures, as it is much harder to be in control of your own destiny in the workplace than at home.

Anxiety and depression are the two most damaging effects of stress and are likely to have an impact on every aspect of your life. They will often manifest themselves in binge drinking, eating disorders or drug abuse (legal or otherwise). Ongoing stress can also lead to cardiovascular disease, as your system remains pumped up and on edge for too long. Digestive problems such as irritable bowel syndrome are not uncommon when you're seriously stressed, as are backache and other muscular complaints, because you are physically tense much more than is good for you. Being stressed does your immune system no favours, leading to a general feeling of malaise and ill-health. If you are experiencing any of the above and the condition persists after you have taken medicinal steps to remedy it, then it could be stress-related.

Get out of there

Keeping a diary of how you feel at work can help hugely when it comes to assessing

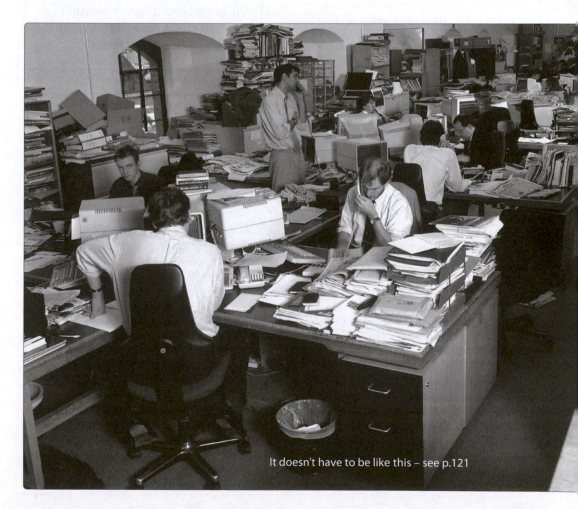

It doesn't have to be like this – see p.121

whether you should be there or not, as it will allow accurate review of your feelings over a period of time.

But if you are stressed-out yet want to stay in the job you're in (at least for the time being), then there are still a number of things you can do to protect yourself – among which eating healthily and making sure you are drinking enough water during the day are good places to start. Particular attention should be paid to the amount of water you are drinking because the modern environment – centrally heated, air conditioned, with a computer screen in close proximity – is dangerously dehydrating.

And don't forget to keep an eye on the amount of coffee you are necking, as not only is it a diuretic (therefore will speed up your drying out), but the caffeine will keep you on edge, which is never the most advisable way not to get stressed.

Expert advice: "Knowing if there is actually something specifically wrong with you or if you are simply over-stressed depends on how well you know your own body and psyche and your level of fitness. People need to take more interest in themselves when they are well, then they would be much more able to tell when something is not quite right – men are not very good at that. If you are worried, or think something might be more than externally caused stress, you should go to your GP." Dr Liliana Risi, GP

Eat to beat stress

Dr Sarah Schenker believes that today's convenience-food-heavy diet is a major factor in the escalating cases of work-related stress:

"People who feel they are suffering from stress, or what they believe to be depression, should look at their diets; the widespread state of low-level, background malnutrition can worsen the effects of fatigue which is a huge contributor to stress.

You could just be slightly deficient in a few vitamins and minerals, and you can remedy that by including a few more fruits and vegetables in your diet. It could be that you're eating a lot of energy-dense food – a lot of fatty, sugary products – and you're beginning to put on weight. Which could easily have the effect of making you feel tired and stressed. So if you replace the bad stuff with healthier food, you'll soon start feeling more energetic.

This is something you probably wouldn't be able to put your finger on and say it's because you're lacking this or that – and that's why you feel fatigued and stressed. In fact you could go for all sorts of blood tests but they wouldn't show it up. It's an overall thing, which can be addressed by looking at what you're eating and working out if you are getting enough all-round nutrition to function at one hundred percent.

Not drinking enough water is another major factor, especially with so many air-conditioned environments and people sitting in front of computer screens all day long – both of which can have a dehydrating effect. Being permanently mildly dehydrated often goes unnoticed, as it's not enough to make you feel thirsty all the time because your body has got used to it, but it's enough to make sure you're operating maybe fifteen percent less efficiently than you could be. Then that becomes the new norm. A work-related malaise could be as simple as dehydration making you feel tired, lethargic and irritable, which will contribute greatly to your being stressed."

There's never any simple solution for work-related stress, but…

Cause of stress	An employee can	An employer should
Demands of the job	Be less reticent in asking questions or asking for help; receive and understand a detailed job description; and prioritize tasks.	Provide adequate training; make sure employee understands how best to carry out tasks; or consider flexible working hours to relieve bottlenecks.
Feelings of not being in control	Plan your working day more precisely; assume more responsibility (without treading on anybody's toes); organize your working environment; try to finish one task before starting another; and resist perfectionism (but, obviously, still do the best you can).	Avoid unreasonable deadlines; provide a clear structure for career development; and encourage smaller units of self-contained teamwork within a large workforce.
Physical environment	Tidy up; stay fit and healthy; make whatever adjustments you can to heating, lighting or furniture; and buy some plants.	Listen to your employees if they say it's not right; renew worn-out equipment or furniture; decorate; and buy some plants.
Personal space/ workstation	Find out what your ideal working ergonomics should be and try to adhere to them (see p.129); keep your space clutter-free and well organized; and change positions frequently .	Carry out regular workstation audits to make sure equipment is as posture-friendly as possible.
Change – in routine or corporate policies	Ask questions of management rather than whisper in corners; put forward your own ideas about small changes; and try to stay optimistic about change – men are actually far less keen on change than women.	Improve communications; be transparent with employees about major changes; involve them in minor changes.
Personal and professional relationships	Report any harassment or bullying – either experienced or witnessed; don't immediately blame others: you might be a pain to work with yourself; and stay away from negative people.	Take reports of harassment or bullying seriously; be prepared to intervene in personality clashes; and pick your management team for people skills as much as work skills.

It's not just what you are eating but where you are eating it. The whole purpose of a lunch break should be as much to do with the break as it is the lunch. Although workplace culture seems to be dictating that more and more of us wolf down sandwiches at our workstations, the need to get a change of environment during the middle of the working day has never been greater.

Getting some real, as opposed to recycled, fresh air will do wonders for your brain, and just looking at something else and interacting with different people will keep you alert. It will also give you the chance to physically walk away from anything that might have been causing you problems and either to think it through clearly or think about something else entirely. Then there's the physical exercise aspect of just walking about for a bit; it will get your blood flowing faster and should burn up a few calories.

Afternoon lows

So many of us, whatever job we're in, will experience mid-afternoon energy slumps, thanks to a combination of the body's circadian rhythm and a dip in blood sugar. It's a situation that can affect both your productivity and motivation, but one that can be addressed. To reduce the slump, eat less but more often, to even out your blood sugar levels throughout the day. Huge, calorific lunches are pretty much a guarantee of afternoon drowsiness. When you eat, you should also mix lean protein and carbohydrate for the most effective energy intake and management. Don't attempt to beat that energy slump with caffeine, as any high gained will be followed by a crash later on. Likewise, avoid sugary snacks or any empty calories. Of course, getting a good night's sleep in the first place will minimize any afternoon low.

Use your holiday time

Getting away from work for longer than a weekend is vital. Holidays need to be taken for all the obvious positive benefits a vacation has to offer, but the time spent away from work gives you the chance to get it totally out of your system and reconnect

Learn to do nothing

One of the reasons we remain so stressed is we don't give ourselves time to think about what has happened that day. Dr Sandra Scott maintains this is a result of constantly stimulated lifestyles.

"Usually people will do anything other than just sit down and think, to simply be left alone with their thoughts, and they are removing a very important aspect of their lives.

Downtime, when you come home at the end of a day, is very, very important. You can come in wound as tight as a spring after the day from hell, and just sit on the sofa and go through it. Think about it, run through every bit of it, try to understand it. While you may re-live some of the pain which will still feel uncomfortable, and it will take a while to get to where you want to be, in the end you will feel a good deal better and probably sleep better.

Now, because technological progress has made our lives so much quicker, many of us have been trained to believe that the smart option in these circumstances is to close the door with one hand, and open the fridge with the other. Get out a bottle of wine, turn the television on and you've got over your day in a fraction of the time. Much more time efficient! That's as may be, but much less effective, as we have just put a great big sticking plaster on the problem and not really dealt with it at all. Things are still unresolved and that will be a big contributor to future stress: the problem continues to lurk under the surface. That half-hour is so important, and it should be claimed back."

Natural stressbusters

Supplement	Effect
St John's Wort	King Calm. Nature's most pacifying herb, containing hypericin which can act as an antidepressant
Ginko	Increases the blood flow through the brain to sharpen focus and improve memory
Calcium & magnesium	Helps muscles to relax
Camomile	Soothes, calms and aids digestion
Celery juice	Lowers blood pressure and can lift the mood to alleviate anxiety
Valerian root	A mild sedative that will help you sleep and quietens the nervous system
Nutmeg	A mild sedative that works like valerian root, but which works much more slowly longer
Kola nut	A minor stimulant, with mood-elevating properties – used to be found in Coca-Cola

with a few of the reasons you go to work in the first place – to have a good life outside it. Even if you just mooch about the house for a couple of weeks.

Try not to take your BlackBerry or laptop with you – or even your mobile phone. Avoid the temptation to keep checking emails. Or if for some reason you have to stay in touch, do so at predetermined times so you are not on permanent call – and possibly from another time zone. You will survive without your work, and, unless you're Jack Bauer, your work will survive without you. You always know when you've had a good holiday, because you feel ready to come back to work.

Stress and the employer

As an employer you are legally obliged to treat stress like any other health and safety issue, and take all appropriate measures to avoid it among your workforce. Should an employee take you to court and prove the stress they suffered was preventable, the compensation that can be awarded will be considerable. Normal sick-leave rules must be applied to stress-related symptoms.

A

Expert advice: "Lunchtimes are the ideal time to start working out. It's easy to schedule a half-hour programme three times a week, so you'll probably stick to it. Exercising in the middle of the day will keep you from eating damaging food at lunch. And because you've had your heart working hard it will boost your energy levels in the afternoon."
Gideon Remfry

Although in the US there are no set-in-stone rules pertaining to corporate responsibilities as regards employees' work-related stress, it is an accepted condition and falls within the bounds of health and personal injury insurance. Thus legal action, taken by employees or by insurance companies against employers after they have paid out on claims resulting from occupational stress, is commonplace and usually successful. Consquently, you will need to take the prevention and treatment of work-related stress very seriously. According to the US Department of Labor Bureau of Labor Statistics, nearly all companies offer access to free stress counselling for their employees, and over half of the major corporations in the US have stress counsellors on site.

Do you know what you're doing?

Making sure you have an accurate, hard-copy job description can save a huge amount of stress further down the line. Knowing precisely what responsibilities and functions your position entails will enable you to approach it

T *Tip: Research has shown that music in the workplace increases productivity and reduces stress levels. Less straightforward though is making sure it's the right sort of music.*

with a greater degree of confidence, meaning you will adjust to it quicker, and reduce any stress levels. Also, if you've got it all written down then there will be far fewer "but that's not my job!"-type conversations.

Your job description should include the basis for and frequency of your performance reviews, what the salary range is for that position, and to whom you will report and who will report to you. Also, be aware of what certain terms mean, and check that they are being applied correctly within your job description: job (an overall term for everything you have to do or are responsible for); task or function (an action or set of actions with a defined outcome); responsibility (making sure certain tasks or

The testosterone myth

Since the 1980s the popular image of striped-shirted City traders "knocking down" serious money in testosterone-fuelled dealing rooms has fuelled the notion that only men could function effectively in such a high-pressure environment. However, research at Cambridge University has found that men are far more likely to get it wrong under these circumstances than women, and that excessive production of the hormones testosterone and cortisol can actually play their part in market fluctuations.

The findings were that when traders go on successful runs, their testosterone soars on a level similar to a winning sportsman, leading to a feeling of invincibility and increased risk-taking – many talked of "being in the zone". This state was found to seriously impair their decision-making abilities, leading to bigger and increasingly unwise trading. Then once things started to take a downward turn, the stress hormone cortisol kicked in to counteract this recklessness and reverse the situation. The same traders would then refuse to take any chances, which would manifest itself in their opting for secure, unprofitable deals, or even not dealing at all. As a result, any downturn of the market would start to accelerate. The conclusion was that women traders, whose behaviour would not be influenced by such hormone surges, could go a long way to creating a more stable economic climate.

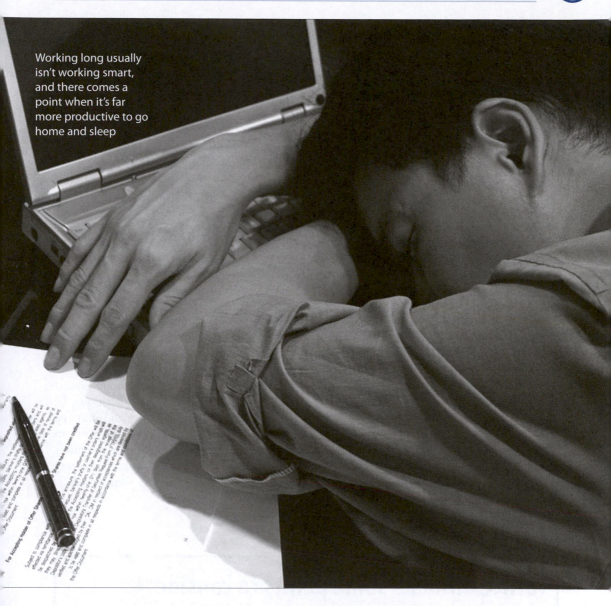

Working long usually isn't working smart, and there comes a point when it's far more productive to go home and sleep

functions achieve their outcome, whether you actually do it or not); and role (a set of responsibilities within a job).

Stress: a last word

Stress will affect everybody in different ways. There is no "cure" for stress as such and the only way to deal with it is to rectify the situation that is causing it. Never be afraid to talk to somebody who's in a position to help – your boss, a union representative, human resources – about whatever is worrying you. Try to keep your working day as ordered as possible: that way you'll feel more in control. Try not to sweat about the small stuff either. Keep things in perspective: realize that some things simply aren't worth worrying about.

Sex and the city

Given that we are spending longer and longer at work, it's perhaps hardly surprising that you are much more likely to have met your long-term partner through work than you would have in previous decades. Office romances have become more and more common. The increasing weight of work in the work/life balance means it's assuming a greater importance in everything we do. Among single men it's starting to become as central to their world as primary school is to a young child. This might, if you're lucky, be accompanied by a more flexible, relaxed and employee-centric work environment, which brings the social aspects of going to work to the fore.

A work environment is actually in many ways the perfect dating agency, as it throws a group of similarly minded, similarly educated people of a similar social status together, then puts them under pressure for some of that time – meaning there's plenty of opportunity to look impressive. (And, admittedly, a fair few opportunities for making a fool of yourself.)

Getting together with somebody from work is arguably a more sensible way of starting a relationship than, say, meeting somebody in a club where what they look like will probably be the sole deciding factor. Prospective couples will have already got to know each other without the immediate bother of trying to "pull" or be "pulled" – thus the chances are they will actually like each other, as well as fancy each other.

Then there is that enormous advantage of knowing you have plenty in common and enough to talk about on a first date to avoid any awkward silences. Is it really any wonder office friendships so often turn horizontal?

If you are an employer

In most cases, an office romance will cause no problems whatsoever. As an employer, it is your job to be aware of what is going on, but you should only feel any obligation to refer to the situation, or offer advice, should what's going on have a potential bearing on the firm – adultery or chain-of-command relationships.

If things do go horribly wrong, and if that could threaten corporate harmony, be prepared to talk to both parties and shift one of them if necessary. But otherwise you can reassure yourself that most office romances turn out fine and may well result in two very happy – therefore productive – employees.

Office affairs – some points to consider

Don't assume nobody else has noticed. Body language has probably meant it's been a talking point for weeks.

A messy break-up will be that much messier if you have to share a coffee machine or ride in a lift with your ex on a daily basis.

Avoid relationships with direct subordinates or superiors. No matter how careful the two of you may be to avoid it affecting your working relationship, it has the potential to cause enormous resentment among others. We are, after all, sometimes talking about people who will go into a strop because somebody else gets a stationery order filled first.

If the affair is adulterous, be aware that a reaction from a wronged party could end up in your place of work.

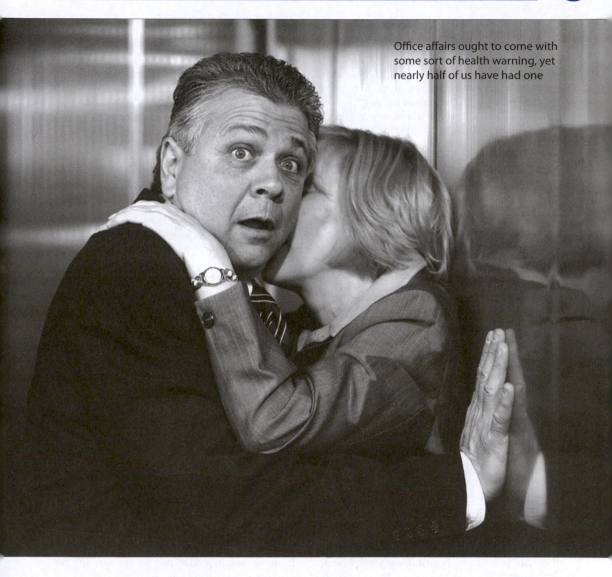

Office affairs ought to come with some sort of health warning, yet nearly half of us have had one

Is your chair killing you?

If you work in an office, the chances are you'll spend at least five hours a day sitting at your desk, probably in front of a monitor. And there's a good probability that it is giving you all sorts of aches and pains, as poor workspace ergonomics is one of the major causes of work-related malaise.

Shoulder, neck and back aches as the result of unhealthy posture contribute significantly to headaches, tiredness and vision problems, as they are usually symptoms of impeded blood supply to the brain. To ensure you are not doing yourself any damage, attention should be paid to your chair, desk and computer screen arrangements.

The top of your screen should be at, or just below, eye level and directly in front of you; the cumulative effects of even minor

133

Dress-down Friday

Many firms actively encourage socializing and organize out-of-office events in the name of team building, allowing colleagues to get to know each other better. In office environments where a suit and tie is still the order of the day, "Dress-down Friday" has played a large part in this, as these casually attired days allow another side of people to show through. However, as your own style reveals much more about you than the standard dark suit, for many people dress-down Fridays have become a sartorial minefield.

Stick to what you are comfortable in, but be careful about just how casual "casual" actually is. Look on it as going to a new restaurant – you don't want to get seated near the toilets for rocking up like a beach bum. Or be pointed at from behind menus for looking too posh. Follow the lead of those who have been at the firm longer than you and dress to their level, but don't let this become a second uniform of clothes you'd never normally be seen dead in, or you'll resent it more than wearing a suit. And never ever show off with expensive designer labels, or people will start to resent you. Blend in and let your performance stand out.

twisting can cause major lower-back pain. The screen should be between eighteen and thirty inches away from you – just beyond your fingertips when you are sitting up straight is a rule of thumb. Wearers of bifocal or varifocal spectacles may even wish to invest in a pair of "computer glasses" that allow you to read comfortably at the distance your screen will be from you.

Your keyboard should be directly in front of the screen, with the mouse kept close to it on your dominant side. It is best to employ a wrist support that will mean the back of your hand is parallel to the desk when operating the mouse.

Your chair needs to allow you to sit in the Ninety Degree Position with your back flat against the chair back. This posture means your upright back will be at ninety degrees to your thighs, which will be at ninety degrees to your shins with your feet flat on the ground. Adjust your chair's height and the angle of its back to achieve this.

It is absolutely vital that the lumbar support in the back of the chair is snug to your lower back to relieve pressure on the base of your spine – if it is not, augment it with a cushion or a folded towel. The seat should firmly support the backs of thighs, with between two and four inches of space

between its front edge and the backs of your knees.

If the chair has arms, they should be adjusted so that your shoulders are neither slouched nor raised when resting lightly on them; this should be just below the level of the desk so your forearms angle upwards slightly. Don't rest your hands on the keyboard or the mouse when you are not actually using them.

Get up, move around and stretch as much as possible, paying particular attention to pulling the shoulders back to counteract the forward posture needed to operate a keyboard. Try "dynamic sitting", which is to deliberately alter your posture every half hour or so, in order not to remain in the same position for too long.

If you're regularly using a laptop at a desk, a mouse is a must, while a proper keyboard and screen will help hugely. Laptops aren't designed for working over extended periods of time and will push you into all sorts of unsuitable positions.

How it all works: the ergonomic workstation

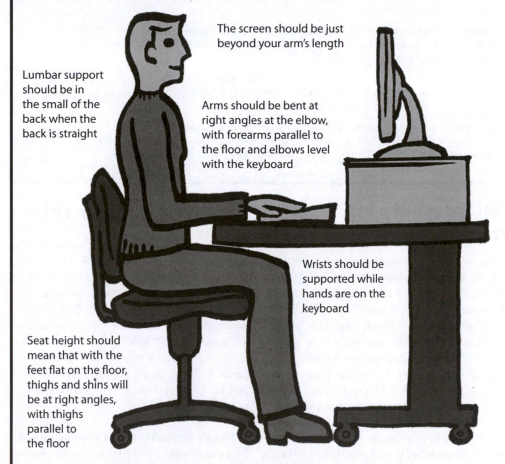

With head erect, back straight and shoulders square, the top of your screen should be just below eye level

Environment should be light, well ventilated or air-conditioned and at a comfortable temperature

The screen should be just beyond your arm's length

Lumbar support should be in the small of the back when the back is straight

Arms should be bent at right angles at the elbow, with forearms parallel to the floor and elbows level with the keyboard

Wrists should be supported while hands are on the keyboard

Seat height should mean that with the feet flat on the floor, thighs and shins will be at right angles, with thighs parallel to the floor

Chair should support the thighs to the backs of the knees

Although feet are flat to ascertain correct seat height, it is best to sit with legs out as straight as possible

Six signs that it might be time to look for another job

The company has stopped hiring and no longer seems to be growing
This is a sure sign that things aren't as comfortable for the firm as they once were.

Good work gets overlooked – and not just yours
Everybody deserves praise for a job well done and encouragement to do even better. If this isn't part of your company's culture you can surely do better.

There is no promotion from within
If the firm is continually making management appointments from outside, they don't appear to trust their existing workforce.

Senior management is shifty about the future or the company's finances
While you can't expect everything to be totally transparent, you should be able to get straight answers to most questions.

Your colleagues seem to have as many problems as you
When that "quick drink after work" regularly degenerates into a marathon booze-sodden moan-fest, it's very likely everybody else is as fed up as you.

Everybody around you seems to be working longer and longer hours
But nobody seems to be getting any more out of the experience in terms of financial reward. This means your firm is quietly cutting back at its workforce's expense.

Tall men have big problems

If you are above average height (5 feet 10 inches), much of the world won't be designed for you. Particularly your workstation. Make sure your computer monitor is raised up to your eye level on a stand, and your chair has back and shoulder support in the right places. Don't be tempted to adjust your viewing position by hunching your neck down into your shoulders, as over time this can push your top vertebrae together, which will pinch nerves and impede the blood supply to your brain. Also, try to avoid chairs with high backs and protruding upper support sections, as they will pitch your shoulders forward. Stretching and moving your neck and shoulders on a regular basis will be particularly important for you.

Trouble at work

Nobody goes through their working life without having a few problems. These could be anything from an unhealthy working environment to a bad boss or infuriating employees; perhaps even bullying or discrimination. You may not want to look for a new job – indeed, why should you? Your problem may not be that big. But it still needs to be resolved. While every problem will be unique, there is a general procedure to be followed:

1. Work out exactly what the problem is
Make sure you are clear about who or what is causing your problem. Make notes or write things down more formally. This will force you into studying whatever it is and may lead you to a straightforward resolution.

2. Can it be sorted informally?

The next step will be to talk with somebody who is in a position to help, such as your foreman, line manager, an HR manager or personnel officer. Although such a talk will be informal, you should take notes to refer to if you have to take it further.

3. Make a formal complaint

Should you go this far you will need to follow your company's grievance procedure – if you don't know what this is, ask for a copy. This will certainly involve making a written complaint that clearly and precisely explains your problem, and the best way to approach this is to set it out in bullet points.

Once your employer has investigated the matter you should be called in for a formal hearing – it is a good idea to take somebody with you (such as a union representative) to this meeting, which is your statutory right.

4. Appeal

If you are dissatisfied with the result of this hearing it is your statutory right to appeal against it. This will usually mean having another hearing with a more senior manager.

5. Outside arbitration

Beyond your own company's grievance procedures, or if you have been dismissed, there are a number of impartial third

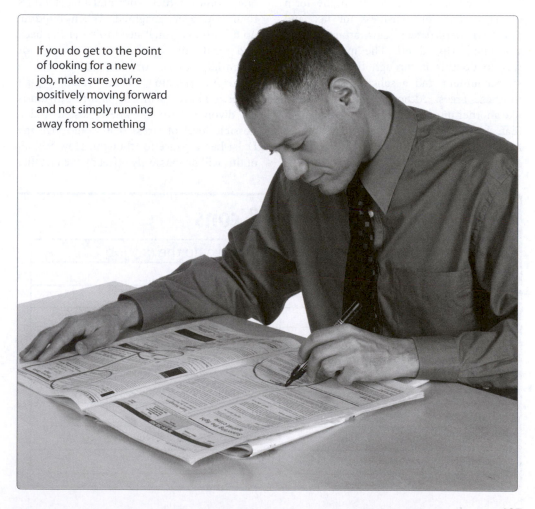

If you do get to the point of looking for a new job, make sure you're positively moving forward and not simply running away from something

parties that can be involved. Conciliation or arbitration services will be potentially less expensive than employment tribunals or civil courts, and you should consult your local Citizens Advice Bureau as to which would be most suitable for your case.

Going it alone

If you do decide you've had enough of working for The Man and opt to become your own boss, you've probably already got to the point at which you've had that brilliant idea, found the gap in the market, written your business plan and found a very understanding bank manager. Now you have to embrace officialdom in the form of registering your business for tax, and any trademark/patent registration to stop you being ripped off. The most reliable way to do this is through the services of an accountant and a solicitor specializing in these areas. Although this may seem like another unnecessary expense, remember that: this probably isn't where your expertise lies; a professional will cover every detail; and you have far too much else to be getting

on with at the moment (if you haven't – you probably should!).

Any solicitor or accountant you are looking to engage should tell you exactly what they will charge you before any agreement is struck. Get this in writing if it is a concern. During the course of your business your accountant will become your best friend, but use him or her sparingly and save yourself money by doing as much of the bookkeeping as you can yourself. Don't simply send in a carrier bag full of receipts and invoices. But if you don't feel your accountant is giving you the best service, find another one. There are plenty more out there.

That was the (relatively) easy part. Now comes harder work and longer hours than you ever imagined. When building up a business, you'll need to be at the beck and call of customers (existing or potential) more or less 24 hours a day and remain self-motivated at all times. There will be more grounds for divorce than you knew existed and a possible level of stress that would give the Dalai Lama pause for thought. However, all of this will be massively offset by the fact that

Self-employed: the pros & cons

Follow your dream	Don't give up the day job
Far more direct effort/reward ratio	Irregular income
Hours to suit	All the hours God sends
You are in charge	There is nobody else to blame
Immense self-satisfaction	Massive frustration if things don't go to plan
No good idea or innovation will go unlistened to	There is nobody to save you from yourself if you get something very wrong
Independence	Stress of shouldering total responsibility
Control over your future	Start up costs
The chance to acquire new skills	Often you'll have to do everything
Potential for vast wealth	Possibility of bankruptcy

Should you get laid off...

Make sure you get what's owed to you
Find out exactly what your employer should be giving you when you leave, then apply for all the unemployment benefits permissible. Don't let any imagined stigma put you off: it's your entitlement.

Explain what's happened to your family
That includes your children, if they are old enough to understand what it means:, they will be affected by this and dodging their questions will only add to your stress levels.

Talk to your bank manager
You may need extended credit facilities or rearranged payment schedules at some point, so it's best to keep your bank in the loop from day one.

Keep to a regular schedule
Get up at a set time, do things according to plans and generally try to keep as much structure to your day as possible. It will help you feel more in control of things. You'll also get a lot more done.

Stay busy
As well as job-hunting, CV-writing and contact-calling, do things around the house. You still need to work, regardless of whether you have a job or not.

Look on the bright side
It sounds trite, but it will greatly help your frame of mind if you look on this juncture as an opportunity to advance your life either by learning a new skill, getting a new job or simply reconnecting with your family.

you are as in control of your own destiny as possible, and all the rewards for your graft or ideas or innovations will come directly to you.

All work and no play

The last few decades have been very tough on men in their working lives. During that time, in almost every area, the landscape has changed to such an extent it's unlikely your dad would even recognize it. We have fewer and fewer opportunities to escape from work and so less time to relieve its pressures. The biggest contributor towards overall chronic stress is a skewed work/life balance.

In today's frantically paced world, information technology has meant we are expected to be contactable at any time. Globalization has meant we'll probably be working with people in different time zones, which has expanded the working day, while longer hours have become par for practically everybody. It means work is taking over the time we spend doing fun things. As the amount of time we have to devote to work-related issues goes up, we need more time away from it to recover, but that side of our lives is actually being reduced.

Re-adjust your work/life balance

The only way to put this right again is to reorganize your approach to all aspects of your life, and, paying particular attention to how you can reduce the work-related side, regain control of how it all adds up. But to do that you've got to be aware of what's going on.

So keep a diary. Yes, this seems to figure in the answer to pretty much everything, but that's because it works – to find out how to change your life you need to know exactly what's going on in it. Over the course of a month, log what you do and how and where you do it on a week-by-week basis, then examine it, maybe with your life partner, to work out what can be redressed.

How to cut back

Better organization, more efficient time management and clearer communications will help enormously to cut the amount of time spent on mundane tasks. Being able to find things, having people understand you, not being late, and logically prioritizing your to-do list will cut the time spent not actually achieving anything. Don't confuse working late with getting a great deal done: the more tired you get, the slower you will be working. It's usually best to pack up for the day and

start again tomorrow, properly refreshed.

Don't be a slave to your BlackBerry or iPhone. While they undoubtedly have all sorts of exciting leisure-time-related features, don't allow yours to shackle you to the office. It has only been three or four decades since cassette-loaded telephone answering machines were novel enough to be considered a superfluous extra: your world didn't grind to a halt if people had to phone you back later in the day. This principle pretty much still applies. On a similar note, if you don't want to take work home with you when you leave, don't bring a bag or a briefcase in with you in the morning.

In your domestic life, split housework to do a little every day rather than spend half the weekend on it. Treat yourself to any labour-saving devices that could save you extra hours here and there, and try to do errands with your partner/housemates/

Make sure the next job's the right job

Once you decide you shouldn't be in a job, start looking for a new one as soon as possible. This in itself can make your working life more bearable, because at least you'll feel in control of your situation. Once you get beyond the theoretical and start applying for jobs or going for interviews, there are a few guidelines that can steer you towards the right one.

Know what you want and don't be afraid to talk about it

If you need specific hours, or have concerns over equipment, or want a certain amount of space, ask about it. Don't be shy about asking to see your potential workspace, or for a rundown of what a typical corporate day involves, because this will help you make your mind up and there will be fewer surprises after you start.

Don't worry about the interviewer liking you

An interview should be a two-sided affair and they should want you as much as you want the job, so give an honest-as-you-can account of yourself and be careful not to agree to or accept less than you had in mind because you think it will increase your chances of getting the job – it probably won't.

If it seems too good to be true, it probably is

Too often the money/old rope transactions will turn out to be anything other than easy, and if a job offers a seemingly huge salary, the chances are you will earn at least that much in terms of sheer hard work, grief or ridiculous hours.

Keep it real

Be yourself at any interview, because if you start playing a part – or get a job because they think you're somebody you're not – you'll have to keep that up for as long as you stay at the firm.

Are you cut out to be the boss?

You are likely to make a good manager if you...	You might be better off in a non-managerial role if you...
Are unselfconscious about telling people what you think they should do	Can make the most of others' ideas or instructions
Assume responsibilities and leadership	Offer valuable support to the decision-making process
Are willing to be hugely flexible when it comes to dealing with problems	See things from a more tightly focused point of view, rather than taking in the big picture
Are a "people person"	Don't feel too confident telling others what to do or that they have made mistakes
Can work or make decisions on your own	Function best as an integral part of a larger unit
Don't mind being where the buck stops	Like to go home at six o'clock, firmly closing the workplace door behind you

family instead of rushing in and out on your free days. It's best to treat housework like work: it is something that can encroach on time you could be enjoying yourself.

Delegate as much as you can in both your work life and your home life, so you don't do more than you need to. At work, trust other people to take their share of the workload. This will improve relations with those around you, as it's fairly insulting to be saying that the only way anything will get done is if you do it. That means taking a day off if you're not well. The world won't grind to a halt and you are doing nobody any favours spreading germs and bad vibes among your co-workers.

On the home front, farm out tasks that you aren't very good at, or haven't time to do: make use of a cleaner, painter, decorator, window cleaner or gardener if you can afford to. It will free up valuable time to spend with your family or on relaxing leisure pursuits.

Explore your options and find out what your firm offers in the way of flexible hours or working from home, and if this cuts down on time spent at work or travelling to work then take advantage of it. If you do work from home, make sure you keep regular office hours for starting and finishing your day and for a lunchbreak; this will stop you blurring the edges between your domestic and professional lives.

Rein in that ego which can so often find you refusing to admit defeat under impossible circumstances. Men are loath to admit they can't do something or that they need help, and will often feel obliged to prove they are working harder than those around them. Even in today's cut-throat corporate culture, where we are led to believe that results must be achieved at any cost, it pays enormously to work smart not hard.

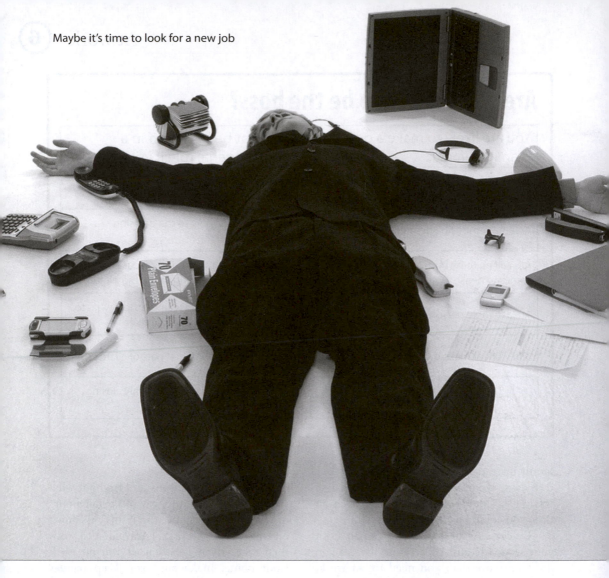

Me time

Set aside "me time" (which could equally be "family time") during the working week, in which your email alerts, your mobile phone and your computer are all switched off, so work cannot find a way through to you. At first it might feel almost like you're playing truant, and you might get a bit twitchy, but ride it out. This time should be reserved for something that will relax you – five-a-side football, taking the kids swimming, watching a couple of DVDs with your partner, dinner with your dad… anything – but make sure you keep that time sacred.

Learn to enjoy doing nothing, and don't spend time off looking for things to do, or, worst of all, feeling guilty about just sitting about. As regards people around you, if you start appearing unoccupied and relaxed, your family will find it much easier to approach you, meaning all sorts of fun will follow.

Do something you've always fancied doing, whether it's learning the trumpet, playing golf, taking an evening class in joinery or training to run a marathon. You'll enjoy yourself, as well as developing a new skill to keep your body and brain ticking over. If you thrive on challenges, set yourself goals that can involve family and friends, targets that only put you under as much pressure as you want

Ten top tips for a less stressful working life

▶ **Tidy up your personal space** Your life will be so much easier if you can find things quickly, and being surrounded by clutter will not help you think in an ordered way.

▶ **Don't be late** Not only will you have less time for whatever it is you have to do, you will be starting on the back foot and you will hugely irritate those around you – why should your time be more important than theirs?

▶ **Ask for help if you need it** Everybody needs help at some point and it's certainly not a "sign of weakness" if it means you get the job done to the required standard.

▶ **Take time off if you are sick** You are not indispensable – nobody is – and those around you would much rather you stayed at home than dragged your semi-functioning, germ-ridden self into work.

▶ **Set achievable goals** There is nothing more frustrating than a lengthy to-do list that gets moved over to the next day time after time after time, as you end up spending the evening thinking about what you didn't do rather than what you achieved.

▶ **Don't let emotions influence professional decisions** If you do they will seldom be the best ones you've ever made, and while it may have been cathartic to write that blistering email, don't actually send it until you've calmed down and read through it again.

▶ **Have a life outside work** You will physically feel better, your family will enjoy your time spent with them and it will help you keep what it is you actually do in perspective.

▶ **Don't take too much crap** If something or somebody is making your life a misery don't suffer in silence, do something about it. Start by talking to your boss or your HR department.

▶ **Get out of there** Physically leaving your workplace at lunchtime, and getting a change of scenery works wonders.

▶ **You can always get another job** Very few people are actually being forced to stay somewhere that's stressing them out on a daily basis and you're probably not one of them. Sometimes even the mere act of looking for another job will make you feel better.

them to. Just remember, you don't have to turn yourself into Miles Davis or Tiger Woods.

Your new-found activities may introduce you to some new friends too. Everybody needs a support system and it might not always be your family. Making friends will expand your perspective on the world in general, as you'll see how other people live their lives. It may shed a new light on how you approach your own.

Lastly, get some sleep. Everything looks better when you've had a decent amount of shut-eye, and it's much easier to behave rationally when you're well rested.

Boardroom benefits

As an employer, paying attention to your employees' work/life balance and helping them keep it on track will bring huge benefits

How to choose a life coach

Go for one with International Coach Federation (ICF) credentials. This is the governing body of professional coaches and sets practice and ethics guidelines.

Talk to several and only consider those you have a good rapport with, as you will have to share a great deal with them.

Opt for a full-time life coach, rather than one who does it as a hobby.

Look for experience, as the more situations they have had to deal with the more knowledge they will have to bring to yours.

Make sure they are very clear about what they offer in terms of time and commitment, and how long they expect you to commit for – three months is the ideal initial period.

to your own time spent at work. A contented, less stressed workforce will give you increased productivity as they will be more motivated, meaning reduced staff turnover. Timekeeping will be better, absenteeism will go down and those who have to interact with customers or other companies will be more enthusiastic about what they have to get across.

Of course, this won't happen by itself. You should consult with your staff on a regular basis to find out what they want, pay attention to what goes on in firms similar to yours and support your management to make sure changes are implemented as intended. If successful, it will do wonders for your stress levels as well.

Life coaches: indispensable or inconsequential?

Life coaching has attracted more than its share of bad press over the last decade or so, but beneath the obvious accusations of superfluous, Californianized mumbo-jumbo, and worries about the lack of regulation, there is a lot of benefit to be had. Especially by men, as they are far more likely to engage a life coach than they are to enter psychotherapy – sixty percent of those in psychotherapy are women; seventy-five percent of life-coach clients are men.

A good life coach will help you look forward to where you should be in the future. He or she will be far more than an expensive personal cheerleader, and should become a dedicated mentor advising you on all matters business and personal. They should help you reach decisions needed to determine and achieve your best goals and, importantly, give you somebody to talk to if things are getting a bit frustrating. It's a bit like having a best friend who actually knows what they're talking about and you don't have to worry about imposing on.

Look upon it as calling in an expert – a bit like phoning a plumber if your hot water system's on the blink.

The best of the web

bis.gov.uk
Formerly the DTi, this is the Department for Business, Innovation & Skies, very useful for both employers and employees as regards to rights, legislation and advice, in the UK and internationally.

cdc.gov/niosh/docs/99-101
The National Institute for Occupational Safety and Health offers a comprehensive online booklet to help identify, cope with and prevent work-related stress from an employee's point of view. Although an American publication, the practical advice is relevant on both side of the Atlantic.

myworklifebalance.ie
Irish-based site that will answer any question you have about how work/life balance can be adjusted within your working life.

healthatwork.org.uk
An NHS-run site dedicated to promoting health and well-being in the workplace.

businesslink.gov.uk
Operating with the Business Link National Contact Centre this offers a wealth of information that will be vital to anybody considering starting up a small business.

hse.gov.uk/stress
Particularly good when offering advice on work-related stress – for both employees and employers – the government's Health & Safety Executive has much information about the working environment.

hmrc.gov.uk
The website of HM Revenue & Customs provides much more than information about tax schedules, and is packed with advice for the self-employed.

coachfederation.org
The International Coach Federation is the professional body that sets the standards and accredits life coaches. If you are considering hiring one this is the best place to start.

dol.gov
The US Department of Labor website has comprehensive advice on US labour laws and workplace ethics for both employers and employees.

In the bedroom

Given the amount of time the average man supposedly spends thinking about sex – around ten percent of his waking life – it's surprising how little so many of us actually understand about it. This chapter sets the record straight on a few myths, and shows that it's not at all difficult to get much more out of your sex life than you do now.

Sex on the brain

In today's cultural and social climate, we are a long way removed from the notion of sex as purely a matter of procreation. Indeed, it has almost become a sport – both a participatory one and, given its prominence in mainstream media, a spectator one too. But it's a sport with an apparently limitless set of arcane rules.

This can be a great deal of fun for all involved, but it also means that many of us spend a great deal of time not so much thinking about sex as worrying about it. Am I getting enough? How do I know if she wants it? Is my technique good enough? Will I stay hard enough long enough? It's a vicious circle: the worry of it all contributes to the stresses and pressures of modern life, which in turn start affecting how you make out in the bedroom. Which in itself might give you even more to worry about.

The pleasure principle

The evolutionary reason orgasms are so pleasurable – for women as well as men – is simply to encourage us to have more of them. It's been that way since Neanderthal times, and is a basic part of the brain's "reward pathway". This is a neurological network, hard-wired to guarantee the survival of the species and ensure that pleasurable feelings result as a consequence of us doing something beneficial. Because an orgasm is the natural conclusion of the act that's fundamental to mankind's perpetuation, the pleasure produced is on a higher level to anything else. It needs to be that good so that we want to do it again.

The orgasm achieves its goal by sending levels of dopamine – the pleasure and desire chemical – soaring in the brain, which stimulates nerves to tingle all over the body. It also communicates with the prefrontal cortex, via a pathway in the brain called the "limbic system", allowing the sensation to be etched onto the memory.

How it all works: sex

Men can produce about 120 million sperm a day, and each takes around two and a half months to fully develop, to the point at which it contains 23 chromosomes, half the genetic material required to build a person. Sperm are made in the seminiferous tubules, about a thousand tiny tubes coiled inside the testes, which, if you laid them out end to end would measure around five hundred metres. Until they are called upon, sperm are stored in the epididymis, a large coiled duct attached to the back of the testes.

To keep all this working as efficiently as possible, the testes need to be at a temperature of around 34°C (92.2°F), slightly below body temperature. This is why, although the testes are internal organs, they need to hang outside the body in the scrotal sac, forming the testicles. The body works hard to maintain the correct scrotal temperature, shrinking the sac to draw them closer to the body if they get cold – in the swimming pool, for instance – and, when they get too warm, relaxing the surrounding muscles to allow the testicles to hang further away from the body – like when you're in the shower.

As a sex act comes to a climax, the testes expand to around twice their normal size and sperm are pushed out of the epididymis, up the vas deferens tube to the twin sacs that are the seminal vesicles. There they mix with seminal fluid to form the milky semen. Seminal fluid is produced within the vesicles and by the adjacent prostate gland. Healthy semen contains around fifty million sperm per millilitre, and around 75 percent of these should be alive, with the majority of these having normal shape and showing forward movement.

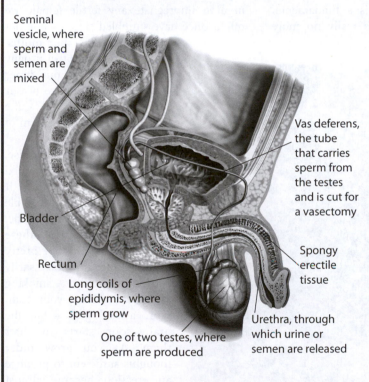

Seminal vesicle, where sperm and semen are mixed

Bladder

Rectum

Long coils of epididymis, where sperm grow

One of two testes, where sperm are produced

Vas deferens, the tube that carries sperm from the testes and is cut for a vasectomy

Spongy erectile tissue

Urethra, through which urine or semen are released

From there the semen is pushed to the ejaculatory duct, where it will be moved into the urethra – this tube will previously have been cleansed by a small emission of seminal fluid, as any traces of urine might kill the sperm. Ejaculation itself is triggered as contractions of the pubococcygeus muscle – the same one you clench to lift the erect penis – the anal sphincter and the rectum combine to push the semen through the urethra and out of the end of the penis.

The average ejaculation is between 2ml and 5ml of semen, and can contain up to 250 million sperm. In the case of unprotected sex, only about two hundred of them would make it to the egg. The rest get lost or die somewhere along the hour-long journey to the woman's fallopian tubes.

Standing up for yourself

Given the right stimulation you'll get an erection. And although the images or sensations that brought it on in the first place will be a matter of personal preference, once it gets stirring there isn't much you can do to control it.

The hard facts

The need to reproduce is a fundamental part of our make-up. It's really no more

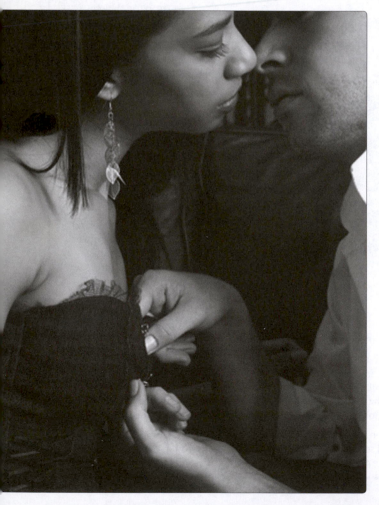

sophisticated than a deep-seated, undeniable urge to impregnate any fertile female we might once have stumbled across while out hunting woolly mammoths. Of course, self-control usually gets the better of our inner caveman, but evidence of our primeval past can still, quite literally, rear up in the form of an inappropriate erection.

Erections happen because, initially, the brain has absorbed an image or sensation it perceives to be so pleasurable it can be filed away as erotic. During adolescence these associations can be pretty random and not necessarily conventionally sexy – smoking a cigarette, seeing your team score a vital goal – but the brain soon starts to filter them. As you grow older thoughts sufficient to produce an erection become almost exclusively related to sex and become a matter of refined personal taste – i.e. your "type".

Once this stimulation has been processed the brain sends messages to the nerves around the base of the penis – this is the first stage of a man's erotic auto-response – and will be registered as that tingling in the loins. These impulses then relax the muscle fibres that are inside the penis, surrounding the corpora spongiosa and the two corpus cavernosum. These are tubes of spongy tissue running the entire length of the penis. The former is central and surrounds the urethra, with the latter positioned along each side. Once the muscles are sufficiently slack they allow the tissues to fill with blood, up to eight times as much as would be there when the penis is flaccid. This engorging with blood is the second stage, and what actually causes the erection.

An erection will be maintained because veins and arteries that would allow this blood to flow out of the penis have been blocked by a combination of stretched internal tissue and the contraction of pelvic floor muscles around the base of the penis. These will keep blocking the blood's return as long as the brain remains stimulated and is sending out the necessary arousal signals.

Once the stimulation is withdrawn, or you have reached orgasm, the messages from the brain change, relaxing the muscles at the base of the penis and contracting the muscle fibres within. This releases the pressure on veins and arteries, allowing the blood to flow away; the erection will immediately start to go down.

After orgasm and the deflation of your erection, the vast majority of men will not be

---

The most likely causes of erectile dysfunction

Diabetes
Heart disease
Obesity
High blood pressure
Smoking
Drinking
Stress
Unhappiness with your partner (either temporary or long term)
Fatigue

---

able to get another one immediately, as the body goes into a refractory phase. During this time it will be normalizing itself after the rigours of orgasm, and will not respond to stimulation until it has done so. This period will be at least ten to fifteen minutes, and becomes longer as you get older.

Er, that's never happened before

Every man will experience some sort of penile malfunction at some point, and as inconvenient or embarrassing as it might be, it isn't really that much to fret about. There is no clinically defined line between "I couldn't get it up last night" and "You have a serious problem". However, a general rule of thumb is that if it persists, or is affecting you more than fifty percent of the time, and you have ruled out the factors discussed below, then you should seek professional help. From a healthcare professional that is.

However, for the majority of men who experience erectile dysfunction (ED) at some point, there are a number of factors to be considered before calling the doctor.

A

Expert advice: "Ejaculations are good to keep the prostate healthy. A recent study at the University of Edinburgh showed that men who had been ejaculating at least three times a week, whether it was by having sex or masturbation, developed far fewer prostate problems." Sarah Hedley

Don't think about it

Back when ED was called impotence, it was reckoned to be almost exclusively a psychological problem. Although more recently it's been accepted that this is far from the case, a significant amount of it will be in your head. The series of messages and triggers to and from the brain that lie at the core of your arousal are such a complex, highly focused succession of impulses that it doesn't take much to throw them out of whack.

Stresses or worries you thought you'd left on the other side of the bedroom door are a major factor, as they will be lurking somewhere in your grey matter, interfering with what you ought to be thinking about. While this can be a temporary situation, linked to equally momentary anxieties, chronic stress will bring about persistent erectile issues, and the only true remedy is to address the causes of the stress.

Erectile dysfunction can also become something of a self-fulfilling prophecy, as immediate worries about getting an erection will affect you in exactly the same way as underlying stresses about work or home life. Nervousness with a new partner or anxiety about being able to "perform" can create a vicious circle of flaccidity, whereby the worry works against the erection, causing more worry, leading to a softer penis ... and nothing will disturb your internal erotic rhythms more than attempting to gain an erection by sheer force of will.

Try to relax. Your partner ought to understand and help you, and, importantly, although it's always a blow to the pride, don't get so caught up in your own distress that you forget there's two of you taking part. Of course, that could be the cause of the problem: if you don't actually fancy the one you're with, or it's a long-term partner you're upset with, very often your body just won't respond.

The lowdown on brewer's droop

A few alcoholic drinks may well be what got you into bed with whoever it is in the first place. But there is a limit to how much "getting in the mood" you should be getting out of a bottle. Although it affects everybody differently, relative to their metabolism and cardiovascular capabilities, hard drinking can mean a soft penis because alcohol increases the volume of blood in your system, depending on how much you've had of it. Although this might seem to be a good thing – the more blood in your penis the harder you'll stand, surely? – it will raise your blood pressure and widen your veins, meaning it becomes increasingly difficult to keep the veins and arteries in your penis closed during the period of arousal. Thus, blood will be allowed to flow out almost as readily as it flowed in, and any stiffness you might achieve will not be easy to maintain.

How much is too much will be a matter of personal experience, and as the only guaranteed way to avoid the droop is not to go over your limit, if you think sex is on the cards then stop drinking. Go on to water, as this will help flush your system out and, being less dehydrated, you'll feel much better in the morning.

Unsympathetic situations

Just as it seems to adversely affect practically everything else, today's lifestyle can also be detrimental to your erection. Obesity is a prime cause of dysfunction, as the extra strain on the cardiovascular system can prevent an efficient delivery of blood to the penis when required; what's more, the attendant high blood pressure will hinder your body's ability to keep blood in the penis to maintain any stiffness. Heart disease is also linked with ED, as deposits in your arteries, or blood pressure problems, can interfere with the blood flow needed to maintain an erection. Likewise, it is a common side effect of diabetes, as the nerve and blood vessel

T

Tip: Most erectile dysfunction is not serious and occurrences of less than twenty percent of the time really do not warrant worrying about.

damage that the condition can cause works against the whole erection process.

Certain medications can bring on ED too. The most common offenders are blood pressure treatments, antihistamines, antidepressants and tranquilizers. If you are experiencing difficulties since being prescribed a particular drug, talk to your

---

Have better sex. For longer.

Something as simple as strengthening and learning to control your pelvic floor muscles can massively increase the duration and enjoyment of your love-making. Sarah Hedley explains how an easy exercise, performed on a regular basis, can have the same effect as Viagra, but doesn't involve buying anything from dodgy websites.

"Pelvic floor exercises were always the domain of women – once you get to thirty, after childbirth and so on, the pelvic floor weakens. However, a study at the University of Bristol in 2004 showed how much benefit they can bring to men. Developing those muscles can help you control ejaculation and lead to multiple orgasms as it will be possible to achieve the sensation of orgasm without actual ejaculation.

It crosses over with the Tantric theories: if you can control the pipework down there then you can control the actual ejaculation and no longer depend on it to achieve the sensation of orgasm. Then, because you haven't ejaculated, your erection won't go down and you can do it again and again. In terms of performance anxiety, premature ejaculation or not being able to get it up in the first place, this can have the same effect as Viagra. Without the side effects.

You isolate the muscle that you use to stop yourself peeing midflow, but you have to make sure you genuinely isolate it – it's important that you don't clench the arse, the thighs or the abdomen, so you focus purely on the pelvic floor muscle. Then once you've isolated it you squeeze and lift the muscle – you should be able to feel your testicles pulling up. Once you've worked out how to do that – and it might take some time – then start doing the movement in sets, just like you would any other exercise. It's best to vary how you do it: ten slow ones followed by five rapid clenches, then repeat that set three times. The next time you do it, build up from that.

You're supposed to do them every day, but I would never advise anybody to do that: it puts pressure on them and they will be less likely to continue to help long term. Just make sure you build up what you are doing; it's probably a good idea to set targets of what you want to achieve."

Age and the erection

The likelihood of experiencing some degree of erectile dysfunction increases in direct relation to your age, as will the frequency and scale of the issue – from minimal through to complete. A forty-year-old man has a forty percent chance of experiencing some ED, an eighty-year-old man has a seventy-five percent chance of experiencing moderate to complete ED, and the probability travels up a sliding scale in between. Of course, extraneous factors such as circulatory problems, lower testosterone levels or taking medication are also more prevalent in older age groups and can play a significant role in the problem.

doctor as soon as possible but don't stop taking the medication. Injury or surgery to the spine or pelvic area can raise the chances of erectile dysfunction too, as either could cause damage to the nerves needed to set an erection off.

Environment can also contribute, and while particular locations – pub toilet, stationery cupboard, mother-in-law's spare room – might turn some people on, they can have the opposite effect on others. And as much as impromptu, alfresco sex might seem like a good idea, if it's a bit chilly don't expect an enormous erection, because when your body gets cold, blood will be diverted away from the extremities to keep the vital organs warm. It's why your hands and feet get disproportionately cold, and why your body won't give priority to delivering the blood needed to raise an erection. This can apply to cold bedrooms as well.

It could be your fault

Keeping yourself fit will maximize your chances of healthy erections, as your cardiovascular system will be operating to the best of its ability. Though don't overdo it, as over-exercising can bring on fatigue, which in turn can cause ED. Stay away from anabolic steroids, which can lead to erectile dysfunction, with the awkward side effect of increased sexual desire.

Alcohol won't help either and the damage smoking can do to your arteries means heavy smokers are far more likely to experience ED than those who don't smoke. Marijuana acts as a suppressant on the central nervous system, as do other recreational opiate drugs; these all interfere with the signals that trigger an erection. Apparently the effects can be

F

Fact: Around fifteen percent of British men are infertile. Yet less than half of that number are likely to have sought help.

Morning glory, what's the story?

The full name for it is "nocturnal penile tumescence" and it's less to do with sexual arousal than the need to go to the toilet. During a decent night's sleep the average man will get three or four erections lasting about half an hour each, with the last one happening near the end of the sleep cycle. While that is occurring, though, the bladder becomes full enough to press against the base of the penis, preventing the blood that has flowed in (to bring on the erection) from being able to flow out again. It will stay like that until you get to the toilet, where you can watch it go down as you urinate. But if your partner thinks it's for them, there's probably no need to disabuse them of this notion.

cumulative, which makes you wonder how Bob Marley managed to father so many children.

Cocaine and other amphetamines will increase the user's feelings of attractiveness and potency in general, but will also cause blood vessels to constrict, limiting the volume of blood that can be pumped into the penis, and increasing blood pressure – meaning it will be more likely to flow back out again. Cocaine also delivers the double whammy of interfering with the production of enzymes that contribute to the erection process.

F

Fact: During an erection the blood pressure in the penis will be at least twice what it is in the rest of your body.

It doesn't have to ruin your night

If you do get yourself into a situation where it's obvious that you're not going to rise to the occasion, get creative and make foreplay

Don't believe the hype

Sex surveys can do more harm than good, as they can put added pressure on people. As Sarah Hedley points out, not everybody who fills them in is being scrupulously honest.

"Plenty of people who fill in these surveys will say 'Oh we do it at least three times a week', but so often that isn't the case – people's libidos, especially men's, taper off as a relationship progresses or as they get older. However, because people read these surveys and take them seriously there follows a tendency for both men and women to tell each other 'Yeah, that's what I do too', because nobody wants to be singled out as not being normal or not up to speed. And as a result, the idea that you're not actually doing it as much as everybody else can be quite intimidating.

People need to ignore the stats; your sex life should be about finding an individual level that you are happy with. You can talk to your partner to find a level that satisfies you both. What is far more important than how many times you are doing it is how many times your partner wants to do it. You have to talk about that, and be honest about how much each of you wants to do it. If you have mismatched libidos – which the vast majority of couples do – then the issue is how you deal with that, not how often you think you ought to be doing it. And the only way you can do that is to talk about it frankly.

For instance, if one partner wants to masturbate because they're not getting enough sex, but that masturbation makes them feel dirty – or if the other partner thinks it's wrong – then you have issues which are as much psychological as they are physical. You need to find a balance between you and your partner and that's far more involved than looking externally and blindly trying to keep up with what you might read about in a magazine. Sexual happiness is about not being stressed, so if anything you are doing in the bedroom is causing you stress then it isn't a good idea. If you and your partner have settled into doing it once a fortnight and you're both happy with that, then why should you care about what other people are doing?

Part of the stress behind all this is that we – and men especially – tend not to talk about anything that might cast doubt on our sex abilities. So it gets swept under the carpet, even when it comes to talking to our partners. But maybe she's totally happy with just doing it once a fortnight; maybe trying to raise the frequency could be the cause of a potential problem. The point is to encourage communication between two people about what they want in order to achieve their sexual happiness, rather than trying to keep up with the rest of the world."

last until you can perform. Or really go to town and turn the supporting feature into the main event; the worst thing you can do is make a big deal out of not getting an erection, as the added stress will do nothing to help.

Every sperm is sacred

It may seem remarkable that while the world's population size is spiralling out of control, sperm counts have been declining since the middle of the last century, both in quantity and quality. In the 1930s, Western men averaged around one hundred million sperm per millilitre of semen, but at the beginning of the twenty-first century this average was nearly half that (at between fifty and sixty million/ml) and continuing to fall.

According to the World Health Organization, forty million/ml is the lowest sperm count that can be considered efficient for conception, and anything below twenty million is technically infertile. In the UK, the number of men with a sperm count of under thirty million/ml currently stands at around 1.3 million. It's therefore little wonder that around half of the problems experienced by couples trying to conceive are the result of male infertility.

Although there is no single irrefutable scientific theory for the "Great Disappearing Sperm Mystery", our modern lifestyle takes much of the blame. Smoking, drinking and drug taking

T *Tip: Although labelled as non-toxic, some commercially available sex lubricants can react with either your or your partner's bodily fluids to damage or kill your sperm. As it will be virtually impossible for you to tell if this is the case, if you are having difficulty conceiving don't use any, or do so under medical supervision.*

all play their parts, while the fatigue and stress resulting from longer working hours don't help – hoping to beat that with an increased coffee intake only exacerbates the situation. Likewise obesity, poor nutrition and a lack of physical exercise contribute to the reduction in both volume and quality of sperm produced.

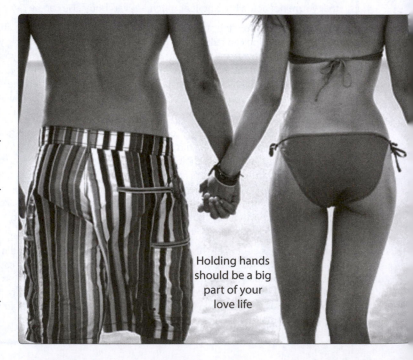

Holding hands should be a big part of your love life

A significant problem though – and one that has been growing for the last fifty years – is what's in the air we're breathing. Lengthy surveys in the US Midwest have shown an inverse correlation between levels of crop spraying and the sperm counts of men living in those areas, while the same reports found that men living in the cities with lower levels of air pollution consistently had the most and the most healthy sperm.

Mythbuster: cycling makes you impotent

There is far more research pointing away from this claim than there is towards it. Yet the notion persists. This is probably largely due to the numbness in the genital area experienced after a long time in the saddle. This is due to restricted blood flow, and may affect the chances of an erection at the time, but seldom lasts longer than half an hour.

Fertility right

Falling sperm counts have not yet reached a point where mankind needs to put itself on the Endangered Species list, but if you are hoping to have children, it's best to do everything you can to maximize your potential.

Sort your diet out The nutrients selenium, zinc and folic acid will help the production of healthy sperm, and antioxidants (particularly vitamins C or E) make sure they stay that way.

Don't worry Although it's not known if stress directly affects the sperm-producing hormones, the effect it has on your body in general will contribute to a low sperm count and reduced sexual function.

Keep cool Your testicles will be at their most efficient if you don't let them overheat: cut down on the hot tubs and saunas, and maybe switch from Y-fronts to boxers.

Stop smoking Cigarettes not only reduce the number of sperm in your semen, but also their health, mobility and the length of time they'll survive after ejaculation.

Cut down on the drinking An excessive alcohol intake will not only lead to ED, but will lower your sperm count and your testosterone levels.

Give up the drugs All recreational drugs will lower your sperm count, but cocaine and heavy marijuana use are the main offenders, causing a drop of up to fifty percent.

Exercise sensibly Your sexual well-being is just the same as your general physical well-being, and the fitter you are, the better everything will function.

Don't drink so much coffee Although it may make you move quicker, caffeine will make your sperm swim slower and reduce their chances of getting to the egg.

Lose a bit of weight Obesity has long been linked with low and/or damaged sperm counts, because it disrupts your hormone production and, when they are surrounded by so much fat, the testicles overheat.

Oops! Sorry about that

Premature ejaculation is the most common male sexual difficulty, and will happen to every man at some point during his life and probably more than once. However, because it is so widespread, unless it's happening on a regular basis, over a period of time, it's not worth worrying about. The causes are pretty much totally random and almost always psychological: anticipation; nervousness; over-arousal; outside stress; fear of discovery; or even fatigue. So there isn't really a "cure" as such, although worrying about it happening might actually bring it on.

Often it's best not to put pressure on yourself to try again, but look for other ways to pleasure each other. If it persists, visit your GP, who may well recommend a sex therapist.

Pornography has a great deal to answer for

As well as being usually quite unpleasant and generally degrading for everybody involved, porn causes its own specific range of problems as it offers such a misleading presentation of sex and sex lives. The following

Expert advice: "Having more sex keeps your heart healthier. Caerphilly University carried out research on one thousand guys over three decades and found there was an inverse correlation between those who were having the most sex and those who were dying of heart attacks. The former group's hearts and cardiovascular systems were quite simply in better nick, because a very passionate twenty-minute session will burn around two hundred calories. Which obviously isn't as good as running. But it all helps."
Sarah Hedley

are the most common misconceptions.

1. I'm not either doing it or thinking about it 24/7

Few men are. Not unless they've really got nothing else to do. In fact, the notion that

Let the Joneses be the Joneses (Pt1)

Not everybody has a more exciting sex life than you. And if they do, so what? Sarah Hedley explains:

"There's a massive pressure these days for people to explore further in their sex lives. Sex shops are increasingly seen as respectable places, while the Internet has made it easier to check out toys and accessories without any face-to-face embarrassment. These days people are often worrying whether if they're not slightly kinky then maybe they're a bit yesterday. There's almost a bit of a burden on people to be able to say 'Oh yeah, I did that' or 'We've tried that'. People are keeping sexual checklists of things they think they ought to have done.

To get over that you've got to make sure you're really comfortable in what you want, and who you are and remain aware that what people are talking about doing might not be what they are actually doing. Then, remember that if people have drawn up this sexual ticklist and are powering through it, then that isn't necessarily sexual happiness. Don't worry about keeping up with the Joneses – what do the Joneses care about you? It's really not about anybody else. It should be up to you what you do."

Be sexy without being sexual

Non-sexual intimacy is an often neglected part of our love lives, Sarah Hedley says. It's important to be able to get intimate with each other without it having to lead to sex.

"Kissing, cuddling and holding hands with a partner is very important, as just the act of being close like that releases oxytocin which is a bonding chemical – it's the reaction that mothers and their kids have. You should do it as often as possible. For instance, when you're sitting and watching television sit together. Don't sit apart on different chairs or sofas, cuddle and hold each other. It's not a substitute for sex, but as another physical expression it's quite an important thing to have. At times when you are stressed about sex, if you still have the physical outlet of holding hands and cuddling then you keep your intimacy on that very private level that only happens between lovers; you maintain that physical bond.

Really, you should do it regardless of what your sex life is like. It will keep your relationship strong: she's also going to have that release of chemicals and is going to feel closer and more intimate with you."

"men think about sex every seven seconds" is a nonsense. According to research, around sixty percent of men think about sex about half a dozen times a day; twenty-five percent think about it no more than ten times a week; for ten percent it's that many times a month; and around five percent of men think about sex no more than once a month.

2. Other women must be much more "up for it" than my partner

Probably not. As men progress in a steady relationship their sex drives remain pretty much on the same level. Women's, however, will often decline progressively as the relationship goes on, and a desire for physical affection rather than sex takes over.

3. It's not very big

It never is if you look down at it – for some reason the rule that makes your feet look bigger doesn't apply to your penis. The average erect length is around 12.9cm (5.08 inches), so don't stress about anything you might have seen in a porno film. Those blokes were never chosen for their acting abilities.

4. I can't keep going forever

Whatever you may have seen on screen or read about or heard about from friends as regards marathon all-night sessions, the average sex act lasts between five and fourteen minutes.

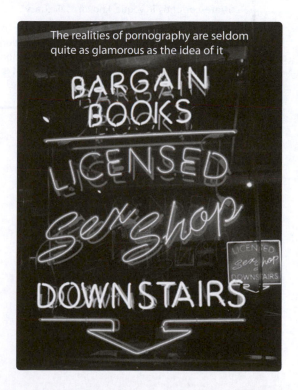

The realities of pornography are seldom quite as glamorous as the idea of it

How it all works: Viagra

Although it has passed into language as your erection's magic bullet, or "Vitamin V", Viagra is actually just a trade name for one of the many brands of sildenafil citrate tablets on the market (albeit the first and biggest selling of them). Developed in the UK by the pharmaceutical giant Pfizer as a drug to treat high blood pressure or angina, the drug's erection-boosting aspect was discovered almost as a side effect. Patented in 1996 and given official approval as an erectile aid in 1998, it went on sale in the US that year and did more than $1 billion's worth of business in its first twelve months.

It works by assisting the tissues within the corpus cavernosum of the penis to relax sufficiently to allow the arteries to smoothly and easily fill up with blood. To do this, a hormone called cyclic guanosine monophosphate (cGMP) has to be present in relatively large quantities, and sildenafil citrate blocks production of the enzyme cGMP-specific phosphodiesterase type 5, which specifically inhibits the production of cGMP. It takes about forty minutes to take effect, and a 50mg dose is usually good for about four hours.

It should be remembered that this medication is not an aphrodisiac; it will only assist with the physical aspect of your erection once psychological arousal has been achieved. Thus the usual erotic stimulation will be required and the notion of a four-hour unprompted boner is best left to the stand-up comedians. Side effects, meanwhile, include headaches, reduced blood pressure, hot flushes, nausea, nasal congestion and blurred vision.

It will come as no surprise that almost as soon as they hit the pharmacies an alternative market for erectile dysfunction drugs emerged, one that was well under the official target age group and rarely suffering from any problems in that department. Bought without prescription, usually online, it is used to either enhance sexual experience or, as is increasingly the case, in conjunction with other drugs to combat their negative erectile effects – there is a mix of ecstasy and sildenafil citrate, currently in vogue, known as "Sextasy".

What may come as a shock though is that there have been, in the US, between five hundred and a thousand deaths per year related to the recreational use of ED medication. Mostly among young healthy men, and mostly for cardiovascular reasons, when used in tandem with other drugs. This is because these combinations of drugs can put enormous strains on the heart, and in the case of amyl nitrate dangerously reduce blood pressure.

5. I'm not very adventurous

Nor are most other men it seems: in a worldwide survey conducted by Durex, 29 percent favoured their partner on top; 28 percent doggy style; and 20 percent good old missionary. Not exactly swinging from the chandeliers, are they?

6. It takes too long before I can do it again

Thanks to the wonders of an editing room, porn stars can hop from bed to bed to bed to bed with barely a pause for breath. In the real world the more you orgasm the longer you're going to have to wait to achieve the next erection. After three or four times it might not happen at all, simply because your brain will have had enough propagating the species for one day and will switch that circuitry off.

A healthy sex life

Remarkably, although education about the dangers of unprotected sex has been a more significant part of governmental public health policies in schools and on billboards since the advent of AIDS, the incidences of sexually transmitted diseases (STD) in the UK have been escalating. Over the last fifteen years,

Buy me and stop one

Method	Involves	Reliability	Pros	Cons
Vasectomy	Vas deferens cut to prevent sperm reaching the semen; local anaesthetic	Around 100 percent*	Never having to worry about contraception again	No protection against STDs; not always successfully reversible
Female sterilization	Fallopian tubes cut or blocked, preventing eggs reaching the womb; general anaesthetic	Around 100 percent	A one-off op; you'll never have to worry about contraception again	More serious procedure than a vasectomy; no protection against STDs; very difficult to reverse
The Pill	Combination of two female-type hormones, oestrogen and progestogen, that prevent ovulation	Around 100 percent	Relatively convenient, allowing for a spontaneous sex life	Must be taken every day; no protection against STDs; side effects can include weight gain and cardiovascular problems; not recommended for smokers
Condom	Latex sheath covering the peni	90–98 percent	Protects against STDs; always available	Unreliable; putting on reduces spontaneity; some find it reduces sensation
Contraceptive injection (for women)	Injection of female-type hormones, similar to the Pill	Around 100 percent	Each injection protects for up to three months; some types protect against cancer of the womb	Remembering to get re-injected; no protection against STDs; can cause some weight gain; takes a while to leave the system after coming off it
The Coil, or IUD (intra-uterine device)	Fitted into a woman's womb to block sperm entry, making womb less likely to accept an egg	97–98 percent	No surgery required; each insertion lasts between five and eight years	Risk of infection; possibility of expulsion; no protection against STDs
Diaphragm with spermicide	Rubber shield, smeared with spermicide cream, inserted into vagina prior to sex	90–96 percent	Can be inserted hours before sex to preserve spontaneity	Relatively unreliable; no protection against STDs; spermicide may cause allergic reaction in either partner

* No method of contraception – other than not having sex – can be described as one hundred percent reliable, because none of them are.

The A–Z of STDs

Condition	Symptoms	Transmission	Treatment	Observation
Chlamydia – infection of the urethra	Painful urination; itching at penis opening; milky discharge	Vaginal, oral or anal sex; very rarely in fingers	Antibiotics – it is a bacterial infection	Symptoms appear a week after exposure; seventy percent of infected women have no symptoms
Crabs – aka pubic lice	Itching in pubic hair and around genitals	Genital contact; an infected person's bed; can be passed on during non-penetrative or protected sex	Specially medicated shampoo	Crabs are not crabs, but tiny insects hatched from eggs laid at the base of pubic hair shafts
Genital herpes – the HSV-2 strain of the herpes virus	Itching in genital or anal area; small circular blisters that burst into painful sores	Contact with a carrier's infected areas – can be passed on during non-penetrative or protected sex	Antiviral medication, although will usually clear itself up within a week	Never fully goes away: symptoms may re-emerge at any time
Gonorrhoea – aka the clap	Thick, yellowish discharge from penis; burning pain during urination; inflammation of the anus	Vaginal, oral or anal sex	Antibiotics – it's bacterial – and if caught early can be cleared up with a single dose	If untreated can lead to infection of the urethra, testicles and prostate; can cause infertility
Genital warts – a symptom of HPV (human papilloma virus)	Small white bumps on the end of the penis; larger uneven lumps in the genital area	Contact with infected skin – can be passed on during non-penetrative or protected sex	Application of prescription creams or liquids; in extreme cases laser treatment or minor surgery	Genital warts can spread to the anus, even if there has been no anal sex

cases of chlamydia have increased by 300 percent, gonorrhoea by 200 percent, HIV by 300 percent and syphilis by 2000 percent. (In terms of significance, however, the last is a tiny figure compared with any of the others.) Each year, over two percent of UK men are treated for an STD. This might not seem like much, but it accounts for some 400,000 people.

Who's Chlamydia?

These increases are massively skewed towards the under-25 age group; in spite of enjoying a much more comprehensive level of sex education than previous generations, the UK has the highest rates of STDs and teenage pregnancy in the EU. It's believed that teens having sex at younger ages, and

The A–Z of STDs cont.

Condition	Symptoms	Transmission	Treatment	Observation
Hepatitis B	Flu-like symptoms; yellowing skin and whites of eyes; weight loss	Unprotected sex; it's spread through bodily fluids	Usually clears up by itself; antiviral medication if it persists	Eighty times more infectious than HIV; if untreated the chronic condition can cause liver damage
Hepatitis C	Flu-like symptoms; yellowing skin and whites of eyes; weight loss	Unprotected sex that involves bleeding, it's spread via blood	A combination of antiviral drugs; regular check-ups in case it comes back	Sufferers should avoid alcohol because of the strain it puts on the liver
HIV – Human Immuno-deficiency Virus	Continuing and escalating propensity for illness	Blood and sexual fluids of an infected person	Antiretroviral medicines slow the transition from HIV to AIDS, but there is no cure	You are very unlikely to become infected with HIV through saliva
Syphilis	Stage One: ulcers on the penis. Stage Two: flu-like symptoms; itching all over; hair loss; white patches on tongue. Stage Three (tertiary): affects the heart and nervous system; can cause mental illness	Vaginal, oral or anal sex with an infected person	A course of penicillin injections	Incidences of syphilis were falling in the UK, but have recently started to rise again; in the US they have been escalating for decades

a widespread notion that HIV belongs to a previous generation, are among the main causes. Youthful drinking and drug taking is also seen as a huge contributory factor to this age group's sexual recklessness, as around 35 percent of teenagers admitted to being drunk or stoned when they first had sex.

Interestingly, while men under the age of 25 are likely to be reasonably well-informed

F

Fact: According to the WHO, there are an estimated 62.4 million new cases of gonorrhoea in the world every year, around 8000 of them in the UK.

about AIDS and HIV, this seems to be at the expense of other STDs. A worryingly large percentage of that age group doesn't even seem to know what many of them are.

Sex and drugs and middle age

In the UK and US, men and women are staying single for longer, and continuing their twenty-something approach to a social life into their thirties and beyond. It's led to a rise in what's known as "risky behaviour" – binge drinking, drug taking, casual sex – among the almost middle aged that is believed to be fuelling the present increase in STDs among older men.

According to World Health Organization research, adult women who, in previous generations, would have brought proceedings to a swift halt if their partner didn't have any protection, are now likely to be at least as drunk and just as liable to instigate reckless sex. Being old enough to know better – one of the most effective preclusions to unprotected sex – arrives later and later, it seems.

That we stay single longer means we will, on average, have considerably more sexual partners than previous generations, which is directly contributing to the rise and spread of STDs among older age groups.

No pain, no problem?

Another important factor in the recent rise of STDs is how easy and relatively painless it is for the lower-level infections to be cleared up with today's antibiotics and antiviral medication. As treatment for men no longer involves a needle and tiny scoop down the urethra, many people are showing such infections less respect. Casual sex is often taken for granted as part of an active social life, with "a dose" being seen as little more than an occupational hazard. The need for precautions is seen as less urgent.

While modern medicinal remedies may be reliable, the big danger that comes with taking frequent courses of antibiotics is the damage that can be done to the bacteria that keep your immune system functioning. Unless care is taken to restore a healthy balance within the gut it could leave your body vulnerable to all manner of other infections.

The best of the web

everydayhealth.com/sexualhealth
Covers all aspects of sexual health, and offers access to articles on the subject.

4-men.org
The more intelligent end of the lad mag approach, which offers plenty of advice for young single men.

Netdoctor.co.uk/sex_relationships
Comprehensive site for men and women, discussing sex and relationships from the emotional point of view as well as the physical.

Brook.org.uk
The website for the Brook Advisory Centres, a charity that has been providing advice and assistance on contraception and sexual health since the 1960s.

realsextips.com
Interesting, varied and generous performance pointers, taking into account the emotional as well as the purely physical.

Ten top tips for a better sex life

▶ **Give up smoking** That nasty habit has a detrimental effect on both your erection and your sperm count.

▶ **Don't worry about not getting an erection** Unless it starts to happen most of the time it's not a serious problem.

▶ **Viagra isn't an aphrodisiac** It won't help you function if the stimulation isn't there to start off with.

▶ **Losing weight will improve everything** It will take strain off your heart, improve your breathing and allow your testicles to keep cooler.

▶ **Don't feel you have to be wildly inventive all the time** Most other people's sex lives are far less interesting than you might imagine.

▶ **Drink water towards the end of an evening** Brewer's droop is not an urban myth, and you will feel better in the morning.

▶ **Take your partner with you if you ever have to visit a healthcare professional to discuss a sexual matter** It concerns both of you, so you should both be there to talk about it.

▶ **Beware of taking Viagra in tandem with other recreational drugs** Such cocktails can have fatal consequences.

▶ **Don't ever admit** your morning erection has nothing to do with your partner's inherent, unturnoffable sex appeal.

▶ **Relax** You're supposed to be enjoying it.

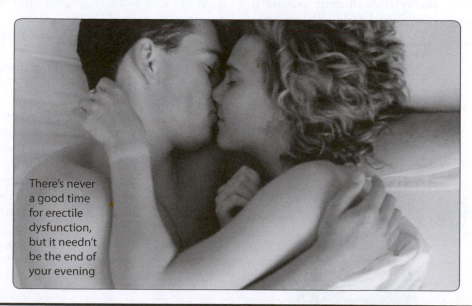

There's never a good time for erectile dysfunction, but it needn't be the end of your evening

In the gym  8

Humanity's bodily energy usage evolved to work pretty much like this: calories taken in equated to calories expended. Even after we no longer used up these calories in catching or digging up the food that supplied them, we still walked places or rode horses. The only labour-saving devices were called "servants", which weren't available to everybody. In today's developed world, however, our day-to-day existence sees many of us expending as little energy as possible, and thus our fuel in to fuel burned ratio has become alarmingly overbalanced. Like it or not, redressing this imbalance means keeping fit.

Why keep fit?

The obvious answer to this question is staring you in the face practically every time you leave your house: virtually everywhere you look there is vivid evidence of the West's growing obesity crisis. Regular exercise is the key to preventing weight gain – together with eating healthily (see Chapter 1) – and will not only keep your weight down, but also reduce your risk of heart disease, high blood pressure and type 2 diabetes.

More than that, it will boost your entire metabolism, meaning everything in your body will start to function more efficiently, causing your all-round health to improve.

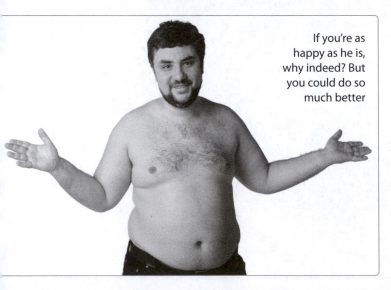

If you're as happy as he is, why indeed? But you could do so much better

This is because exercise is part of what we are supposed to do as human beings, so by making sure you're getting enough you are simply functioning correctly. However, given that so many of us continually operate somewhere below par, just getting up to normal levels of fitness can make a huge difference. An exercise routine will also help you sleep as you will be physically tired and have less nervous energy keeping you awake.

How it all works: fitness

When people talk about measuring how fit a person is, they are talking in terms of cardiovascular (heart and lungs) efficiency, which will be gauged by his VO₂ max measurement. This represents the maximum volume of oxygen he can make use of to power his muscles in one minute, and it is measured in millilitres of oxygen per kilo of body weight. The higher the figure, the higher your performance is likely to be, as oxygen is the key to effectively converting the carbohydrates you have consumed into the energy needed to power your muscles.

Energy is produced from carbohydrate or fat becoming fuel for the working muscles, but before these nutrients can be delivered to and utilized by the muscles they have to be converted into a substance called adenosine triphosphate (ATP). This process is the "burning" stage and requires oxygen to happen. As you exercise – or do anything, for that matter – the oxygen from the air you inhale is delivered to the bloodstream via the lungs, meaning the oxygen-rich blood cells can be transported to the muscles that need it. Once arrived, it metabolizes with the carbohydrate, which has now been broken down into glycogen and glucose to produce the ATP which actually makes the muscles work. A by-product of this intra-muscular process is carbon dioxide, which is removed from the muscles by blood flowing in the other direction. It is taken to the lungs where it is discharged into the atmosphere as you breathe out.

As exercise intensifies, the demand for oxygen to metabolize increasing amounts of fat or carbs will increase proportionately, which is why you gasp for air when you raise the effort you are putting in. This means VO₂ levels have to increase, and as they do your cardiovascular fitness improves – the lungs provide more oxygen and a stronger heart delivers it to the muscles quicker.

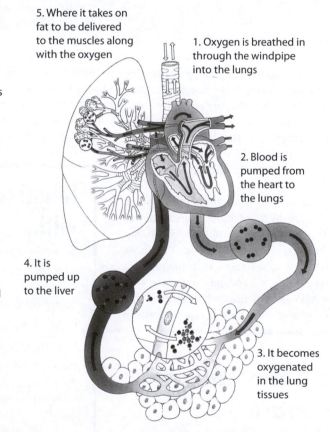

5. Where it takes on fat to be delivered to the muscles along with the oxygen

1. Oxygen is breathed in through the windpipe into the lungs

2. Blood is pumped from the heart to the lungs

4. It is pumped up to the liver

3. It becomes oxygenated in the lung tissues

You can raise your VO₂ max with aerobic training that increases in intensity and endurance over a period of time, during which your stamina levels will rise appreciatively. However, there will be a limit to which you can take it, and if after about three months you are no longer noticing any improvement you have probably reached it.

F

Fact: Overall, 60 percent of American men do no exercise activity at all, which compares with 50 percent in the UK; this is against 40 percent (US) and 29 percent (UK) of women. The figures also show, in each country, men under thirty are twice as likely to exercise as those over fifty.

There's also a huge psychological benefit to keeping fit. The increased blood flow will boost the oxygen levels in your brain, making your thinking clearer – it's not by accident that you'll find yourself able to better think things out on a good hard run. Exercise releases endorphins, the brain's feel-good neurotransmitters, which can promote an "exercise high". Equally, the act of physical movement or having to think about an activity (as you do in a competitive sport), can dominate the brain to the degree that you forget the tensions and problems of the day. And when you've finished working out, those same tensions won't seem so immediate or pressing. All this will conspire to reduce your stress levels – indeed, research has shown that regular exercise can relieve the symptoms of mild depression and persistent anxiety.

But I haven't got the time

The real problem with keeping fit in today's society is that people have too many excuses not to bother. By far the most popular single barrier to keeping fit is time, or the lack of it, and this tends to be cited as a reason for not keeping up with a fitness plan as much as it does for not getting started on one in the first place. The thing to do is to sort out something that fits in with your life rather than which causes you to make huge amounts of changes. That way, provided you accept that there is going to be some element of disruption, you are far more likely to logistically be able to do your exercise, and also much less likely to resent the time it's taking from all the exciting things you could be doing instead.

There are so many options when it comes to keeping fit, and such a vast array of practical and affordable home gym equipment available, it's virtually impossible not to be able to find something that can fit in with your life. Running can be done at any time, almost anywhere. Most gyms and swimming pools have extended opening hours; many keep-fit classes, martial arts clubs and five-a-side football squads hold lunchtime sessions; or you could always buy a bike to get around on, and in the process end up saving yourself some time.

Regular exercise will...

Raise your overall energy levels.

Stimulate your brain and increase its activity.

Contribute to lowering your stress levels.

Reduce everyday aches and pains.

Help you sleep better.

Keep your heart and lungs healthy.

Get rid of excess calories that would end up being stored as fat.

Boost your overall health, meaning fewer niggly coughs and colds.

Improve your sex life as you will be more energized in general.

Increase your confidence, as you will feel better about yourself.

Activity	Pros	Cons	Expense
Cycling	Excellent cardiovascular exercise; the quickest way to get around our cities; cuts down on fares; you can cycle practically anywhere at any time	Will not develop upper body or arms; inconsiderate fellow road users; exhaust fumes; a bike is stolen every seventy seconds in the UK	Once you've bought the bike it can actually save you money
Running	Excellent cardiovascular exercise; you can do it anywhere and at any time; it can be used to get you from A to B	Wear and tear on the joints can cause problems later in life; if you run to work, you'll need to take a shower	A good pair of shoes will set you back about £80 ($150); after that all you need is shorts and a shirt
Rowing	Excellent cardiovascular exercise; good for all-round conditioning; being on the water can be very relaxing	You'll need a large body of water and a boat	Hiring a boat or joining a rowing club needn't be too expensive
Karate	Good for cardiovascular exercise, strength and flexibility; boosts confidence; encourages mental discipline; has a spiritual side	You'll need to join a club; steep learning curve; requires a strong dedication over a long period of time	Club fees are seldom overly expensive; a gi (suit) will cost about £40 ($25)
Basketball	Good cardiovascular exercise and improves coordination; sociable; relatively easy to find somewhere to play	You can't play by yourself; the injury rate among leisure-time basketball players is high	A ball and a decent pair of high tops. Other than that you can wear your regular gym kit
Walking	Mild cardiovascular exercise – excellent for seniors or those starting exercising; you can do it anywhere, at any time; will get you from A to B without needing a shower	It might not be intense enough for everybody to use it as their main form of exercise	It can save you money on fares; no initial outlay needed
Football (soccer)	Reasonable cardiovascular exercise and improves coordination; sociable; easy to find somewhere to play; practically everybody in the world can play it	Because it's unlikely you'll play more than once or twice a week, it should only be part of a fitness plan; the injury rate among Sunday footballers is high	A ball and suitable footwear
Tennis	Excellent cardiovascular exercise and improves coordination and reactions	You can't play by yourself; there are relatively few facilities (compared with football and basketball); many public courts shut for the winter	A racquet, balls and appropriate shoes if you use public courts; joining a club could be costly and you will need all the gear

A

Expert advice: "If you're going to do one thing towards getting fit then it should be breathing. Sit down and take three minutes a day to get diaphragmatic breathing back into the body. Most people, through stress, breathe through their chests and not very deeply, but breathing exercises help in that they aid your posture, energy levels … everything. Once you can get them to work it'll make a difference in so many other areas and provide the best basis for getting fit."
Gideon Remfry

In the beginning, look to spend about three hours a week on your keep-fit schedule – that's an amount of time pretty much anybody can spare. Split that up into chunks of no more than one hour and no less than thirty minutes, then allocate a convenient time of day, such as early morning or lunchtime, and look for an activity and location that will fit in with what you do. Importantly, though, once you have arrived at what you are going to do, make sure you genuinely incorporate it into your schedule so you look at it as being as much an intrinsic part of your routine, just as taking a shower in the morning is.

I've tried a gym, but it didn't work out

This has become increasingly commonplace as a reason people don't keep up with a fitness regime, and it can be as much a fault of the gym itself as it can be of the individual. In the first instance, gyms too often fail to keep up the level of instruction members receive when they have just joined, and after half a dozen or so visits, newbies are left to

T

Tip: Don't be swayed by a gym that seems populated with bodybuilders. An over-muscled physique is not something most people are trying to achieve, and it simply isn't relevant to the majority of members. Also, too often that gym's staff will devote their time to these guys as they might be entering competitions from the gym, or they just see them as a good advertisement.

Find the time

According to our fitness expert Gideon Remfry, there is no reason at all why you can't make time to work out.

"Everybody has time to keep fit. If anybody says they don't, then that's a time management problem: they should sit down with their weekly diary and note all those times when they've wasted an hour or half an hour doing something useless – or doing nothing at all. They've got to literally plan out their week and pinpoint all the spots when they have downtime and then ask themselves: 'What's the easiest way to do this? Shall I do this at home? Shall I join a gym? How best can I factor keeping fit into my life to make it work?' I guarantee there's nobody out there who hasn't got thirty minutes, three times a week."

get on with it by themselves. Not only can this be dangerous, but it's demoralizing as you might keep on doing the same things for too long, as they don't know when or how to advance their routines.

In the case of the individual not getting something out of it, going to a gym and working out with weights or on machines in a crowded, noisy and brightly lit environment simply might not be right for them. This isn't unusual and is perfectly understandable – you might not relish the showing-off factor that will never be too far away at these temples of the body beautiful. Perhaps you feel more confident working out by yourself, or you may simply be better suited to a different way of keeping fit. The problem is that you probably won't find out you aren't the ideal candidate for gym membership until you've actually joined one.

Choose carefully when considering which gym to join and read the small print on any contract – make sure you can stop your payments if you opt out, because there have been many horror stories of people locked into twelve-month deals when they thought they could get out after three.

I can't afford it

Keeping fit can cost as much or as little as you want it to. At the affordable end of the scale there is walking – to work, to college, to the shops, to the pub, and so on – anywhere you'd normally drive or get the bus. Walking at a medium-to-brisk pace can burn between 280 and 320 calories per hour, and that figure rises considerably if there are hills involved. It won't cost you anything and will even save you money if it's a journey you'd usually make on the bus. Running or cycling involves minimal initial outlay on a decent pair of trainers, a good bike and perhaps some sensible clothing, but it won't cost anything more after that. All you need to go swimming is a pair of trunks and the cost of admission to the local baths, where you should also be able to find details of municipally run gyms and keep-fit classes, which shouldn't cost you an arm and a leg. Any activity that will require a huge investment in kit ought to have facilities for you to borrow or hire equipment before you decide to commit to the activity. If you are not offered this helping hand, look for a more amenable club or fitness centre.

I don't like team sports

Then don't do them! Team sports are brilliant for those who want to attach a social (or competitive) element to their keeping fit, but they are definitely not for everybody. There is so much choice on offer that you really don't need to feel you have to join just the local football team or cricket club.

It wasn't making any difference

Be patient; anything as beneficial as getting fit is worth waiting a little while for. Don't expect to see differences immediately as it will take three or four weeks for your body to start noticeably changing shape. But, if you are following your plan correctly, your fitness levels will have been improving from the very first session. Simply stick at it and, as well as looking better, you'll find you can perform whatever exercise you have taken on a little better and easier each time. Then before too long it will be time to pick up the pace or increase those weights.

It hurts

Although the phrase "No pain, no gain" is usually a self-delusion covering up the fact you're doing something wrong, there will always be a certain amount of physical discomfort following a good session of physical exercise. When you start a programme, the chances are you will be

Fact: 41.3 million adult Americans (13.1 percent of the population) hold gym memberships, compared with 1.4 million in the UK (2.4 percent); but the UK figure does not take into account the huge number of people who use local authority leisure centres on a regular basis.

exercising muscles – and specific parts of muscles – you haven't used much in the past. So there will be a degree of soreness afterwards; your muscles will have suffered microscopic internal tearing.

However, this will ease up as you use them more and more, and to minimize post-workout discomfort, or risk of muscle damage while exercising, make sure you follow the warming up and cooling down routines as described on pp.177–178. Don't let a bit of stiffness put you off.

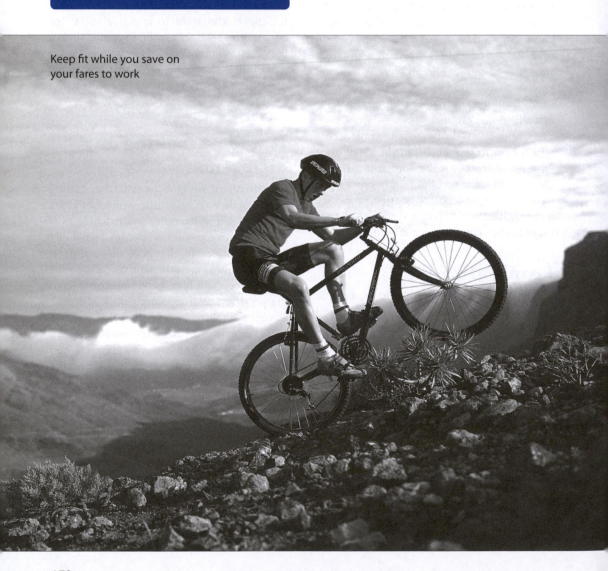

Keep fit while you save on your fares to work

B

Best investment: heart-rate monitor A vital piece of kit if you want to train smart as well as hard, these send a signal from a band around your chest to a digital readout on your wrist. They allow you to monitor your cardio improvement, to check when you have warmed up, or to regulate your intensity levels.

Most can be set to warn you if you stray outside prescribed limits, and incorporate stopwatches and lap-timers. Top-of-the-range models store your previous performances and with some you can even download data onto your computer.

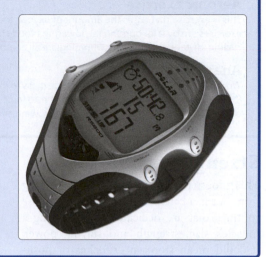

The elements of a fitness programme

For an all-round healthy and fully beneficial exercise programme to work it needs to boost your cardiovascular levels, increase the strength and size of your muscles and improve the flexibility of your joints and tendons. For this it needs to incorporate three elements: aerobic exercise, strength training and stretching.

Some activities will provide all of this as an intrinsic part of the training; organized clubs will make sure all are covered in each class's schedule. But under some circumstances you may need to incorporate some extra routines, for yourself, at the beginning or end of an activity.

Aerobic exercise

This is the continuous, heart-pumping, fat-burning variety of exercise that involves working the large muscles in the legs, arms and trunk, and should be the basis for every exercise routine you take on. Regular cardiovascular exercise will strengthen your heart, increase your lung capacity and lower your blood pressure. All of this goes a long way to preventing heart disease, while it is also the best form of exercise for keeping your weight down.

Beyond that, the immediate effects of a good aerobic workout are to help you release stress after a hard day; lift your mood, as it releases endorphins in the brain; and improve your cognitive powers, thanks to increased oxygen flowing through the brain. In the long term, an aerobic exercise schedule improves bone strength and boosts the immune system; also the increased overall stamina boosts your sex drive and makes life in general seem a bit easier. Plus you will be less likely to suffer from osteoporosis or chronic muscle pain in later life as you will be strengthening your bones and promoting the growth of capillaries within your muscles.

Running, cycling, walking, swimming, rowing and elliptical training are all good aerobic exercises, as is dancing or anything that involves constant movement, such as squash or basketball.

Aerobic exercise

This is exercise that raises the amount of oxygen the body can process to power the muscles. Such exercises are best for burning fat, lowering blood cholesterol and increasing endurance. Sports like cycling, distance running or swimming are all aerobic.

Anaerobic exercise

Workouts that build strength and muscle mass to increase strength, these would be used to train for events that require explosive power, brute force or those which do not last more than a couple of minutes – sprinting, weightlifting or throwing events benefit from anaerobic training.

Strength training

This doesn't necessarily mean pumping iron, but is a catch-all term for any exercise routines that are dedicated to increasing a muscle's size, strength and staying power. It could mean stomach crunches or push-ups, as well as bench presses or deep squats. Strength training will cause the most obvious alterations to your body shape and tone, which can do wonders for your self-esteem. Also it will help you enormously with other exercise routines you are doing, as you will last longer and be able to perform better.

Health-wise, strength training helps combat muscle loss which, for an average man, will be between six and eight pounds every decade after his twenties. It will also increase bone density as everything gets stronger to cope with the additional load bearing, which will help to relieve the joints and go a long way to preventing arthritis or reducing the pain arthritis causes. Putting on a bit of muscle will help keep your body fat down too, as maintaining a pound of muscle requires more energy that maintaining a pound of fat. Thus your metabolism increases – you'll be working out even when you're sitting still. Most importantly, though, strength training as applied to your body's core, or torso, is one of the best remedies there is for the lower back pain that seems to afflict so many men past the age of thirty.

It's never too early to start

One of the biggest problems with men's approach to keeping fit is we don't get into the habit soon enough. Too many of us stop right after we leave school and don't start again until much later. Gideon Remfry explains:

"Guys over thirty are the most likely to start worrying about general fitness because that's when things start to really change for them and they're taking on a different body shape. Men of 35 will suddenly realize they're about 40 pounds heavier than they were when they were 25 and they're taking trousers with waists that are suddenly 4 inches bigger. While it's a good thing they're doing something about it at that point, it would have been so much easier and better for them if they'd started ten years earlier. Or kept up their fitness levels from the time they left school.

The trouble is that so many men don't really consider fitness for fitness' sake when they're young, and unless they get involved with a team sport or take up some sort of specific activity, then their fitness efforts tend to stop dead as soon as they finish school. It has been getting better during the last few years as there is so much more opportunity to keep fit – so many more home gyms, so many more health clubs, so many more local authority gyms and classes – but it's changing slowly. It's still something men need to positively address."

If your regular fitness routine doesn't incorporate all-round strength training you should include at least one session a week of something that does. Swimming, weight training, circuit training, martial arts and boxing are all good strength training activities.

Flexibility

Unless you are doing yoga, Tai Chi or a martial art, it's unlikely stretching, or any sort of flexibility training, will be incorporated into your routine. So it's all the more important you do some. As a long-term prospect, stretching improves overall flexibility and mobility, and allows improved blood flow through the joints, all of which is a vital safeguard against the aches and pains brought on by ageing. It will also improve your balance as you get older, because a supple body's movements will be more fluid and more easily able to correct anything that gets out of line.

F

Fact: any exercise is better than nothing so if, when you start off, short periods suit you better, do them instead of doing a scheduled hour. But do this with a view to increasing the lengths of these periods as you get fitter.

Your resting heart-rate (in beats per minute)	Your level of fitness
80–100	Grossly unfit
70–80	The UK average, but still unfit
50–70	Fit
30–50	Extremely fit

In the short term, stretching as part of your warming-up routine will reduce the risk of you injuring yourself, as your joints will be looser when you subject them to the stresses of exercise. If you stretch immediately after you've finished, as part of your cooling down routine, it will leave you better prepared for your next session.

Choosing a fitness regime

When it comes to deciding what you want to do to keep fit you will be pretty much spoilt for choice. But that doesn't mean you should take your decision lightly. To arrive at your ideal activity, ask yourself the following questions.

Weightlifting rules

Make sure you are thoroughly warmed up before you start.

Have somebody with you if you are attempting challenging weights.

Rest between each set.

Be careful not to dehydrate.

Keep the correct posture – if you are forced out of it, the weight is too heavy.

Stretch comprehensively after a weights session.

Type of diet	Calorific requirement	Composition of intake
Standard healthy diet	2800 calories per day	50% carbs, 20% protein, 30% fat
Weight loss diet	2500 calories per day	40% carbs, 35% protein, 25% fat
Endurance training diet	3000 calories per day	60–65% carbs, 15% protein, 20–25% fat
Strength training diet	3500 calories per day	60% carbs 25% protein, 15% fat

What do you want from it?

If you are looking to lose weight you'll need to take up a specifically cardiovascular activity, such as an aerobics class, or look for a sport with a high calorie-burning aspect to it. Your local authorities (and Google) are sure to help you locate commercial fitness classes in your area.

If you simply want to improve your general levels of fitness and maybe increase your body strength a bit, a mixture of aerobic exercise and strength training will be ideal, and the best place to find that is in a well-supervised gym. Once again, start with your local municipal leisure services, then try the internet.

To tone up your body, weight training will represent the best value. To achieve this you could join a gym, but it can be done at home with minimum inconvenience and expense if you invest in a set of basic weights (see p.184). Or, if you want to take part in a competitive sport, think about what you actually like, what you used to be good at and what you think you might be able to handle at your time of life. Then, do some research to see what is available in your area.

Is a personal trainer worth the money?

Yes, according to Gideon Remfry. And he's not just saying that because he is one...

"Men seeking to get fit – especially if they've not done anything since they left school – should go and get a good, well-qualified, reputable personal trainer. That way they'll get a whole lot more out of their training because they will get it right straight away. Even if they don't stick with him or her forever, they'll stand less chance of getting injured, will stay better motivated and – because the trainer will be able to address all sorts of areas of the workout they otherwise wouldn't have known existed – their training will have much more focus and do them much more good.

Also, they will get access to the newest technology and the newest training techniques, because a good personal trainer will keep up with what's going on in the world of fitness and see how it can be applied to their clients. It's also worth going to see a nutritionist, to get advice on what you should be eating to complement your programme and what supplements you should be taking.

Of course, there are some pretty terrible trainers out there who will do you more harm than good. It's best to go on personal recommendation and for a limited period of time at first."

If you are going to take on a personal trainer, the best way to find one is through a friend's recommendation. Then make sure they have a knowledge of basic physiotherapy. And ask for a trial period before committing long term.

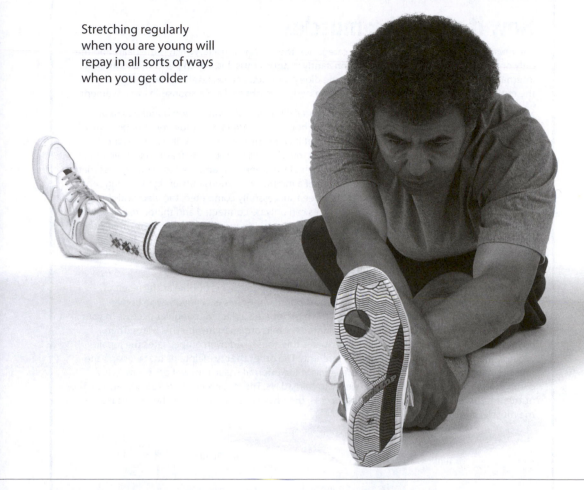

Stretching regularly when you are young will repay in all sorts of ways when you get older

What sort of person are you?

Some people get on much better at a gym than others, and this is perfectly understandable – if you're a bit shy about any visible lack of fitness, a neon-lit room full of adrenalized, Lycra-clad beautiful people won't be your idea of a good time. And that's even without negotiating communal changing rooms and showers. An activity less open to public scrutiny such as rowing or walking might suit you better.

Team sports are good if you're looking for the social side of keeping fit, as the camaraderie following a fierce game of football or basketball can be the perfect end to a session. If you see yourself as more of a solo player, martial arts will give you a club atmosphere but allow you to compete on your own, while tennis, cycling or skating are activities you could do with

F

Fact: The reason you feel like stretching when you wake up in the morning is because your tendons and ligaments will have tightened up during the inactivity of sleep.

How it all works: muscles

The muscles in your body fall into three categories: the **cardiac muscle**, which is the heart and the only one which expands and contracts constantly; **smooth muscles**, which perform unconscious internal functions like moving food along the digestive tract; and **skeletal muscles**, which cover the entire skeleton, make up around half of the body's weight and are responsible for movement.

Skeletal muscles are made up of long, strong, parallel fibres that connect two bones across a joint and are contracted powerfully to move the body and its parts. This movement begins with a thought, then, once the brain has decided what it wants moved and how, it sends electrical signals along the nervous system to the relevant muscle. This prompts the filaments within the muscle's fibres to cause it to contract, moving one of the bones it is attached to. It's a process that can take place thousands of times in the space of a minute, with thousands of signals being sent to different muscles. After the movement has been successfully completed, the electrical signals are switched off and the muscle relaxes. Muscles can only be contracted and therefore will only produce a movement in one direction, but each is paired with another muscle on the other side of the bone, which moves the body part in the opposite direction – as one contracts the other relaxes. The stronger and more powerful a muscle is, the faster and firmer the contractions will be, thus the movement is more powerful.

Science is unsure as to why muscles grow bigger and stronger (hypertrophy) as the result of progressive resistance training, but the two most popular theories each involve the body's capacity for regeneration. The first is that as the muscles are subjected to regular overuse in your workout, they are internally damaged by hundreds of microtears to the internal fibres. Then, as your schedule progresses, the brain anticipates this abuse and overcompensates the repair process, increasing the muscle's bulk and strength. The other theory maintains that working the muscles hard speeds up and makes more efficient the internal tissue renewal cycle – muscles completely renew themselves every twenty to thirty days. This means an increased demand on the nutrient reserves used to carry out this process – they swell in volume and, as they are situated in the muscle, it grows in size.

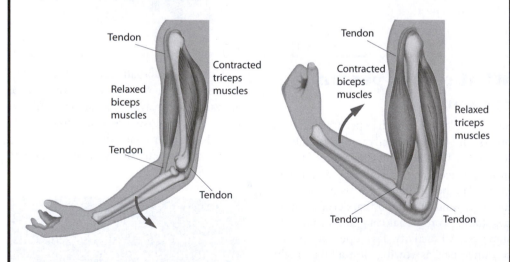

B

Best investment: running shoes

Owning a good pair of running shoes means you will never be too far away from an invigorating cardiovascular workout. And even if you have no intention of taking up running seriously, they will be worth what you paid for them. While it may be tempting to go for the occasional run (or jog to warm up for something else) in your tennis shoes or high tops, please don't. Inappropriate footwear is one of the most common causes of running injuries. If you are considering running as your main keep fit activity, then it is impossible to over-stress the importance of good, well-fitting shoes.

There is no "best"

Only the best shoes for you. So don't be influenced by advertisements or other people.

Buy them

at a specialist running shop, where they will watch you run and assess what type of shoes you need.

Shop for them

as late in the day as you can, because your feet could expand up to half a size during the day.

They should feel

comfortable and supportive immediately – if you think you are going to have to break them in, they're too small.

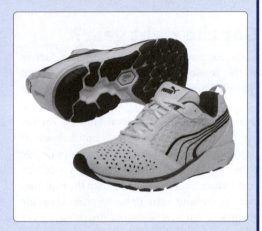

your partner if you're deciding to get fit together. If you're a more solitary type, then running is an ideal pursuit – it allows you to take off by yourself for hours on end at more or less any time you like.

How much of a routine can you cope with?

Team sports, clubs or regular sessions at a gym or leisure centre will mean you'll have to fit in with their set times, which may not suit you. If you can't guarantee you will be able to attend most sessions or games, at least during the first three months, you should look for something with a more flexible schedule. This is because if you start missing classes or not turning up for matches so soon, you will not form the exercise habit

and probably drift away from it, or you will so irritate your teammates that they will drift away from you.

Getting started

Once you've decided what you want to do and where you're going to do it, actually getting started is going to be quite a major event. It needn't be a traumatic one, though.

Are you well enough?

Unless you are over sixty, asthmatic, arthritic, suffer from uncontrolled high blood pressure, are on medication, have a family history of heart disease or are under your doctor's care for an existing medical condition, you shouldn't need to clear it with your doctor before you start your programme. As long as you start slowly you won't do yourself any harm. Push yourself just beyond your limits each time (only just), increasing the amount of time and effort you are putting in as those limits get higher. If you can't manage the half-hour sessions straight away, then that's no problem – schedule fifteen, or even just ten-minute sessions to start off with and work up from there. Crucially, remember to warm up properly before you start.

Got the right gear?

Make sure your kit fits before you arrive at the session. This is especially important when it comes to shoes, but the rest of what you're wearing needs to be comfortable too. It shouldn't chafe anywhere, and must allow full movement for your activity – but it shouldn't flap about to an irritating or dangerous degree either. Clothing should be made of a specialist performance fabric that will keep the moisture away from your skin, to be evaporated on the garment's surface – unlike anything as old school as cotton, which will collect sweat, weigh you down, rub and disrupt your body's temperature regulation.

Stay on track

Don't expect to see too many huge changes in your physique too soon. This can be a major

demotivator, so set yourself achievable short-term goals: shed two pounds each week; run for ten minutes; and/or cycle all the way to work. Then reward yourself in some way when you reach them. Stay focused on your programme as a long-haul project, regularly marking your achievements along the way.

Be prepared to adjust your diet, whether you are working out to lose weight or not. Losing weight through a combination of diet and exercise will involve cutting out the fat and cutting down on the carbohydrates, forcing your body to burn fat to power your muscles. If you are not trying to lose weight but want to improve your fitness levels, you will need to increase the amount of complex carbohydrate you eat in order to provide that extra energy.

Drink water before, during and after your workout and, once you have finished, don't forget to cool down.

What's the worst that could happen?

If you are careful and follow the correct procedures before, during and after you work out, you should be reasonably injury-free. You are bound to pick up something, though. These are the most likely occurrences:

Ankle sprain

A sharp pain in the joint, caused by the tearing or stretching of the ligaments due to suddenly twisting the ankle into an unnatural position. Remember the acronym PRICE (see box p.196) and stay off that foot as much as possible for at least two weeks.

Cramp

A contracted muscle that goes into spasm as the result of fatigue, dehydration or salt deficiency. Gentle stretching and deep

A

Expert advice: "If you're doing resistance training, to recover as efficiently as possible you should drink a really good protein shake drink within ten minutes of stopping your workout. Natural Super Red and Super Green are the best and can be found in any fitness or nutrition store."
Gideon Remfry

Choosing a gym

If you've decided to join a gym, here are some things to consider before you sign on the dotted line

• **Check the opening hours** and make sure they are going to be convenient for you.

• **Check out the journey time from home or work**, as the more awkward the trip is, the less likely you are to keep going.

• **Make a couple of visits** at different times of the day or week to get an overall feel of the place. It's best to do so without an appointment, and be wary if they object to you looking around more than once.

• **Does it have all the equipment you think you will need?** A good gym should have a wide selection of resistance machines, free weights and cardio equipment, including treadmills, bikes, elliptical trainers, rowing machines and stair climbers.

• **Is it crowded?** You want the place to be buzzing and not deserted, but it is not a good sign if people have to wait for machines at certain times.

• **Is it clean?** Not only should the changing rooms and the showers be hygienic, but if there is a low standard of general cleanliness and tidiness it could be unsafe.

• **Are there sufficient changing facilities?** Just as the gym itself may get crowded, it will be frustrating if you are bumping into people in the changing rooms or have to wait for a locker or a shower.

• **What are the staff like?** Are there enough of them? Are they sufficiently attentive and knowledgeable? Do they look fit themselves?

• **Will they let you try the gym out before you sign up?** There's no reason why they shouldn't.

massage along the muscle fibres will relieve the stiffness; make sure you rehydrate.

Delayed onset muscle soreness

Your muscles start aching at least 24 hours after you've finished exercising because of the microscopic tears in the fibres caused by the unusual strain you have been putting them under. This will be particularly acute for people who are just starting an exercise routine, and old hands will feel it when they try something new. Treat with PRICE, gentle stretching and massage.

Groin strain

Tearing or straining of the large muscle that runs down the inside of the thigh, due to overstretching or sideways stretching of the leg, which results in swelling and soreness. Stop your activity immediately and treat with

Mythbuster: you can "spot reduce" to lose fat from a specific area

Burning fat is an overall body experience, and it cannot be targeted. One persistant myth is that of "spot reduction" – targeting a specific part of the body and exercising it alone. Although it might appear that doing hundreds of sit-ups and stomach crunches is blitzing your belly fat, what you are doing is toning your stomach muscles so that it all tightens up – any fat-shedding that is going on is actually happening everywhere. If you really were able to spot reduce then people who ate too much would all have thin faces.

The muscle will have either been moved too violently while not sufficiently warmed up or it's been put under too much strain. Stop what you are doing, apply PRICE and try to stay off that leg for a few days; don't attempt to exercise again until you can stretch your leg out gently with no pain. Wear a support around that thigh – a bandage or compression shorts – for your first couple of comeback sessions.

Knee ligament damage

Pain and swelling from inside the knee; may be the result of an unnatural sideways or backwards movement that has ruptured or stretched the ligaments holding the joint together. Stop what you're doing immediately and apply PRICE. Stay off that leg as much as possible for the next two weeks, icing frequently for the first few days, and if there is no improvement seek medical advice as you may need surgery.

PRICE. Don't attempt to work it off as you could do yourself much more damage.

Hamstring damage

Sharp pain down the back of the thigh as muscle fibres have been torn – how great the pain is will depend on the severity of the tears.

What to do first

When starting an exercise regime there will be three aspects to it: what you eat, what you do and, importantly, what you don't do. Gideon Remfry breaks it down:

"As regards working out, nutrition has to complement your exercise: you have to eat properly if you want to get properly fit. It's vital that you take on the fuel to get you through it and absorb the nutrients you need to make sure your system functions properly under the stress of working out – and to make your muscles grow. If you were putting the wrong fuel in your car it wouldn't go very far, especially if you wanted to put your foot down. And something's liable to break down.

Then there has to be a really good rest cycle in between workout sessions, because you have to make sure you are fully recovered before the next time you train. The rest cycle is probably the most missed component among men trying to get fit, because they've set themselves slightly overambitious targets or are trying to get fit or lose weight within a certain time frame. This isn't necessarily about being sedentary either, but if you're going to hammer it in the gym then you have to alternate it with light exercise, and this goes for resting in between sets as well as getting rest days in between sessions. The rest period is the only time when your body is going to get the chance to regenerate.

Overtraining is a common problem, especially among younger men who think they are invincible, who believe the more they work out, the more benefit they will get from it. But the reality is they are far more likely to do themselves damage. Every time you do some sort of resistance training, what you're doing is something the muscles aren't used to, so they are having to overcompensate. To do that, they will break down and rebuild and regenerate bigger and stronger to cope with the load you're throwing at them. They can only do that while you're resting."

What to do next

Gideon continues his advice for those starting off on a fitness programme:

"When you start an exercise programme, give yourself six months then take a look at yourself and evaluate where you've got to. You have to do it consistently, and do it for a small amount of time but over a long period: then you'll start to see results. The problems come when the very goal-fixated go into a programme with a definite idea of what they should be doing and what they want to achieve, and they hammer it for two weeks and end up in a lot of pain. They often get into so much pain that they don't go back to it at all, or don't go back for a few weeks and then they're back to square one. Or, at the other extreme, they don't go often enough or do enough when they do. So there's not nearly enough of a result at the end of it and they get dispirited with the whole idea. You have to find that happy medium.

That said, goals are very important on two distinct levels. Anybody will stay motivated much better if they have a target to aim for – to lose a stone or get rid of that gut – rather than just starting to do exercises and seeing where it takes you. Then there is a deeper level, at which goals help you keep real records of what your progress is, and that will keep you improving as well as keeping you motivated.

During that initial period, don't pay too much attention to the scales. When you start to lose fat and increase lean muscle tissue, you'll also be increasing your bone density and blood volume, so your weight will actually go up. However, there will be very little change in your body shape initially; you will have got slightly smaller at the same time as that weight increase. So you have to look at it long term; ignore the scales in the beginning."

Lower back pain

Pain in the small of your back or at the top of your buttocks is usually symptomatic of something else, such as tight hamstrings or weak abdominal muscles, or, if a distance runner, a bad posture. Massage the painful area and treat with PRICE, then address what might be causing the problem. A good trunk-stretching and loosening session before exercise can help prevent lower back pain.

Side stitches

This stabbing pain just underneath the ribcage is caused by the jolting of your internal organs, straining the ligament that holds the liver in place. Deeper breathing can prevent it, and as a remedy push your fingers up under your ribs to lift your liver, or stretch that side out with the corresponding arm over your head.

F

Fact: Failure to warm up is the biggest cause of injuries among amateur sportsmen and casual keep-fitters. This is because the body will be too tight when it is called into vigorous action and something – usually a muscle or a ligament – has to give.

Before and after your workout

If you take the correct steps before and after you work out, not only will you be much less likely to injure yourself, but your body will perform better, thus you will get more out of your routine.

Warming up

This does exactly what it says it does, by bringing up your body to the ideal operating temperature for exercise. Plus it loosens the muscles and will provide a zone for you to get ready mentally for the tasks ahead. It is absolutely vital to warm up before you start exerting yourself; if you pitch yourself straight in, then your cardiovascular system won't be able to deliver the oxygen required and you'll struggle.

Also, a cold, tight muscle is much more susceptible to tearing than a warm, loose muscle – not warming up properly is the number-one cause of injuries among amateur sportsmen and gym users. Your warm-up routine should consist of three parts, carried out in this order:

1. Pulse warmers

Light jogging or jumping or skipping, slowly gaining in intensity, to raise the cardiovascular levels. This allows increasing amounts of oxygen to be transported by a faster blood flow, which in turn expands the blood vessels in the active muscles, meaning the tissue becomes looser. It will also raise the body's internal temperature ready for action.

2. Dynamic stretching

A series of slow, controlled movements that loosen joints and increase mobility by gently stretching out the muscles, tendons and ligaments. It will cut down the risk of sprains and strains and make your joints better prepared to move efficiently. Dynamic stretching includes rotating the hips, knees and trunk – in both directions; flexing the ankles; loosely swinging straight arms; and turning the head from side to side.

3. Skills rehearsal

As the final part of your warm-up, practise the movements you will be using during your activity. This will reactivate the neuron path from brain to muscle, or "muscle memory", and put you in the right frame of mind.

Cooling down

This end-piece to a session is often shamefully neglected and has two major effects: it will go a long way to preventing stiffness later in the day; and will prepare you for your next workout or event. It falls into two parts:

1. Tapering off

This is like warming up backwards, as it allows the system to gradually return to normal – cardiovascular levels drop, adrenalin production stops, etc – and is important to remove any surplus lactate from your muscles. Lactate is produced in the muscles as a waste product of carbohydrate metabolization, and normally your high pulse rate while exercising will pump it away. If you stop dead, however, any excess stays there to produce soreness.

PRICE

This acronym is a reminder of steps that are a universal cure for all *minor* sporting injuries.

Protection Stop playing, take weight off any injured joint and wrap it up if necessary.

Rest Don't try to run or work off an injury; rest up until you no longer feel pain.

Ice Icing an injury reduces swelling, numbs pain and speeds up the internal healing process.

Compression A tight bandage will support an injured limb and help bring down swelling.

Elevation Raising the injured area – preferably above the level of the heart – will reduce swelling.

Keep it safe

- Make sure you are in good physical condition and don't work out or play sport if you are ill or injured.
- Wear the correct clothing, and protective gear if required.
- Stay hydrated.
- Don't take part in any exercise if you have had less than five hours' sleep the night before.
- Always warm up before starting.
- Understand and abide by the rules or guidelines for whatever you are doing.
- Rest between sets or matches and allow recovery days in your schedule.
- Listen to your body – if you are in pain it's telling you to stop because something is wrong.

2. Static stretching

This involves putting gentle pressure on muscles to, quite literally, stretch them out, and over time it will permanently extend and loosen the fibres. The idea behind this is to make future workouts easier, rather than to affect your recovery from the session it follows, but it's carried out now because it is much easier and safer to stretch a warm muscle. Static stretching involves stretching the major muscles just past their point of comfort and holding it for twenty or so seconds. Always achieve a static stretch with very gentle pressure rather than a bounce.

Hydration, hydration, hydration

When working out, running, or playing sport, the golden rule is to keep your fluid levels topped up, as nothing will affect your performance more or put you in more danger than starting to dehydrate.

Once you are warmed up and into your routine you will start sweating – this is because one aspect of your system has raised your body temperature a few degrees while another part of you is producing sweat to try to cool you back down. As you can't stop yourself sweating, you have to constantly replenish the fluid you are losing. If you are perspiring freely you should be drinking water at a rate of about 200 millilitres (six

What are you drinking?

There are three different types of sports drinks. They all contain carbohydrate, electrolytes and water, but each has different advantages.

Isotonic: the ratio of carbs and electrolytes to water is much the same as what is already in the body, so it will be absorbed at the same rate as water.

Hypotonic: this has less carbs and electrolytes so is absorbed quicker for speedy rehydration, but has less energy replacement properties.

Hypertonic: more carbs and electrolytes than isotonic, therefore will be absorbed slower but will be of greater aid to recovery.

B

Best investment: weight set

Keeping a set of weights at home removes any last vestiges of excuses for not working out, as you'll be able to put in half an hour or so any time you like. Although what you're likely to buy and keep at home is unlikely ever to be enough to turn you into Mr Universe, it will be plenty for you to get good toning or for a mildly cardiovascular workout. Also, the companies that make weights for home use have finally got wise to the idea of them being in your house and have designed some very nice-looking pieces of kit.

Go for a set with a bar as well as dumbbells so you can do squats and presses too. Look for quick change collars, rather than anything involving keys: you will appreciate the trouble saved in between exercises. Buy a set with as many different weights as possible to allow maximum flexibility. And invest in a weight training instructional book; don't just hurl yourself into it.

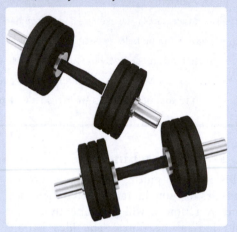

fluid ounces) every twenty minutes or so – increasing that amount if the weather is warm. Keep this intake up regardless of whether you think you need it or not, as if you wait until you feel thirsty you are already in the first stages of dehydration. After you have finished, continue drinking water at the same rate for about an hour.

Sports drinks

These are a blend of carbohydrate, water and electrolytes, and can prove more effective than plain water – especially if you are in an endurance event – because the carbohydrate content will provide energy and help your body to absorb the water quicker.

Sports drinks come in three types: isotonic, where the dilution of the carbs and the electrolytes in the water is about the same as your body, so it is absorbed at the same rate as water; hypotonic, which has less carbs than the above, and therefore won't provide so much energy but will be absorbed quicker;

and hypertonic, where there are more carbs than either of the other two. Hypertonic drinks are best for energy replenishment but will be absorbed the slowest and are very good for post-workout recovery.

The medicine cabinet

A decade or so ago, sports and body-building supplements were the slightly shady preserve of the professional. Now they are big business among many regular gym members and Sunday sportsmen.

As that spectacular ripped body becomes an increasingly must-have fashion accessory, and the desire to win burns as brightly among weekend warriors as it does in the professional competitions, it seems everybody's looking for an edge. For many, that boost comes in powdered form, or as capsules, gels or super-thick shakes. The sports nutrition-supplement industry

The effects of dehydration

Body weight lost through sweat	Stage	Symptoms	Effect
1–2 percent	Normal	None	Won't affect performance
2–4 percent	First stages of dehydration	Thirst and dry mouth	Reduced endurance
5–6 percent	Reduced aerobic capacity and rising body temperature	Raised heart-rate and shortness of breath	Exercise will become harder and decision-making will suffer
7–9 percent	Dangerously high body temperature and blood thickening through lack of oxygen	Difficulty breathing and impaired vision	Loss of balance, dizziness and overall weakness, meaning working out is virtually impossible
+10 percent	Potential heat exhaustion	Confusion and possible hallucinations	Blackouts and collapse as your system is on the verge of shutting down

in the UK has expanded dramatically, and is now worth some £100 million annually, with many amateur athletes and gym rats spending over £100 per month on supplements. The retail aspect is no longer the preserve of gym chains and health food shops either, with supermarkets and pharmacies accounting for half of all sales. The sports supplement industry has entered the mainstream. But do you really need those supplements to achieve the results you want? And is it really worth it?

T Tip: Make your own sports drink with water, fruit juice, sugar (or powdered glucose) and salt. A good isotonic mix is 500ml (17 fl oz) with three large spoons of demerara sugar and a pinch of salt. Alternatively, you can substitute fruit juice, or squash stirred into the water, for the sugar.

Muscle growth

The reason many of us will work out is to increase muscle size, while the majority of amateur sportsmen – footballers, rugby players, tennis players and so on – will usually benefit from a bit of extra muscle strength. Muscles are made up, pretty much, of pure protein. Therefore it will come as no surprise that the biggest-selling sports supplement, worldwide, is muscle builder in the form of flavoured protein powder, which is mixed with water, milk or fruit juice to make shakes.

Tip: Getting off the bus or train a stop or two early and walking the remainder of the journey can really add up, in exercise terms, over the course of the week.

Whey protein is the most popular – whey being the liquid by-product run off when cow's milk is turned into cheese. It contains very high levels of branch-chain amino acids, which are vital for metabolizing protein to build lean muscle tissue. Whey protein comes as concentrate or isolate. Whey protein isolate has a considerably lower calorific value, and is more expensive than concentrate, but its increased protein purity makes it by far the most popular choice.

It is fast-acting, and so a shake could be consumed first thing in the morning, another sipped during the day and one more immediately after working out. Each shake should contain around 40 grams of protein powder.

Casein is another milk-derived protein, again sold as powder and mixed into shakes, but this is far slower-acting than whey. As it will go on releasing protein into the system for up to eight hours, between twenty and forty grams should be consumed before bed, meaning your muscles get nourished while you are sleeping. Neither whey nor casein should be taken by anybody with a dairy allergy. They should opt for the soy- and egg

Supplement	What it does	Foodstuffs it is found in
Chromium	Helps insulin process carbohydrate to produce energy, build and repair muscles and burn fat.	Broccoli; grapefruit; black pepper; brewer's yeast; cereals
EFA (Essential Fatty Acids)	Maintains joints; improves stamina; speeds recovery between training sessions.	Fish oil; vegetable oil; olive oil; nuts
Magnesium	Without it the other electrolytes potassium and calcium cannot be absorbed into the body to prevent muscle cramps; assists in burning glucose for energy.	Leafy green veg; whole grains; nuts; pulses
Vitamin C	Repairs damaged cartilage; protects the joints from inflammation when under stress.	Fruit; leafy green veg
Vitamin E	An anti-oxidant protecting muscle tissue from damage during exertion by retaining key proteins within the fibres; this will also aid recovery	Vegetable oil; seeds; nuts; leafy green veg
Zinc	Increases blood cell reproduction, to boost tissue repair and speed recovery	Liver; red meat; seeds; yoghurt

white-based alternatives.

Protein powder is not cheap, and many believe it doesn't represent good value for money, as the average Western diet contains more than enough protein to support the exercise regimes required to build big muscles.

Performance power

Creatine is a substance produced in the body in relatively small amounts but which, when delivered to the muscles via the bloodstream, forms adenosine triphosphate (ATP), a highly effective energy-bearing molecule. ATP levels can be raised by introducing creatine monohydrate with two five-gram doses per day (after working out and before bed) as a supplement over a period of several days.

After about a week the muscles will be flooded, meaning the body will have greater stores of instant energy to boost explosive performance – creatine metabolizes much faster than glucose. Body-builders will use creatine in conjunction with protein to help them do more "reps" (repetitions) with heavier weights to more efficiently build muscle mass. "Stacking it" with carbohydrate in this manner greatly speeds up the absorption rate.

Nitric oxide increases the blood flow to the muscles, facilitating the delivery of creatine and other nutrients. This is vital to muscles that are put under the sort of stress involved in pumping iron. Nitric oxide is also favoured by body-builders as an improved blood flow ultimately allows muscles to be pumped up to spectacular dimensions.

F

Fact: Although many older (or old school) body builders swear by liver tablets, if you are taking a good quality multi-vitamin and whey protein you do not need them.

Fat shedding

The two most popular of the three most popular anti-fat supplements are fat burners and meal replacement products. They only work within an established cardio and dietary programme and function by boosting or assisting what is already being done – after all, if they worked by themselves, nobody would be fat.

Meal replacement products (MRPs), a blend of mostly protein, vitamins and minerals and some carbohydrate, do pretty much what you'd expect. They replace meals by offering most of what you need and nothing you don't, in a handy sachet or as powder to be made into a shake. While these can be a valuable substitute for the occasional missed meal during a

Which whey?

Whey protein is the most popular muscle building supplement on the market, but there are two types – whey protein concentrate and whey protein isolate. Whey protein concentrate, usually makes up the bulk of commercial supplements, as it is less expensive than whey protein isolate, which is of better quality as it has a higher biological value. That means isolate is more pure, containing between 90 and 98 per cent protein, compared to whey concentrate's 70 to 85 percent purity, with the rest being fats and lactose. Most readily available whey supplements are largely concentrate with some isolate mixed in – the more isolate the more expensive it will be but it will also be more effective.

T

Tip: Always buy established brand supplements from reputable retailers. Avoid the unfamiliar labels and the unknown internet suppliers, regardless of what bargains they might be offering. Your biggest risk won't be that they'll do you harm, but that they won't do anything.

training schedule, they shouldn't replace eating properly, as regular food contains a host of vital micronutrients that will not be duplicated in these supplements.

Fat burners, or thermogenics, nearly all contain some permutation of caffeine, cayenne, aspirin and ephedrine, which will stimulate the metabolism to boost the fat-burning properties of your own cardio routine. Pills with the greatest proportion of ephedrine (a powerful amphetamine) will boost it to such a degree you may not need the cardio. The drawbacks, however, are edginess, shakes and palpitations. The most recent generation of thermogenics contain thyroid regulators, targeting the hormones that control metabolic rate. These are best avoided as not nearly enough research has been published as to their long-term safety.

Appetite suppressants, the third popular option, should not be considered, as your body needs to eat for nutrition: tricking it

into ignoring hunger pangs is never a good idea. This is even more relevant if you are regularly playing sport or working out.

It's difficult to offer recommendations for any of the quick weight-loss supplements on the market, as fat burning has always been a fairly straightforward matter of balancing calories consumed with energy expended, in a way that still allows for healthy and nutritious eating.

Carb loading

This refers to an entirely safe and natural method of increasing your body's store of energy in preparation for an endurance event such as a marathon or triathlon – or even a ninety minute football match. During the three days before the event, increase the proportion of carbohydrate in your diet by about half, while leaving the overall calorie count the same – this means around seventy percent of your diet should be carbohydrate, with around twenty percent of it protein and ten percent fat.

Done over this short space of time, your body will store the extra glycogen created in the muscles and the liver, leaving you greater energy reserves to draw on when competing. Keeping the protein intake the same is important too, because protein slows down carbohydrate's metabolizing, meaning the energy stored will last even longer. When taking on this extra carbohydrate, do it gradually over the course of each of the three days, and change your eating patterns to six small meals a day rather than three big ones, with the option of taking the carbs

Anabolic & catabolic

The former refers to the metabolic process that causes the building of body tissue, and can be applied to anything, not simply steroids; catabolic is the complete opposite as it is applied to the breaking down of tissue to provide a release of energy. The two are balanced inside the body during day-to-day life to provide energy and to repair and regrow damaged tissue, but to gain muscle for sports participation or body building, the anabolic side must be given preference.

Supplement	Function	Format	What's in it	Potential dangers
Carbohydrates (simple and complex)	Energy provision; engineered for quick absorption and slow release	Drinks; gel	Glucose; fructose; fine ground oats; barley starch; waxy maize starch; D-Ribose	Weight gain; potential obesity
Creatine	Muscle gain; strength increase; tissue repair; speeds recovery from injury; reduces mental fatigue	Capsule; drinks	Occurs in tuna, salmon and beef, but creatine supplements will be synthesized	Diarrhoea; potential kidney damage
HMB (Beta-Hydroxy beta-methylbutyrate)	Minimizes muscle breakdown to promote muscle growth; burns fat; increases endurance	Capsules	Found in alfalfa, catfish and grapefruit, but supplements will be chemical	No known side effects
Hydration drink	Replenish carb and electrolyte levels to increase endurance	Drink	Glucose; sodium; potassium chloride; water	Weight gain
Multi-vitamins	To keep up with the increased demands for nutrients brought about by sporting activity	Tablets; liquid	Different multi-vitamins will be designed to suit specific needs, thus ingredients will vary – check the packaging	When taking multi vitamins it's tempting to neglect eating properly and so miss out on the important micro-nutrients in real food
Nitric oxide	Increases blood flow to the muscles, pumping them up; boosts explosive power; can raise endurance levels	Tablets; powder	It's a chemically synthesized product of one part nitrogen to one part oxygen	Nausea, vomiting and diarrhoea. Avoid if you have high blood pressure
Protein	Speeds metabolism; builds muscles; burns fat; aids tissue repair	Powder for shakes; bars; ready-mixed drinks	Most will be whey or milk (casein); for the lactose intolerant there is soy or egg white	Gout; weight gain; kidney damage
Testosterone enhancer	Increases testosterone levels to increase strength, build muscle and enhance libido; reduces body fat	Capsules	Zinc, Magnesium and Vitamin B6 (ZMA); or extract of Tribulus terrestris	Repeated tests have shown testosterone enhancers to be almost totally ineffective

When to take a supplement

When	What	Why
Upon waking	Water/sports drink; multi-vitamin	You will have been dehydrating while you sleep, it's important to replenish those fluids
Breakfast	Protein shake; fibre	Establish the conditions for muscle growth early in the day; internal health
Mid-morning	Carbs and some protein	Five small meals a day are much easier to metabolise than three large ones
Pre-activity (30 mins beforehand)	Amino acids – preferably beta-alanine	As a protein "building block" this will ready the body to grow muscle and repair tissue during and after exercise
During activity	Isotonic sports drink	You will absorb this quickly and it is has a high calorific value for energy replenishment
Post-activity	Protein shake mixed with water; hypertonic sports drink; glutamine	The drink and the water will rehydrate you and replenish carbs; the protein and the glutamine (an amino acid) will speed recovery
Lunch	Carbs, protein and fibre	For energy, post-activity muscle maintenance and body protection
Mid-afternoon	Carbs and fruit	For energy and micro-nutrients
Dinner	Lean protein, carbs, vegetables	To keep up the supply of amino acids and to take on some fibre
Evening snack	Slow-action protein such as casein	For gradual release of amino acids to the muscles during the night

on as energy drinks. Ideal foods for carb loading include wholewheat bread and pasta, porridge, peanut butter and brown rice.

Can you believe the hype?

Nutritional or dietary supplements and ergogenic aids in the UK are not classified as drugs or medicine, therefore do not have to conform to MHRA (Medicines and Healthcare Regulatory Agency) regulations. Instead, they come under the Food Safety Act, the Food Labelling Regulations and the Trades Descriptions Act. This removes the rigid scientific testing that will have preceded any new drug launch to make sure it is both safe and delivers what it promises, then will continue to monitor the product once it goes to market. This means, despite many sports supplements' quasi-scientific jargon and audacious claims, they need only have been officially scrutinized as stringently as a packet of cheese slices. Only if a product proves to actually be harmful or misrepresenting its ingredients on the labelling or its capabilities on the packaging, will a government agency intervene. It's worth noting, *vis-a-vis* the Trades Descriptions Act, the hyperbolic claims most make about results are quotes from satisfied third parties rather than the manufacturers themselves.

Endurance enhancing

Apart from the obvious carb-rich energy drinks, the previously discussed nitric oxide can also aid endurance as it boosts blood flow delivering oxygen to the muscles more efficiently.

HMB (Beta-Hydroxy beta-methylbutyrate) is a tested endurance enhancer. It will raise an athlete's maximal oxygen consumption, delivering more oxygen to the muscles for longer, thus raising performance length and levels. It also reduces the likelihood of metabolic acidosis (when your body builds up too much acid) by delaying blood lactate accumulation.

Recovery boosting

Creatine and protein both assist recovery, as they deliver the high-quality protein needed to rebuild muscle, while hypertonic energy drinks will replace carbohydrates and enzymes used up during participation.

Amino acid supplements – particularly glutamine and arginine – not only reduce the muscle damage brought on by intense exercise, but greatly boost your body's recovery powers afterwards. As essential components of muscle tissue, amino acids speed the repair of internal tears and bruising exercise, reducing post-workout soreness.

T

Tip: Protein bars are not an effective way to supplement protein due to the amount of sugar and other carbohydrate, meaning they will contain a relatively low amount of high quality protein.

They stimulate the release of growth hormone (to rebuild muscles after the stress of working out or sport) and of insulin to reduce fatigue. Amino acids will also assist in wound healing and combat the suppression of the immune system often brought about by debilitating physical activity.

Steroids: they're growing

According to the drug education service Frank, there are an estimated 150,000 regular abusers of illegal anabolic steroids in the UK, a fast rising figure that includes a disproportionately large amount of men under 25. The NHS claims the problem is now so rife in some areas that over half the

Ten top tips for getting fit

▶ **Build keeping fit into your routine** Make it an intrinsic part of your life. Keeping it as some sort of optional extra will only encourage you to miss sessions.

▶ **Set yourself goals** But make sure that, although they will stretch you, they are achievable goals. Then reward yourself when you attain them.

▶ **Be flexible about it** Don't adopt an all-or-nothing approach. If you have to miss a session don't worry, just put a bit extra into the next one.

▶ **Don't overdo it** Overtraining is common among beginners and can sneak up on you without you realizing. It can lead to all sorts of injuries, bring on fatigue and eradicate any exercise-related feeling of well-being.

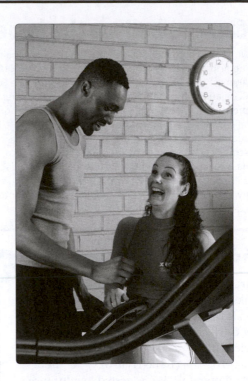

▶ **Don't expect immediate results** You are in this for the long haul and it will take time for you to start to see changes in your body shape or attain a noticeable increase in fitness – be patient!

▶ **It's supposed to be fun** If you're not enjoying whatever activity it is you've started, then stop it and do something else. There's masses of choice out there, and if you're not motivated by what you're doing you're unlikely to keep it up.

▶ **Anything is better than nothing** If you can't run then walk, and if you can't walk for thirty minutes, walk for fifteen. Everybody has to start somewhere, so don't get discouraged

if you can't work out like a madman from day one.

▶ **Sneak in some extra exercise** Take the stairs instead of the elevator or get off the bus early and walk the rest of the distance, or dump the power mower in favour of an old-school push model.

▶ **Hang with a fit crowd** Find yourself some like-minded friends, or, better still, encourage the friends you've got to keep fit with you. You'll have more fun, and you're bound to end up motivating each other.

▶ **Eat correctly** You will have the energy to work out and the nutrients to speed recovery. This will probably mean alterations to your diet even if you were a healthy eater to start off with.

The best of the web

keepfit.org.uk
Website of the Keep Fit Association, a body supported by Sport England, which offers advice and guidance on all aspects of keeping fit, either at home or as part of a class.

buiding-muscle101.com
An American site dedicated to weightlifting; although its primary purpose seems to be to sell you stuff – videos and supplements, mostly – it has a vast amount of tips, instruction and advice.

runnersworld.com or **runnersworld.co.uk**
Everything you need if you're going to go running or are already doing so. Packed with fitness and training routines, technique tips, gear guides and injury advice, it also has a lively runners' forum and a comprehensive race calendar.

mensfitness.co.uk
The website of the magazine of the same name; includes exercise, nutrition, weight loss and gear-buying advice, and even offers an online personal trainer.

menshealth.com
The website of the magazine that claims to offer "tons of useful stuff", and it isn't lying. Every aspect of fitness for men is dealt with here.

fda.gov/food/dietarysupplements
The US Food and Drug Administration provides excellent overall advice on dietary supplements.

senr.org.uk
The Sport and Exercise Nutrition Register accredits properly qualified sports nutritionists and should be the place to start looking for professional advice.

UKAD.org.uk
The UK Anti-Doping Agency offers a wealth of information about what can and can't be legally taken to improve performance.

---

needle exchange users are not junkies but on steroids, and that on Merseyside, for example, they are treating four new steroid abusers for every new heroin addict.

Anabolic steroids are factory-made substances that approximate the male sex hormone and stimulate muscle growth; they are illegal unless on prescription. Even aside from instant disqualification from sports, the stigma of being branded a cheat and possible criminal prosecution, steroids are bad news. The most common side effects are liver tumours, jaundice, hepatitis and a hugely increased risk of prostate cancer, while steroid abuse will also lead to fluid retention, acne, and extreme and often violent mood swings known as "roid rage". Add to that the prospect of infertility, shrinking of the testicle, high blood pressure, an increase in LDL cholesterol and the distinct possibility of growing man boobs. Is that extra couple of inches on your biceps really worth that much?

On the treatment table

If you play any sort of sport, you will at some point get hurt. That's pretty much a given. What you do to minimise that risk or cope with injury afterwards, though, is entirely down to you.

No gain, no pain

What sport you do will have little bearing on the likelihood of your getting injured during the next twelve months – a collision sport such as rugby actually carries a lower risk of injury than football (soccer). In fact, you are more likely to injure yourself during such apparently gits as running and golf than rugby; they're deceptively dangerous pastimes.

There are, however, specific dangers attached to different disciplines, as you might expect. Back pain is most common among golfers. Football players are most likely to suffer foot, ankle and knee injuries. (The injury rate for playing football on grass is nearly twice that of playing on an artificial surface.) In tennis it's damage to the shoulder joints and the tendons and ligaments of the forearm (known as tennis elbow – no surprise there). Cricketers, on the other hand, are most likely to strain their hamstrings. And bowlers are nearly three times as likely to get injured than the average member of their team.

Most sporting injuries are not serious and can be dealt with on the spot, or treated at home. But it is seldom the case that anything other than minor knocks or aches can be "run off". A general rule is that if you can't walk on it, you shouldn't run on it either. If pain persists after treatment on the sidelines, drop out of that session. Should you take time to rest and treat your injury, but experience a recurrence of the pain when you return to your sport, the injury has not yet cleared up: you should rest until it has. If pain persists without you returning to the sport, despite home treatment, your injury is not healing at all and you should seek immediate professional help.

For persistent or recurring injuries it is worth examining your technique or your equipment, because awkward movements could be putting unnecessary stress on joints or tissue, while faulty, worn-out or ill-fitting equipment may not be protecting you properly.

Another common cause of chronic injury is repeated overuse of certain muscles, or RSI (Repetitive Strain Injury) – relatively widespread among tennis players and cricketers. Pushing yourself too hard in training or simply not taking enough time out to recover between games is also a sure path to the treatment table. It's worth informing one of your teammates (or a competition official) if you have a pre-existing medical condition or are on any medication, just in case something serious happens to you and they need to call the paramedics.

Following are the most common sporting injuries and how best to treat them.

Feet & ankles

Ankle sprain

A stretching or tearing of the ankle ligaments, brought on by sudden twisting of the joint or landing awkwardly. Probably the most common injury in amateur sport.

Symptoms

Pain and stiffness of the joint; inability to bear your weight. Bad cases will swell up with noticeable bruising.

Treatment

PRICE (see overleaf); if the sprain is severe enough to show bruising or pain is not easing after a couple of days, see your doctor.

A joint

All the body's synovial joints work in much the same way, with the same essential components.

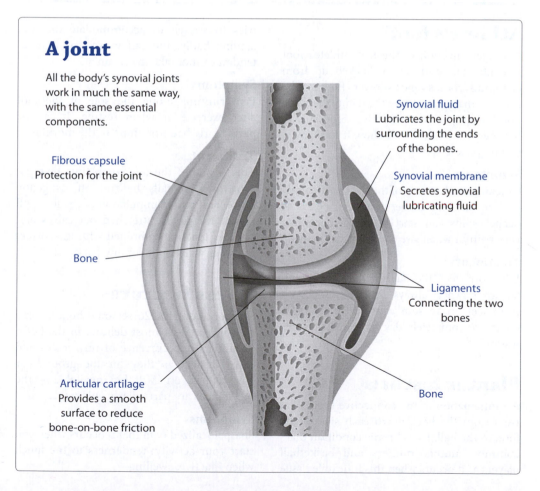

Fibrous capsule
Protection for the joint

Bone

Articular cartilage
Provides a smooth surface to reduce bone-on-bone friction

Synovial fluid
Lubricates the joint by surrounding the ends of the bones.

Synovial membrane
Secretes synovial lubricating fluid

Ligaments
Connecting the two bones

Bone

PRICE

Referred to many times in this chapter, PRICE is a very useful acronym to remember: it is a great treatment for the majority of basic sporting injuries. It is also one of the most straightforward:

Protect: make sure the injury suffers no further damage; this will probably mean withdrawing from the exercise in question.

Rest: to allow the damaged muscle, tendon or ligament to heal, use it or put weight on it as little as possible.

Ice: an ice pack will relieve short-term pain and reduce internal swelling.

Compression: a tightly-wrapped bandage will reduce swelling and can help immobilize an injured joint.

Elevation: raising an injured area to above the level of your heart will stop blood collecting there, reducing swelling and easing pain.

Note: when icing up an injury, keep the ice pack on it for no longer than fifteen minutes, let the area's temperature come back to normal, then re-apply, as too long an exposure could damage your skin.

Athlete's foot

A fungal infection of the feet, athlete's foot is contagious and can be picked up from changing rooms and shower floors. The bacteria that cause it love the damp, therefore not drying your feet properly – especially in between your toes – will allow it to thrive if you do pick it up.

Symptoms
Cracking and soreness of the skin, particularly underneath and in between the toes. The deeper splits can start bleeding, becoming very painful when sweat gets inside them.

Treatment
Dry your feet thoroughly then dust with talcum powder; always put clean socks on clean feet; make sure your sports shoes or boots are completely dry from the previous session.

Plantar fasciitis

An inflamation of the connective tissue that runs from the heel, down each side of the foot, to the ball. Its a chronic condition that's common among runners and basketball players as it occurs when this inflexible tissue tries to stretch to accommodate the foot landing badly; the calf muscle or Achilles tendon cannot take the strain.

Symptoms
Pain running along the sole of the foot after exercise or when resting. It can be particularly bad first thing in the morning.

Treatment
This is one of the few complaints that can sometimes actually be run off, as gentle movement and manipulation of the foot will loosen the tissue; stretched out calves and Achilles tendons combined with the correct footwear will stop it coming back.

Stress fractures

The foot contains 26 separate bones, some of which are the most delicate in the body, meaning the occurrence of tiny cracks and chips in feet as they hit the ground, or are stepped on, will be inevitable – the metatarsals are particularly vulnerable.

Symptoms
Sharp, localized pain that reoccurs when you start your activity; tenderness to the touch when inactive; swelling.

Treatment
PRICE; no sporting activity until it is completely healed, which should be between four and sixteen weeks; on returning to activity, runners should check their shoes for adequate cushioning.

Tibulis posterior tendinopathy

Stretching of the tendon that runs behind the ankle to connect the muscles at the bottom of the calf to the underside of the bones of the feet. It's common in runners who over-pronate (that's to say, roll their feet inwards).

The ankle and foot

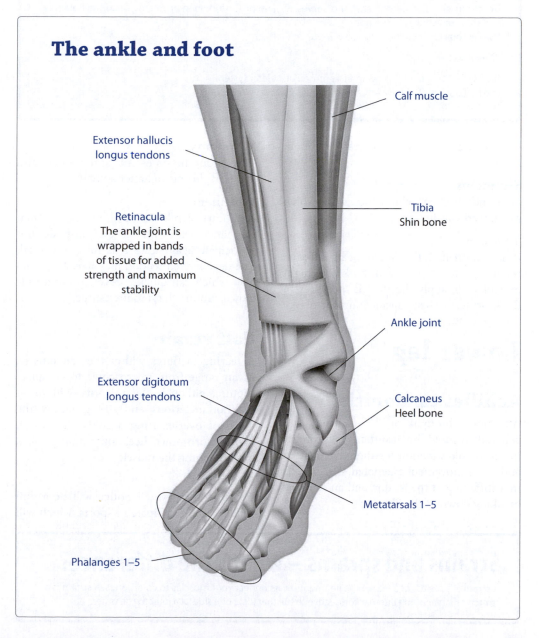

Calf muscle

Extensor hallucis longus tendons

Tibia
Shin bone

Retinacula
The ankle joint is wrapped in bands of tissue for added strength and maximum stability

Ankle joint

Extensor digitorum longus tendons

Calcaneus
Heel bone

Metatarsals 1–5

Phalanges 1–5

Who does what

Physiotherapist

Carries out physical therapy to ensure efficient, maximum and pain-free movement of all parts of the body, usually following an injury.
The Chartered Society of Physiotherapy: www.csp.org.uk

Osteopath

Treats muscles, ligaments, joints and nerves, RSI and posture-related problems, restoring balance and smooth running to the body.
The General Osteopathic Council: www.osteopathy.org.uk

Chiropractor

Treats disorders of the spine and the muscularskeletal system.
The Federation of Chiropractic Licensing Boards: www.fclb.org

But it occurs in all sports where the feet are stretched.

Symptoms

Pain and swelling behind the ankle, which gets progressively worse.

Treatment

If left untreated the tendon can rupture, requiring surgery, so if you think you might be suffering, apply the PRICE measures in the short term, then consult your doctor.

Lower leg

Achilles tendonitis

An injury brought on by overuse, and generally caused by insufficient flexibility in the Achilles tendon for the range of foot and ankle movement attempted. This results in a stiffening of the tendon and an eventual breaking down of the fibres.

Symptoms

The tendon becomes stiff and swollen, and will hurt during and after activity.

Treatment

If it hurts while engaged in sports, then stop and treat with ice and rest; do not participate again until it is fully recovered. The degenerated tendon may have tiny tears in it which can quickly develop into a full-blown rupture that requires surgery.

Calf strain

A tearing of fibres within the calf muscle, it can range from microscopic to complete rupture, although the majority will be at the not-so-serious end. It's generally the result of over-exerting a cold calf muscle, or the worn-down heels on running shoes overstretching the muscle.

Symptoms

The first thing you'll notice will be a dull ache as you participate in sports, which will

Strains and sprains – what's the difference?

A **strain** is a stretch or a tear of the ligaments that connect your muscles to your bones. A **sprain** is a stretch or a tear of the internal connective tissue that joins one side of a joint to the other.

get progressively sharper as the tears start to open up.

Treatment

PRICE; lay off the sport until you are sure you're recovered; make sure you warm up and loosen calf muscles to prevent reccurrence.

Shin splints

Also known as medial tibial stress syndrome, this applies to problems of the muscles, bones or tendons at the front of the leg between the knee and ankle. It's caused by over-exerting yourself in training or failure to warm up properly. Will be made worse by running on hard surfaces.

Symptoms

A dull ache down the inside of the shin bone, increasing as damage goes untreated.

Treatment

PRICE; no sport for a couple of weeks; and cut down the intensity on your return.

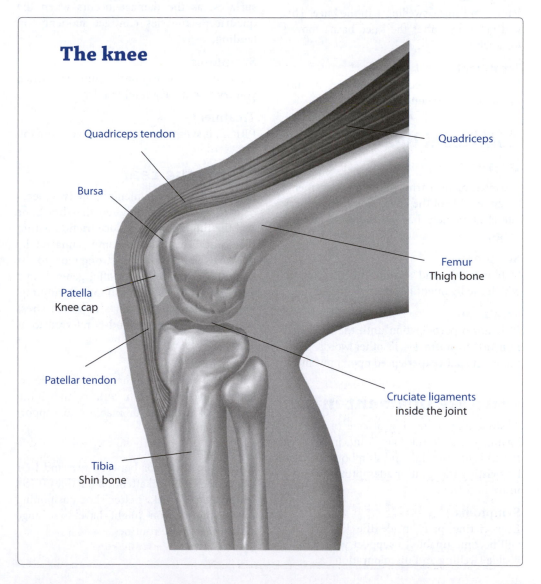

The knee

Quadriceps tendon

Bursa

Patella
Knee cap

Patellar tendon

Tibia
Shin bone

Quadriceps

Femur
Thigh bone

Cruciate ligaments
inside the joint

Knees

Knee bursitis

Bursitis describes the swelling of the sacs of synovial fluid that internally lubricate the joint as it moves and it can affect any joint. But it is most common in the knees and is brought on by impact to the joint when running or jumping.

Symptoms

Pain – and some swelling – in the knee. This will get worse after the knee hasn't moved for a while.

Treatment

PRICE; if pain recurs on return do not participate until you are pain free.

Collateral ligament injury

A stretching or tearing of the thick ligaments on either side of the knee joint, from a sharp lateral movement beyond the joint's natural range.

Symptoms

Stabbing pain and swelling on the side on which the ligament has been damaged.

Treatment

PRICE; no participation until the tissue has returned to normal – in other words, when there is no pain experienced upon movement.

Cruciate ligament injury

A stretching or tearing of one of the two ligaments inside the knee joint, in between the ends of the thigh and shin bones, caused by twisting the joint or attempting to have it move backwards.

Symptoms

Excruciating pain inside the knee, which will become unable to support your weight; visible swelling and discolouration.

Treatment

PRICE and resting up for anything up to two weeks; if you feel no improvement then you have a tear rather than a stretch, and that may require surgery.

Knee tendon damage

Small tears, stretching or a complete rupture of the patellar tendon, which connects the kneecap to the shin bone. It's most common in sports that involve jumping on hard surfaces, as the damage occurs when the quadriceps muscles contract suddenly on landing.

Symptoms

A swelling at the top of the shin; pain when you try to put weight on that leg.

Treatment

PRICE; if symptoms persist, see your doctor.

Meniscus tear

Damage done to the menisci, the two pieces of cartilage that sit between the shin bone and the thigh bone to reduce friction within the joint. They can become damaged by twisting the joint or by a strong blow to the knee. This can also occur after general wear and tear in sports such as football, running, jumping or skiing – sports in which stress is put on the knees – and is referred to as *patellofemoral syndrome*.

Symptoms

Pain and swelling at the side of the knee; clicking sounds from within the joint; locking of the knee or inability to support your weight.

Treatment

PRICE; no sport for between two and four weeks; seek medical attention if it doesn't feel better after a week. Better shoe cushioning can help. But you might have to change sports or exercise routines.

Patellar dislocation

The kneecap (patella) slips out of the grooves that hold it in place; this is common in sports that involve stop/start running, jumping and kicking.

Symptoms

Pain and swelling around the knee; you may even hear a cracking sound when the knee is flexed.

Treatment

In most cases it can be massaged back into place, then treated with PRICE; do not participate for a couple of weeks. Working to strengthen your quadriceps will help you avoid this, as they hold the kneecap in place.

Thigh & hips

Hamstring pull

A tearing of the fibres in the muscles running down the back of the thigh, it's usually associated with explosive bursts of speed, when the muscles have been put under sudden and excessive stress.

Symptoms

Swelling and bruising at the back of the thigh; in severe cases it will impossible to contract and expand the muscle to bend the knee.

Mending a broken bone

Ruptured blood vessels

Blood clot

Mesh of fibrous tissue

New bone forming

New dense bone

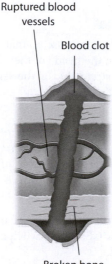
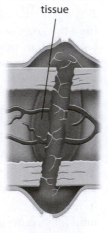
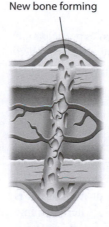
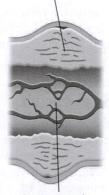

Broken bone

Reconnected blood vessels

Immediately
Almost at once a blood clot forms to seal off leaking blood vessels within the bone

A few days later
Fibrous tissue replaces blood clot

Two weeks later
A spongy bone substance (callus) forms on the fibrous tissue, connecting the ends of the break

Three months later
Dense bone has formed from the callus; the blood vessels have regrown

Treatment
PRICE and stay off the leg completely if possible; if, after a few days, stretching out the muscle to straighten the leg is painful, seek medical advice. When returning to participation, wear a support bandage or cycling shorts to compress and support the recovered muscles.

Iliotibial band syndrome

Swelling of the thick band of tissue that connects the hip bone to the shin bone, running down the outside of the thigh and knee. A common overuse injury, brought on by too much running or insufficient rest periods between participating in running-heavy sports, resulting in a swollen iliotibial band rubbing against the knee.

Symptoms
Pain at the outside of the knee, sometimes continuing up the thigh.

Treatment
Ice and rest; when you return to participation start off gently, and make sure the band gets stretched out during your warming-down exercises.

Labral tears

The labrum makes up the cartilage that lines the hip socket to prevent friction within the joint. It can get damaged through sudden stops, changes of direction or jumping. It is also common in martial arts where extreme movement of the hips is par for the course.

Symptoms
Swelling around the hip; pain in the hip or groin radiating to the buttock; a clicking sound or pinching sensation within the joint.

Treatment
If you think you have a labral tear, seek medical attention immediately.

Quadricep strain

Football's ubiquitous "thigh strain" occurs largely when sprinting or employing an explosive burst of speed; the muscles along the front of the thigh tear due to over-extension.

Symptoms
Tightness of the thigh muscles; sharp pains that will be greater the more serious the strain.

Treatment
PRICE; deep tissue massage; non-participation for anything up to a month, or until it no longer hurts to sprint – although more gentle running might be possible during this time.

The groin

Groin strain

Tearing of the adductor muscles that run from the groin down the inside of the thigh, caused by an over-stretching of the leg or sudden changes in direction.

Symptoms
A swelling and tenderness at the top of the inside of the thigh, where the leg meets the torso; pain during lateral movement of the leg.

Treatment
Do not attempt to "run it off". This will make it much worse; PRICE; non-participation until fully recovered.

Hernia

Most common is the abdominal hernia, occurring when a section of the small intestine pushes through the weakened muscle wall in the groin area, caused by explosive twisting, turning or bending. It's most common in tennis.

Symptoms

A stabbing pain in the groin area, which may get sharper when exercising, coughing or sneezing; you might even be able to feel a lump where the pain is occurring.

Treatment

In most cases you'll be able to push the lump down, with the section of intestine returning to where it should be, inside the muscle wall; then rest for a while and return to activity gradually. If it will not push back, seek medical attention.

Trochanteric bursitis

A running injury, caused by over-use, that happens when the greater trochanter, the fluid-filled sac (or bursa) that eases friction between the glute and the top of the thigh bone, becomes swollen.

Symptoms

Tenderness from the hip down the outside of the thigh; pain when running; sharp pain when bending or twisting.

Treatment

Rest and ice.

Arms & shoulders

Rotator cuff injuries

A tear (tendinopathy) in the muscles or tendons that surround the shoulder and upper arm, rotator cuff injuries are brought on by over-use or sudden movement of the arm above the shoulder – common in volleyball, swimming, tennis and baseball.

Symptoms

Sharp, severe pain, weakness and limited movement of the shoulder joint.

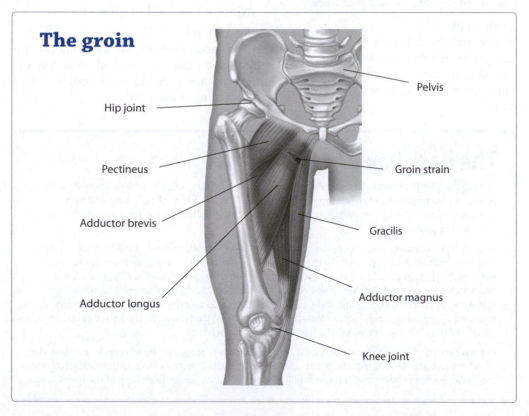

The groin

Pelvis

Hip joint

Pectineus

Adductor brevis

Adductor longus

Groin strain

Gracilis

Adductor magnus

Knee joint

Treatment
PRICE in the immediate term; non-participation, when the arm may initially need supporting with a sling. Muscle tears may require surgery.

Shoulder joint inflammation

Either inflammation of the bursa between the shoulder's bones and muscles; or swelling of the soft tissue inside the joint (frozen shoulder). Both are repetitive strain injuries common in sports that involve lifting the arm above the shoulder.

Symptoms
Both of these complaints will cause pain when the arm is raised and will limit movement. Inflammation of the shoulder bursa will reduce arm strength and may cause swelling; frozen shoulder may cause pain when reaching behind your back.

Treatment
PRICE for the inflamed bursa and heat and gentle movement to loosen the frozen shoulder. In each case do not participate until movement can be performed without pain.

Elbow bursitis

Inflammation of the elbow bursa, brought on either by a knock or repetitive sharp movement, common among tennis players or bowlers in cricket.

Symptoms
Painful swelling at the point of the joint.

Treatment
PRICE and non-participation until arm movements are pain free.

Tennis elbow

Also known as or "golfer's elbow" or "thrower's elbow", this is an inflammation of the forearm tendons where they attach to the upper arm bone, just above the elbow. Tennis elbow affects the outer side of the arm, golfer's the inner, and thrower's both sides. The injuries are the result of resistance met by the wrist joint as the ball is struck or the arm whips to release whatever is being thrown.

Symptoms
Pain and swelling in the joint at the corresponding spot. In bad cases this can extend down the forearm and lead to a weakening of the wrist.

The back box

With the exception of bruised or strained muscles, or spinal damage, the vast majority of back pain as a sporting injury manifests itself as either sciatica or lower back pain, and will be a symptom of something else. With sporting back pain, it's usually unlikely the pain is in the same place as the problem.

Sciatica is the compression or irritation of the sciatic nerve, a main channel of the nervous system that runs from the lower spine down the legs to the feet, and brings on a numbness or tingling in the buttocks that can radiate down the back of the leg to the feet. It comes about as a result of a misaligned pelvis; tight hamstrings, glutes, calves or iliotibial band; damaged or misaligned vertebrae; or an awkward running style. Lower back pain is usually the result of a bad running style; tight hamstrings or glutes; or weak abdominal muscles that allow the back to soak up too much of the shock transmitted up the legs when you run or jump.

In each case you'll need to locate and treat the cause of the problem. In the interim, to alleviate the pain from sciatica, keep as mobile as possible, take painkillers if you have to and gently stretch out the spine. For lower back pain, treat with PRICE, massage and a gentle stretching of the lower back.

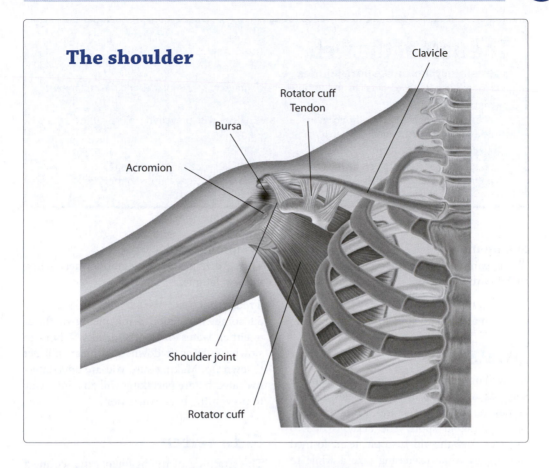

The shoulder

Clavicle

Rotator cuff
Tendon

Bursa

Acromion

Shoulder joint

Rotator cuff

Treatment
Immobilize the forearm; regularly apply ice to the affected area for two or three days; non-participation in sport for several weeks.

Wrist sprain

See ankle sprain (p.195): the symptoms, causes and treatment are almost identical.

Wrist & hand tendon injuries

An inflammation of the sheath enclosing the two tendons that control the thumb, this is a repetitive strain injury common in sports involving gripping, squeezing and pulling, particularly tennis, rowing and skiing.

Symptoms
Sore wrists and pain along the thumbs, sometimes extending along the inside of the forearm.

Treatment
PRICE and non-participation until there is no more pain.

Other common complaints

Cramp

The sudden contraction of a muscle, lasting anything from a few seconds to a few minutes, brought about by over-exertion, dehydration or salt deficiency.

Symptoms
Sharp pain in a particular muscle and the inability to move it.

Treatment
Gentle massage and stretching; rehydration.

DOMS

Delayed onset muscle soreness is, as the name suggests, a soreness in your muscles. DOMS comes on between 24 and 72 hours after participating in sport. The delay is due to the fact that the microscopic tears formed in muscles while exercising take a while to break down sufficiently to cause discomfort. Unexercised muscles are far more susceptible to this tearing, which is why DOMS is common after a lay-off, or when taking up a new sport.

Symptoms
Aching and soreness in the exercised muscles.

Treatment
PRICE; gentle massage and stretching.

Heat exhaustion

You don't have to be exercising in tropical conditions for the body to overheat: a combination of dehydration and excess sweating will drastically raise the body's internal temperature.

Symptoms
Thirst, dizziness, disorientation, headaches, nausea, fatigue.

Treatment
Sit somewhere cool; drink plenty of fluids – either water or sports drinks – but sip slowly; gulping it down may mean it'll get thrown up. Making sure you are adequately hydrated before partaking will go a long way to preventing heat exhaustion.

Side stitch

The straining of the ligaments that connect internal organs to the diaphragm, notably the liver, it is usually brought on by a jolting running style or if your breathing is too shallow – therefore not depressing the diaphragm fully and not completely extending the ligaments.

Symptoms
Sharp pain on one side, just below the ribcage.

Treatment
Slow down (or stop). Push your fingers up on the lower right side of your stomach to lift the liver; breathe deeply; stretch out the ligaments by raising your right arm straight above your head and leaning over to the left, hold, repeat on the other side.

Ten top tips for prevention and recovery

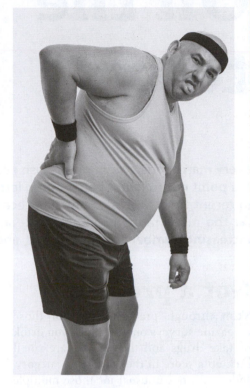

▶ **Warm up properly**, as the vast majority of strains and sprains occur in tissue that was pressed into action while still cold.

▶ **Warming down** is also vital to disperse unused lactate in the muscles and prevent stiffness from setting in.

▶ **Get in shape** before you start a new sport, as a fit and healthy body is less likely to suffer self-inflicted injury.

▶ **Don't rush back** after an injury. Take your time and follow any recommended programme to get back to your previous level of activity.

▶ **"No pain, no gain"** doesn't always apply: pain is your body's way of telling you all is not right.

▶ **Wear the right footwear** So many ankle and knee injuries occur because the feet are not supported properly or given enough grip.

▶ **Check your technique** Performing actions incorrectly is a frequent cause of muscle strain or joint wear and tear.

▶ **Stay hydrated** Dehydration will hasten tiredness thus bringing on a range of fatigue-related injuries.

▶ **Don't overdo it** Make sure you take adequate time for rest and recovery between activities – this period will increase as you get older.

▶ **Get professional help** if the pain won't stop.

On the town

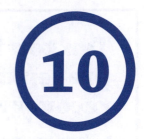

Every man needs a night on the lash every now and again. Even men that make it a point not to might benefit from letting their hair down once in a while. But in recent times "occasionally" has become "regularly" or even "every night" for far too many men, meaning drink- and drug-related issues are affecting an increasing number across the world, and in the UK in particular.

Got a problem?

Skim through practically any of those magazine surveys on how much you drink or take drugs and the chances are you'll rack up a score in the "problem" category. Indeed it's not unusual for those multiple choices to make even the most restrained among us feel uncomfortable about our indulgences. But as killjoy as they may seem, they make a valid point. Alcohol, nicotine and most illegal drugs are toxins and those ticked boxes ought to make you recognize that any amount greater than None At All will be doing a degree of harm. Therefore, the idea that you should actually enjoy/look forward to/derive some sort of benefit from introducing a poison into your system has to be addressed in some sort of way.

However, as apparently unnecessary as drinking, smoking or taking drugs might be – and, let's face it, you'd need a Sid Vicious-level IQ to truly believe anything different – it's naïve to assume everybody's going to give them up completely. Prohibition didn't work back in the first part of the twentieth century, and in the War on Drugs the authorities are being outfought in every major city across the world.

Indeed, current figures show that, in the UK, one-third of all men drink over the recommended limit of 21 units of alcohol a week, while twenty percent of us worry we drink too much and one in six admits to regularly binge drinking, which is officially

Measure for measure

A unit of alcohol equates to half a pint of regular strength beer, a small (125ml) glass of wine or a single measure of any spirit, and the recommended consumption for men in the UK is 21 units per week (it's 14 for women). These days, however, drinkers need to take extra care if trying to stick to these guidelines. Strong ales or lager can supply more than one unit of alcohol per half pint; many pubs and bars now serve wine in 250ml glasses; and wine in general has increased in strength from eleven or twelve percent to fourteen or fifteen percent.

How it all works: the drunkometer

Every drink you take during a night out has a cumulative effect, slowly disrupting different aspects of your system until it more or less shuts down and you pass out. Everybody's tolerance levels to alcohol will be different and they will go up the more regularly you drink. The sequence presented here is for the casual/social drinker. It assumes one drink every 25 minutes or so, and as it takes the liver almost an hour to process one unit of alcohol, drinking at this rate quickly builds up.

This sequence assumes two units per drink, as most men in a social drinking situation will be drinking pints of beer or large glasses of wine.

First drink	The instant effect you'll feel from downing that first pint is a small amount of alcohol passing directly from your stomach into your bloodstream. As most of it passes into your small intestine, this will be mild and short term.	Alcohol/blood approximately 25mg/100ml
Second drink	Brain activity is starting to decrease as the alcohol affects the frontal cortex, where conscious thought is processed, which means your inhibitions start to disintegrate. You are probably talking too loudly and are unaware of it.	Alcohol/blood approximately 75mg/100ml

UK legal drink/driving limit 80mg/100ml

Third drink	As logical thought centres get further suppressed your confidence soars and you'll know very little fear. The booze will be working on your cerebellum by now, throwing your coordination out – slurred speech, wonky balance, misjudging of distances – but because of your new-found confidence, you'll probably find it quite funny.	Alcohol/blood approximately 120mg/100ml
Fourth drink	As alcohol suppresses the anti-diuretic hormone vasopressin, your kidneys will direct fluid straight to your bladder and you'll be popping to the gents with increasing regularity. Coordination will be very poor, but confidence will be so great you'll be convinced you are actually doing better than normal – it's why so many people will drive very drunk but wouldn't dream of getting behind the wheel when just a bit pissed.	Alcohol/blood approximately 160mg/100ml
Fifth drink	Your lack of inhibitions will be such that your emotions swing to extremes – enthusiasm, aggression, affection, misery… Or you could start to feel maudlin, as the alcohol's depressive qualities suppress the production of glutamine, one of the brain's stimulants. You may well be staggering too.	Alcohol/blood approximately 200mg/100ml
Sixth drink	Your central nervous system will be greatly affected, slowing down communication between brain and muscles, meaning everything you do or say will be sluggish – not that you'll be making a great deal of sense at this point. You should also be feeling hungry as frequent urination has been depleting your system and blood sugar levels will be falling.	Alcohol/blood approximately 240mg/100ml
Seventh drink	Confusion and disorientation sets in as the brain and central nervous system are on the verge of shutting down. Drowsiness and overall tiredness will result as increased glucose from the sugar in the alcohol means massively raised insulin levels have removed nearly all your blood sugar. You may start throwing up as your body finally rebels against the poison you've been feeding it since you left home.	Alcohol/blood approximately 280mg/100ml
Eighth drink	The brain ceases all conscious activity and you pass out. There will be so much alcohol in your bloodstream it may take a couple of days to clear, and you will definitely fail a breathalzser test the next morning.	Alcohol/blood approximately 300mg/100ml

defined as more than twelve units in one session. The trick is to keep recreational intake under control and to know when and how to cut back or stop if it starts getting out of hand – to use it without it using you.

What those limits are is going to be a matter unique to every individual's metabolism and circumstances, and a broad-brush approach will never be too practical when judging what constitutes a "problem". In practice, that will be when your actions-under-the-influence start adversely affecting other people like your family, your co-workers, your friends, fellow road users, the police, the health service, society in general. After all, if your habitual substance abuse isn't impacting on anybody except you and yours – that is your health, your bank balance and your liberty – why should anybody else care? You might believe, if that's the case, that it's not even a problem.

But because it can be a scarily short step from merely behaving like a jerk to staggering around the street, shouting at traffic, it helps enormously to understand what it is you're doing to yourself. That way you will have the best chance of staying in control.

Fit to drink

Much like anything else, going on the lash will be much easier for your body to cope with if it's in good shape. If you eat healthily, there will be far less rubbish floating around in your system for your liver to have to deal with as it sorts out whatever toxins are contributing to your good night out – this

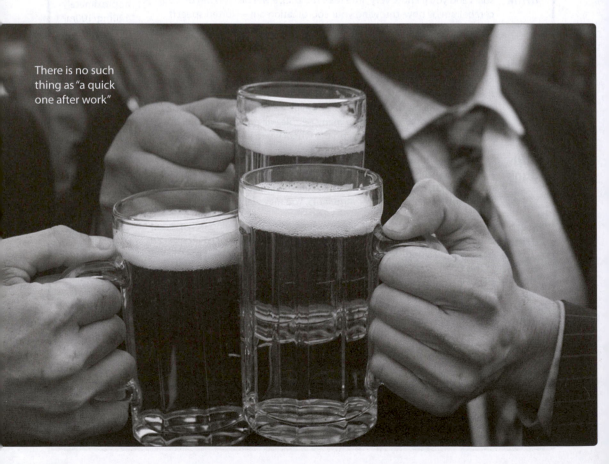

There is no such thing as "a quick one after work"

will ease the next day's hangover too. A good strong heart, at the centre of a healthy cardiovascular system, will make sure that toxins are processed and despatched as efficiently as possible. And not being overweight will minimize strain on your liver when it puts fat conversion on hold to process the poison you've just brought to it.

It's because professional athletes are so much fitter than us mere mortals that they can survive going on benders with few apparent performance problems. It's also why so many of them get into trouble with drink or drugs when their playing careers are over – they carry on at much the same levels, but are no longer fit enough to cope with it.

Provided you look after yourself for the rest of the week, there is no reason why one night off from such responsible behaviour will do you too much harm. Indeed, it will do you good to be able to relax and not worry about what's best for you for an evening. Provided, that is, one night doesn't turn into two or three, and if you find yourself feeling the effects to an increasing extent you address the issue before it gets out of hand.

Fancy a drink?

The chances are you do. In Britain, like so many other Western countries, alcohol oils the wheels of many machines. We think nothing of hanging out in the pub, or sealing a deal over lunch, or ordering a decent bottle

F

Fact: In vino veritas – with the drastic lowering of the inhibitions, tactful behaviour or self-preservation disappears, and around the fifth drink, are replaced with a dangerous compulsion to tell the truth.

of wine on that potentially awkward first date. If imbibed responsibly it is unlikely to do you too much harm. After all, our love affair with beer dates back six thousand years, to when the Ancient Egyptians and Mesopotamians began brewing, and civilisation does not appear to have collapsed yet.

First the good news

Everybody is aware of strong drink's relaxing qualities. Recently though, it's been found to have physical benefits too. And this isn't merely the "glass of red wine a day" mantra. A British survey of 20,000 moderate drinkers – one or two glasses of wine or pints of beer per day – found there was no difference in health between the exclusively beer-drinking and exclusively wine-drinking halves, and both showed the same improvements over the teetotal sample. In other research, moderate drinkers have consistently scored higher on the "how healthy do you feel?" charts.

Dying for a drink

During the last thirty years the alcohol-related death toll in the UK has more than doubled, with a rise of twenty percent in the first five years of the twenty-first century.

In the UK in 2010, the number rose again. An average of 25 people per day died through excessive drinking and there were over one million admissions to hospital for alcohol-related complaints during that year, up more than twelve percent on 2009.

Eight percent of British men will have a problem with alcohol at some time in their lives. In the US, that figure is eleven percent.

How it all works: the liver

The largest, heaviest organ in the body, the liver is also the most complex – after the brain, obviously – and carries out over 1000 functions, around half of which are vital to keeping us alive.

The three main duties are the storing of fat extracted from food and its controlled release into the bloodstream as cholesterol; the chemical processing of nutrients that have been taken from food and metabolizing them into a usable form for delivery around the system; and the filtering out and breaking down of toxins that have found their way into the bloodstream, such as alcohol. It also manufactures the bile used to break down fats in the small intestine, produces and regulates the proteins needed for blood clotting, converts excess glucose into glycogen and stores it ready to provide energy bursts, and creates the factors that form the basis of the immune system.

It manages all of this by processing oxygenated blood that is delivered from the heart, via the hepatic artery, and nutrient-rich blood arriving from the intestines through the hepatic portal system. This is a network of capillaries and blood vessels that feed into the hepatic portal vein at the base of the liver. All the body's blood passes through the liver, and at any point it will contain around thirteen percent of it.

Once inside the intricate lattice of veins of the liver, blood passes through thousands of tiny lobules, themselves made up of billions of cells called hepatocytes, which are miniature chemical processing plants. They extract food's nutrients and fats, modify them into usable form and store them to be despatched to tissue and organs around the body. They will also distribute the oxygen delivered from the heart. Once everything has been removed, the blood is pumped back to the heart via the largest vein in the body, the inferior vena cava.

4. Once in the liver the toxins are filtered out before the blood flows back to the heart

1. Alcohol is taken into the stomach and the intestines

3. It is delivered to the portal vein, which feeds it into the liver

2. It is then absorbed through the walls into a series of blood vessels and capillaries

The lobules in the liver will also cleanse the blood, removing bacteria and damaged blood cells and filtering out toxins. These it processes into a form that can be passed back into the intestine to leave the body in faeces or urine. It's this that is related to alcoholic liver disease, as removing the high concentration of toxins in alcohol occupies far too many of the liver's resources and capabilities.

Expert advice: "If you keep yourself fit and look after yourself you'll stand a better chance of getting away with going on the lash. If you have a high basic level of fitness and your everyday nutritional level is good, then you're going to bounce back much quicker. Your metabolism will work much faster, therefore you're going to get the toxins through your system much more quickly, and if your nutritional level is high and you've got a good level of antioxidants in there, then that's going to cure a lot of the lingering problems you get from going on the lash. You're going to get away with more, big time, and while that shouldn't be the biggest plus point of getting fit, it's certainly one of them."
Gideon Remfry

Science has yet to fully explain why modest amounts of alcohol – a poison, after all – seem to promote several different types of good health. For a long time the idea of Mediterranean men living longer and healthier lives was attributed to the diet and air quality as much as the regulation red wine, but more modern findings are isolating the drink as being equally beneficial. (This is a finding of large study groups rather than scientific research.) Moderate drinking has cardiovascular benefits, as it seems to raise HDL (good) cholesterol and lower LDL (bad) cholesterol, while test subjects have also experienced fewer incidents of high blood pressure compared to that of teetotallers. The antioxidants in red wine are believed to help protect against cancer, while it is the richest known source of reserpine, a substance that activates protein metabolization and in doing so could increase longevity.

There's also good reason to drink before, during and after a meal. When the Italians first coined the word *aperitivo* toward the end of the eighteenth century to describe an alcoholic drink taken before a meal (it means "opener") they were formalizing a tradition that dated back to the ancient Egyptians. It was they who discovered that such a drink before a meal stimulated gastric juice production to increase the anticipation and digestion of food. The right wine with a meal can heighten the perception of different tastes on the tongue, particularly sweetness or spices, and will take the edge off the sharpness of overly acidic dishes. Whoever invented the *digestif* after the meal knew what they were doing too, as small quantities of alcohol can help break food down in the stomach to aid digestion long after the plates have been cleared away.

Get something in your stomach

Have that fry-up *before* you go out drinking, rather than mopping up remaining alcohol after the event – there won't be much left in your system by now anyway, hence the hangover. Fatty foods serve to line the stomach more effectively, thus slowing down the absorption of alcohol into the bloodstream. This will mean you'll get drunk slower and your system has more time to process the toxic, hangover-inducing by-products, meaning you won't feel so bad in the morning. It is a custom in southern European countries to swallow a spoonful of olive oil before a night on the drink, for precisely this purpose.

Getting drunker younger

More and more people in their twenties and thirties are being treated for alcohol-related liver disease, a condition which was previously almost exclusive to the middle-aged and elderly. The toll among women is rising faster than among men, but that's no reason to feel at all smug as, according to the World Health Organization, the UK's level of drink-related disease is twice the worldwide average.

Too much of a good thing

The key word in all of the above is "moderation" because it's when responsible or occasional drinking becomes heavy and/or regular that alcohol's true toxic nature reveals itself. Quite apart from potentially destroying any relationship or home life you may have, removing your means to earn a living and easing you over on to the wrong side of the law at some point, there's also the physical cost.

Alcohol abuse will seriously damage your liver. Everybody knows that. But how it can creep up on you and quickly become very serious indeed is less widely acknowledged. One of the liver's vital functions is filtering toxins out of the system, those internally produced and introduced from outside – like alcohol. Thus, when large amounts are taken on board, it neglects other operations to cope with this poisonous overload, and the first to be affected is the regulation of fat in

F

Fact: If alcohol, as a drug, was up for consideration for legality today, it is so dangerous in terms of the damage it causes to people and society, it would almost certainly not get passed.

World-class drinking

Alcohol consumption around the world is rising, although in France and the US it is falling. Currently, the per capita average of alcohol drunk in developed, non-Muslim countries across the world is just over five litres per annum. Here's how much the world's biggest-drinking nations are putting away:

Germany 19.2 litres per annum (the most in the world)
Luxembourg 15.5 (second)
Ireland 14.4 (third)
France 14.2 (fourth)
UK 11.2 (ninth)
Australia 9.8 (fourteenth)
Russia 9.29 (eighteenth)
US 8.3 (twentieth)
Canada 7.8 (twenty-third)
Japan 7.6 (twenty-fifth)

Source: World Health Organization

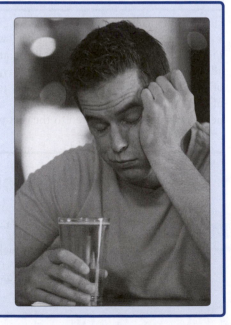

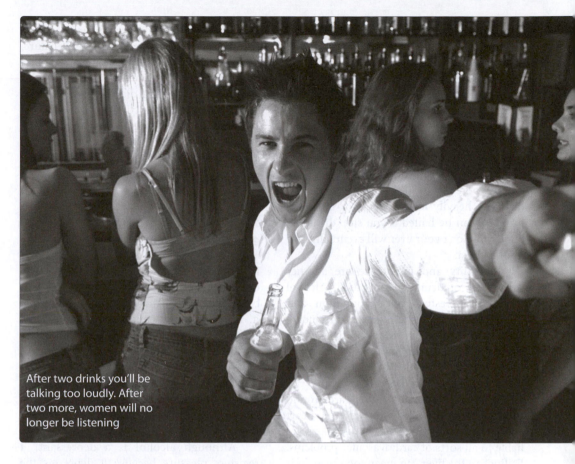

After two drinks you'll be talking too loudly. After two more, women will no longer be listening

the bloodstream. Fat will be held back for processing later, but if large amounts of alcohol are regularly coming in, the fatty deposits build up to dangerous levels, causing fatty liver disease. It swells the liver, causes discomfort in the upper abdomen and is a reliable first physical sign that you are drinking more than your system can handle. This will be experienced by every heavy drinker, but will clear up as soon as you cut down to more sensible levels.

The next stage is alcoholic hepatitis, which comes about after the liver is so overworked and clogged up over a period of time it can no longer process all the toxic elements being shipped in. Cell damage and tissue inflammation will result. Around one-third of heavy drinkers will suffer from this condition, of which the symptoms include abdominal pain, nausea, headaches, jaundice and fever. Again, it is not permanent, and will reverse itself if you

M

Mythbuster: you sober up the next day by sweating out alcohol

Exercising wearing a bin bag or sitting in a sauna won't remove any alcohol lingering in your bloodstream, but it will make you feel a great deal worse as you will be further dehydrating yourself.

stop drinking completely for an extended period – six months – but if ignored it can easily lead on to cirrhosis.

Alcoholic cirrhosis comes about after years of heavy drinking, and is the result of persistent damage that has resulted in scar tissue building up inside the liver, meaning it has become progressively less efficient. Cirrhosis is a permanent, irreversible condition suffered by between ten and twenty percent of those who have been drinking heavily for ten years or more. Its progress can be halted if you stop drinking, but if you don't your liver will eventually give up the ghost.

Infertility and impotence are another side effect of drinking too much. Alcohol can inhibit testosterone production and interfere with the testicles' sperm-producing cells, while its suppression of the central nervous system will impede the complex set of responses needed to bring about and maintain an erection (see p.144).

Whereas moderate drinkers are around fifty percent less likely to suffer a heart attack than non-drinkers, heavy drinkers are liable to all sorts of cardiovascular problems. Failings in the liver can mean too much fat is getting into the bloodstream, which can raise blood pressure and even cause heart failure. Alcohol's high calorie content can lead to obesity and all of its attendant cardiovascular complaints, including diabetes, which won't be helped by a malfunctioning liver.

And if all of the above wasn't quite enough, persistent alcoholic assaults will attack your stomach lining, causing sharp pains and maybe even ulcers.

From social drinking to antisocial behaviour

If drinking too much is so bad for us, why do nearly all of us do it on a fairly frequent basis? The simple answer is because we like it. It's part of the "positive reinforcement" trait of the human brain: our minds are hard-wired to make us want more of anything we find particularly agreeable. The brain's reward pathways are remarkably easy to access, prompting us to increase the amount of stimulation involved to achieve more pleasure.

Although alcohol is a depressant, it registers pleasure because it depresses the parts of the brain that restrain our behaviour and feelings, to allow a usually enjoyable state of abandonment. (Alcohol is categorized as a sedative-hypnotic type drug, along with Valium, Librium, Seconal and Rohypnol). As the system becomes used to this state

F Fact: According to the WHO, 2.5 million deaths per year are directly related to alcohol.

The cost of a drink in Britain

The NHS spends £3.75 billion per annum on alcohol-related conditions, spending that has more than doubled in the last ten years. Drink-related crime and public disorder costs the police and the judiciary in the UK around £10 billion a year – it is estimated that half of all violent crimes involve alcohol.

UK employers estimate they lose around £7 billion per year through drink-impaired performance or absenteeism caused by drink – that's between three and five percent of all absences, adding up to eleven million "sickies" being taken each year.

of affairs, however, it builds up a tolerance and requires larger and larger doses to achieve the same effect, and will push us into administering them. Which is where the health problems start.

There's also a psychological "tolerance" aspect to this, whereby behaviour becomes progressively more outrageous, as general drunkenness levels increase often without the drinker being aware of it. Standards get recalculated for what is acceptable on a night out, an escalation which can have a herd-like mentality as people see what others are

T

Tip: Black coffee will not sober you up. All a caffeine fix does is turn a sleepy drunk into a wide-awake drunk, which will probably cause more problems, unless, of course, you're trying to get him off your sofa and out the front door.

Twelve tips to cut down on the drink

1. Start the evening off with a big drink of water
It'll quench your thirst and stop you downing the first in one and going straight on to the second – if that happens your inhibitions will be instantly lowered and you'll be likely to drink more.

2. Drink water alongside your drink
This will help with the hangover and the next point.

3. Drink slower
This one's not rocket science, and if you're gulping down glasses of wine then switch to beer.

4. Miss yourself out of your own round
That way you won't have to make a big deal about refusing a drink.

5. Don't stand at the bar
It's much too easy to buy more drinks or for the bar staff to offer you one.

6. Avoid salty bar snacks
Their whole purpose is to make you drink more.

7. Have a couple of days off a week
Even if you have cut down the amount you drink, a couple of teetotal days will prove you're in control.

8. Be the designated driver
If your friends have any instinct for self-preservation they won't let you drink too much.

9. Don't keep booze in the house
Otherwise you'll drink it at some point.

10. Stop hanging out with people you only ever meet in pubs
The chances are all you really have in common with them is drinking, so it's all you're ever going to do with them.

11. Arrive later if you're meeting in a bar
By turning up at eight instead of seven you'll probably save yourself three drinks.

12. Get a hobby
But not collecting beer mats.

Help is at hand

addaction.org.uk
Britain's largest specialist drug and alcohol treatment agency, offering help and advice to anybody who has a problem or has to deal with somebody who has.

alcoholics-anonymous.org
The international AA site, explaining how the organization works and where to find a meeting.

aa-uk.org.uk
Alcoholics Anonymous have a 24-hour helpline: 0845 769 7555.

al-anonuk.org.uk and **al-anon.alateen.org**
The support service for the families and friends of alcoholics, or for those affected by somebody else's drinking – the latter is aimed at young people.

getting away with and, drunkenly, follow suit. Then, when enough people are carrying on like that, "normal" becomes redefined.

Beyond recreational drinking there's another more insidious level of alcohol abuse, at which being drunk becomes a desired default setting. This used to be largely the preserve of the less outgoing who needed "dutch courage" to put themselves at ease, and who found their tipsy-self to be preferable to their usual comparatively flat-self. Nowadays, however, it appears far more widespread, among both men and women.

Twenty-first-century men are becoming so stressed maintaining a decent work/life balance that the bottle is an increasingly convenient pressure release valve. Once again, through the reward pathway mechanism, life as viewed through the bottom of a glass can become far too desirable a situation – it's no coincidence that the areas of Britain with the highest levels of alcoholism are the more deprived parts of the country.

Curb your enthusiasm

Provided you're not a fully fledged alcoholic, in which case you should seek professional help (see box above), cutting down your drinking to a reasonable level isn't all that hard. It's mostly a matter of changing habits and altering the sort of behaviours that for a long time have been drink-related.

Old enough to know better

Binge drinking and persistent overindulgence is far more common among the young. This is largely because, as men grow older so their work/life balance shifts and career, domestic and relationship responsibilities preclude the behaviour of their youth. It's just as well, because although moderate drinking has been shown to help protect against heart disease, with age comes a reduced tolerance to drink and drugs. It's simply because, as the body ages, it becomes progressively less able to break harmful substances down, thus the prospect of liver disease rises as toxins linger longer to do more damage. You'll also feel worse the next morning, as less poison will have been processed while you sleep, and that sleep will be of greatly reduced quality.

Although working harder to keep fit will hold this off, you will start to notice the adverse effects increasing from your mid-forties onwards. Then by the time you hit your sixties, you should even be reducing levels of indulgence that were previously considered "responsible".

Not unlike rewriting your eating plan or giving up smoking, the key to cutting down drinking is to address the situations in which drink is a (if not the) vital component.

The biggest hurdle for British men though, is pub culture and the kind of heroic associations that go with drinking far too much. Too often what, logically, ought to be a simple matter of announcing that you're on the Diet Coke, turns into a night of humorous remarks directed at you about your sexuality, gender and whether or not you've got "a dose". Often it can be far less painful just to get sloshed.

However, if you're prepared to put a bit of effort into it you can climb on the wagon without looking like a complete girl.

Climbing aboard the wagon

In the beginning, give up by stealth. Tell as few people as possible you're giving up/ cutting down, and make as small a deal as possible of it as this immediately removes pressure. If you make an announcement, it will become a recurring topic of conversation and you'll end up having to think much too much about the drinking you're no longer doing. Also, if you do slip off the wagon it's probably

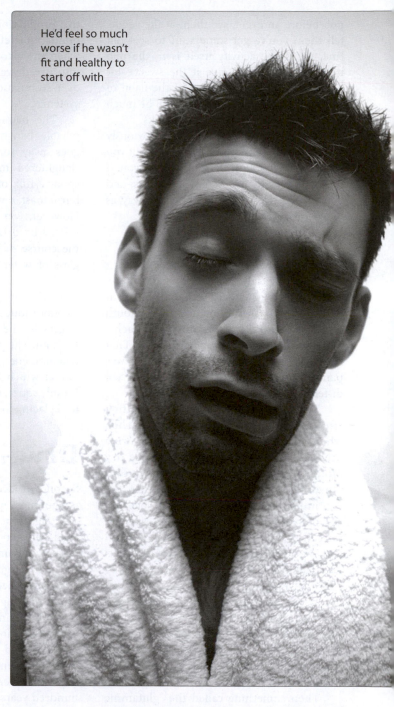

He'd feel so much worse if he wasn't fit and healthy to start off with

best not too many people know about it. To get out of situations when you know you'll drink, make excuses that have nothing to do with not drinking – don't meet friends in a pub before an event, see them at the venue, tell them you've got some stuff to sort out first. Or if the activity itself is in the pub it's probably best to give it the swerve for a while, until you've got out of the habit of drinking so much – that way you'll be much more confident about refusing drinks.

When you do come clean, obviously you're going to endure a bit of abuse, but you should expect your friends to support you. If they don't it's their problem not yours, and you should drop them in the same way as you're dropping the booze.

Anatomy of a hangover

The morning after is never particularly pretty, and the standard legacy of a decent night on the lash can include a dry mouth and eyes, fatigue, irritability, headache, nausea and lack of concentration. That hangover will be hard to shift, as it was painstakingly constructed by a number of different alcohol-related factors.

The most significant is the dehydrating effect caused by the ethanol in the alcohol, which has been causing increased urine production. This will account for the dry mouth and raging thirst as you strive to rehydrate yourself. It is also behind the continually throbbing headache, because the dehydrated brain has shrunk slightly, retreating a little from the inside of the skull and stretching the connecting membranes. Any feelings of sickness will be a lingering effect of last night's alcohol acting as an irritant on your stomach lining. Blood sugar will be low because the liver will have been overworked and it is struggling to restore the correct glucose levels. This causes general fatigue, reduced concentration and a fuzziness of thought.

Then something called the "glutamine rebound effect" tops things off with an acute sensitivity to light and sound, restlessness, anxiety and trembling hands. This happens because drinking suppressed the production of glutamine, one of the brain's most effective natural stimulants, so when the alcohol dissipates the body goes into overdrive to replenish it, resulting in over-stimulation of the senses and nervous system.

The bad news is that the only truly reliable hangover cure is to wait until it goes away (or you could try not getting slaughtered in the first place), so forget spoons full of Marmite, cayenne pepper, burnt toast, raw onions or the hair of the dog. However, you can minimize the next day's misery by drinking plenty of water during the course of the evening, and try a large glass of water or a hypotonic sports drink just before going to bed. The next day, eggs, being rich in cysteine, will help get rid of the alcohol-induced toxin acetaldehyde, which lingers in the liver, impeding its function. Fruit juice helps too, as the fructose provides a natural energy boost and will speed up the rate at which the body rids itself of toxins. Freshly squeezed juice will also go a long way to replacing lost nutrients.

Drug-related

Second to alcohol and tobacco, marijuana is the most popular drug there is, with over eighty percent of the UK's population aged between fifteen and thirty admitting to having sampled it at some point. And the drug arguments continue to rage. Is smoking weed ultimately more harmful than smoking cigarettes? Or, if there are far more drink-related deaths than those attributable to cocaine, shouldn't booze be banned? And wouldn't nicotine be banned if its staggeringly addictive capabilities had been discovered today instead of a few hundred years ago?

All this, while making good taproom conversation, is conjecture and the idea that one particular drug is not quite as dangerous as another does not make any

The UK law on drugs

	Drugs	For possession	For dealing
Class A	Ecstasy, LSD, heroin, cocaine, crack, magic mushrooms, amphetamines (if prepared for injection)	Up to seven years in prison or an unlimited fine or both	Up to life in prison or an unlimited fine or both
Class B	Amphetamines, cannabis, methylphenidate (Ritalin), pholcodine	Up to five years in prison or an unlimited fine or both	Up to fourteen years in prison or an unlimited fine or both
Class C	Tranquillizers, some painkillers, gamma hydroxybutyrate (GHB), ketamine	Up to two years in prison or an unlimited fine or both	Up to fourteen years in prison or an unlimited fine or both

The specific and separate points covered by the Misuse of Drugs Act 1973 are:

- To possess a controlled substance unlawfully (a small amount for "personal use").
- To possess a controlled substance with intent to supply (large amounts).
- To supply or offer to supply a controlled substance – even if there is no charge made for it.
- To allow premises you occupy or manage to be used for the purpose of drug taking or drug supply.

of them a good idea. The only difference worth considering between tobacco and alcohol and those drugs listed below is that the first two are legal and the others are not. They'll all kill you if you do too much of them and our inherent reward pathway systems form habits in much the same way for all of them. But the two legal ones are much more widespread – hence the higher fatality figures – therefore they are dealt with here in greater detail.

Adulteration alert

Although fags and booze have much higher numerical fatality and hospitalization rates, proportionately the illegals lead the way, largely because they are totally unregulated and nobody really knows what they are taking. Unless you grew the weed yourself, that is. Cocaine and heroin will be cut with all sorts of white powdery stuff from chalk dust to baby milk to rat poison and most of that will end up in your lungs or your veins. No wonder instances of pneumonia and pleurisy are so high among otherwise healthy cocaine users, and hepatitis isn't uncommon among intravenous drug users. Bad ecstasy is all too common, and the make-up of each batch of pills will be something of a lottery as far as the buyer's concerned. Plus the environment in which so many illegal recreational drugs change hands or are taken – nightclub toilets, for instance – is never likely to promote good health.

However, if you still think there's something cool about drug abuse, it's probably best you're aware of exactly what the most popular of them are capable of.

Coke-crazed Britain

Britain has become the world's cocaine-consumption capital. In 2010, 7.7 percent of adults admitted having used it compared with an EU average of 3.4.

- Of people aged between fifteen and fifty, 2.7 percent are regular users, which, for the first time, has overtaken the US, where the figure is 2.4 percent.
- Cocaine use in Britain has doubled in the last five years making it the second most popular of all illegal drugs.
- Since the beginning of this century the price per gram has more than halved, from £70 to £30.
- One-quarter of all heart attacks among the under-fifties in the UK last year were cocaine-induced.
- Roughly fifty percent of British cocaine users end up with a habit that they can't control.
- Twenty-two percent of all requests for help with drug problems last year were cocaine-related.

Why does anybody do it?

Every developed country has a drug problem. In some it's more acute than in others, but every country that can afford one has got one. For example, according to the WHO, in the UK 82 percent of people aged between fifteen and thirty have smoked marijuana at some point; in Australia, overall drug usage has levelled off, but methamphetamines are on the rise. The US has five percent of the world's population, yet consumes fifty percent of the world's illegal drugs. On an average day one-third of German adults will binge drink. Yet, remarkably, everybody knows it's not doing them any good.

How habits can form

Habitual use, or addiction, goes beyond the reward-based psychology of the casual user and is more about the coming down after whatever high has just been experienced and how to avoid it. After a drug's active ingredient has got into your bloodstream via the lungs, the stomach or intravenous injection, it rapidly invades the nervous system to affect parts of the brain and the cardiovascular system. It'll produce a high

Expert advice: "The most popular illegal drug at the moment is cannabis: around thirty percent of young people in the UK use it. Studies have shown that, among young people, there's an increase in sexually risky behaviour when cannabis is used due to increased hedonistic behaviour and them being less likely to take precautions. It would appear that, while under the influence, they have less appreciation of the consequences of their sexual risks; it seems for many they just don't care or the pleasure in the moment trumps the risks. They need a clear wake-up call so that they cannot remain in effective denial." Dr Sandra Scott

that will soon start to wear off, initiating a comedown that the brain will seek to avoid. This is when cravings to get high again start up, and they will be of different strengths and persuasiveness depending on the drug and the individual. Although this is actually the body returning to normal, it's no longer what the brain believes is best compared with the high.

Crack cocaine is particularly effective in this way, producing an intense high followed by a brutal comedown, meaning the user immediately wants to get high again. And, scarily, up there on much the same level of addictiveness is nicotine.

Aided by other chemicals used in cigarette manufacture, nicotine produces an instant elevated heart rate and a rush of euphoria, which stops as soon as you finish that cigarette, meaning you'll be starting to come down and will want another one

F *Fact: Cocaine and heroin prices in developed countries have been falling steadily for 25 years, pretty much in inverse proportion to the increase in their usage.*

almost straight away. Heavy smoking elevates the notion of what "normal" is, hence during the time without a cigarette – which is what you should naturally be like – you feel awful.

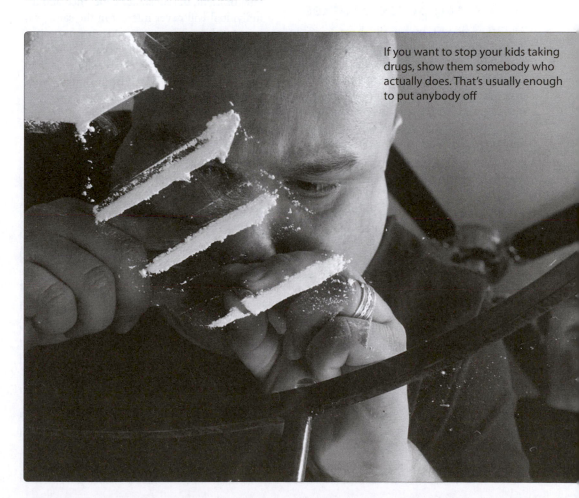

If you want to stop your kids taking drugs, show them somebody who actually does. That's usually enough to put anybody off

Rubbish at football, great at skinning up

Regular marijuana use among 15–34-year-olds during 2010:

UK 26 percent are regular weed smokers
US 24 percent
Spain 22.3 percent
Czech Republic 18.8 percent
France 15.9 percent
Australia 12.2 percent
Canada 7 percent
Japan 5 percent

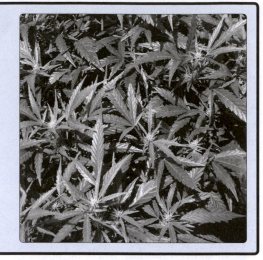

Addictive personalities

Addiction doesn't necessarily have to mean drugs or drink. In the modern world addictions to such things as pornography, food, gambling, adrenaline rushes or self-mutilation are not uncommon. But while these cases are on the rise, science is far from in agreement about the root cause of addictions and why some people become addicts when others don't. Because the environment, the substance concerned and the individual will never interact in the same way in more than one case, pinning down specifics has proved difficult. Opinions are split between it being a disease and a personality trait, with the former being favoured by the international medical community.

This is more a matter of default rather than positive research though, as the theory of the "addictive personality" becomes

A nutritionist writes:

"The problems brought on by drink and drug abuse are twofold. The first is that it makes it much more likely you won't take in the nutrients you need, because you are unlikely to eat healthily under those circumstances due to time, convenience, money or just because you feel unwell. Then, as you recover from the hangover or after-effects, you are unlikely to be receiving your requirement for vitamins and minerals from your diet. Food that you are eating is more likely to be high in fat, salt and sugar and nutritionally inferior. If you are going over the top on a regular basis, you are going to be missing out, nutritionally, especially on nutrients like vitamin C, potassium, folate, beta-carotene and vitamin E that are supplied from fruit and veg and whole grains.

The second problem arises from the fact that more of the body's reserves of vitamins and minerals are needed to protect the body from cell damage caused by the abuse – drink and drugs weaken the immune system, deplete levels of vitamins and minerals in the blood and body tissues and these are not likely to be replaced by eating healthily.

You have to pay particular attention to what you are eating under those circumstances, otherwise you'll be causing a lot more damage on top of what you are already doing to yourself."

Dr Sarah Schenker

Drugs: the choice is yours

The drug	The facts	The high	The comedown
Marijuana	The dried leaves of the hemp plant; smoked	A sedative that produces a dreamy state, heightening perception of sounds and visuals	Lack of coordination and inability to judge distances (driving stoned is riskier than driving drunk); hunger pangs; lowers sperm count; long-term demotivator
Cocaine	Powdered, chemically obtained extract of the leaves of the coca plant, once used as an anaesthetic; snorted, smoked or injected	A rush of energy; intense feeling of well-being; massively increased self-confidence	Risk of stroke or heart attack; numbs tissue in between nostrils to the degree it may fall out; crashing comedown; insomnia; aggressive behaviour; long-term use causes paranoia, anxiety and depression
Crack cocaine	Cocaine purified and reduced down to solid pellets; smoked	More instant, more intense rush than cocaine	High lasts less time; comedown crashes harder; immediate craving for more; long-term use can cause paranoia and suicidal depression
Speed	Amphetamines, a chemically manufactured central nervous system stimulant; swallowed as powder or tablets	Speeds up cardiovascular system to boost energy and keep you awake; rush of euphoria	Can lead to depression and irritability when not speeding; prolonged use can cause insomnia and malnutrition as it suppresses the appetite
Heroin	Chemically refined from the opium poppy; smoked or injected	A dreamy, woozy state of euphoria	Quickly addictive; painful comedowns; risk of HIV and hepatitis from injecting; prolonged use damages liver and kidneys
LSD	Chemically manufactured lysergic acid diethylamide; swallowed as tablets or liquid	Mind-altering "trip" that distorts perceptions of sound, shapes, colour, time, movement, space, relativity…	A bad trip can be a terrifying experience; long-term use can cause paranoia, depression and radical mood swings
Ecstasy	Chemically manufactured methylenedioxymeth-amphetamine (MDMA); swallowed as tablets or liquid	The "love drug", combining speed's energy boost with a dreamy, huggy euphoria	Raises the body's internal temperature dangerously high; risk of heat stroke; serious dehydration; the amphetamine content can cause insomnia and malnutrition

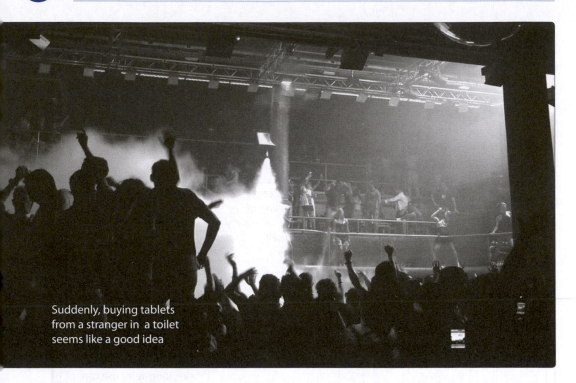

Suddenly, buying tablets from a stranger in a toilet seems like a good idea

difficult to sustain in the light of some aspects of addicts' characters being shared but equally as many not; and plenty of people exhibit all the characteristics of an addict without becoming one. The most notable conclusion to be reached by extensive research into personality was that alcoholic men were slightly more likely to have an alcoholic father, but at the same time huge numbers of sons of alcoholics didn't develop a drink problem.

There may be trouble ahead

Quite apart from the internal harm that can result from somebody's habitual

Help is at hand

na.org
The international Narcotics Anonymous site, explaining how the organization works and where to find a meeting.

ukna.org
Narcotics Anonymous' UK-specific site; the helpline number is 0845 373 3366.

nicd.us
The National Institute on Chemical Dependency is an American Christian, non-profit agency offering advice, counselling and treatment centres for addicts and those affected by addiction.

familiesanonymous.org
An international organization offering support and information for those affected by the drug or alcohol addiction of others.

overindulging, there is a great deal of collateral damage to be done, as, once under the influence, the likelihood of risky behaviour soars.

Thirty percent of all unplanned pregnancies in the UK in 2009 were conceived when both partners were drunk or stoned, a rise of twenty percent over the previous two years, and around half of all STDs were contracted under similar circumstances, a rise of over fifty percent. In 2011, over seventy percent of all hospital admissions on weekends were drink/drug-related; and the rise of binge-drinking, often combined with drug-taking, exacerbated by extended opening hours and cheap supermarket booze, has made city streets at night a far less safe place to be. According to the Home Office, in the UK, 46 percent of all violent crimes in the UK were alcohol-related, while in 58 percent of all assaults by a stranger, the victim claimed the perpetrator had been drinking.

Perhaps the most worrying figure though is that 44 percent of the victims of violent crime were drunk themselves, a statistic that rose to 65 percent when it was narrowed down to assault by a stranger. So regardless of how mild-mannered and happy a drunk you might be, you stand a much greater chance of getting involved in trouble if you've had a few drinks. Be extra careful out there.

No smoke without harm

Although still more socially acceptable (just) than swigging from a tin of super-strength lager or shooting up, tobacco smoking is the world's number-one dangerous addiction. Currently just over one-third of all adult men in the entire world are hooked on cigarettes. Smoking kills one in ten adults globally – that's one every six seconds – and WHO figures indicate this will rise to one in six by 2030. In the UK, tobacco smoking is recognized as the number one cause of preventable illness, and in 2006 was responsible for 114,000 deaths.

F

Fact: Less than ten percent of men who contract lung cancer survive the disease.

Smoking will:

Lower your sperm count and decrease the frequency and rigidity of your erections.

Vastly increase the likelihood of heart disease, a stroke and high blood pressure.

Cause irreparable damage to your lungs.

Reduce the elasticity of your skin, leading to a prematurely aged appearance.

Increase the amount of LDL cholesterol in your bloodstream.

Make you feel the cold more because it destroys nerve endings just below the skin.

Introduce such toxins as arsenic, cyanide and formaldehyde into your body.

Leave you with much less cash then you might have otherwise.

As well as causing lung cancer, it can lead to cancer of the mouth, throat, kidneys and pancreas.

Be a quitter

It won't be easy to give up cigarettes, but it is far from impossible and will be much more manageable if you take these guidelines on board.

Stop dead
Don't try to phase it out. You'll just be putting off the day you actually stop – if you can cut out cigarettes during the day, you can do so in the evening too.

Stay out of pubs
Drinking and smoking for you will go together like, well, beer and snout, and your resolve will be so much less when you've had a couple of drinks.

Change your habits
Vary your routines to avoid the situations in which you always used to spark up.

Change your friends for the time being at least
Don't hang out with people who smoke as it will be very hard for you a) to ignore how relaxed they appear; b) to think about anything other than smoking; c) not to inhale secondary smoke and remind your body what it's missing; and d) refuse cigarettes offered.

Don't tell people you've given up
That way your not smoking won't come up in the conversation every time you meet them.

Give up when you are relaxed
Not in the run-up to exams or moving house or getting married, or just after a parent has passed away, or at any other high-stress time.

Sort your fridge out
You will start eating/snacking more, so make sure you've got plenty of healthy, non-fattening snacks readily to hand.

Keep fit
You will put on weight when you stop – it's natural because nicotine is an appetite suppressant – so take up running or going to the gym. It will reduce any weight increase and give you something else to think about.

Drink plenty of water
It will help get the residual toxins out of your system.

Treat yourself
Save the money you would normally spend on cigarettes to pay for a big treat (you'll be amazed how quickly it adds up) after a couple of smoke-free months.

Smoking is directly responsible for around 40,000 lung cancer deaths a year in the UK, but it is far more varied a killer than that as the carcinogens in cigarette smoke also cause cancer of the stomach, throat, mouth, kidneys and pancreas. Smokers have a 75 percent higher chance of cardiovascular problems than non-smokers and smoking causes 30,000 deaths by heart attack or stroke each year. Smoking does this by thickening the blood and reducing the amount of oxygen being carried, meaning the heart has to work much harder and the risk of clotting goes up. Also, it will increase the level of LDL cholesterol, which can affect the blood supply to extremities and damage blood vessels in the brain through a condition known as ischaemia.

Then quite apart from the smoke itself damaging your lungs, it creates a condition where they are less likely to look after themselves even when you're not smoking. The persistent introduction of hot smoke to your airways destroys a percentage of the tiny hairs that act as filters to keep out particulates we might breathe in during the day. With them no longer functioning as they should, it is much easier for pollutants to get in and cause serious lung damage including pneumonia, shortness of breath, and a susceptibility to infections.

Then there's what smoking will do for your looks as it activates an enzyme that destroys the protein collagen. As this is what gives your skin its elasticity and allows it to stretch and contract as your face changes expression, keeping it looking plump and healthy, without collagen the skin stretches but doesn't snap back. This leads to wrinkles and folds, and skin will appear flat and parchment-like, with no natural glow. Knowing all of this, it's hard to imagine why anybody ever thought smoking would make you seem cool.

Giving up

Acupuncture

By inserting needles at specific points under the skin, blockages in a person's *chi* (life force

The Smoking World Cup

- China: 67 percent of men are smokers
- Russia: 65 percent
- Turkey: 63 percent
- Philippines: 60 percent
- Japan: 51 percent
- Israel: 47 percent
- France: 38 percent
- Germany: 36 percent
- US: 29 percent
- UK: 23 percent
- Worldwide average: 34 percent

Source: World Health Organization

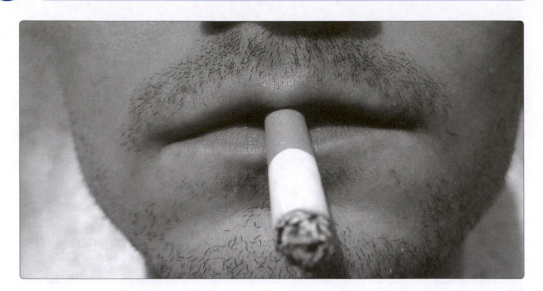

flow) are cleared. It is most commonly used to treat chronic pain, but has a high success rate in helping people overcome addictions.

Hypnotherapy

Once in a trance the subject will be convinced that smoking is not a good idea and one that shouldn't be indulged in again. Often this can trigger unpleasant sensations when smoke is inhaled. Reasonably successful, but there is a high proportion of charlatans out there, so choose a hypnotherapist by personal recommendation or via the National Council for Hypnotherapy (hypnotherapists.org.uk).

Natural help

The following herbs and natural remedies won't make you give up, but they will help enormously to get you through the miseries of coming off a particular dependency.

Smoking	Ginger; cleanses your bloodstream	Cubeb berry; repairs damage done to lung tissue	Kola nut; calms the nerves to help relieve anxiety
Drinking	Evening primrose oil; helps restore balance of essential fatty acid	Turmeric or milk thistle seed; repairs and rebuilds the liver	Valerian root; boosts the nervous system
Cocaine/ amphetamines/ ecstasy	Ginseng; energizes and fights fatigue	Turmeric or milk thistle seed; repairs and rebuilds the liver	Kola nut; calms any feelings of anxiety or paranoia, and provides an energy boost
Heroin	Magnesium; reduces anxiety and keeps you calm	Garlic; removes residual impurities from the blood	Turmeric or milk thistle seed; repairs and rebuilds the liver

Nicotine substitutes

Patches, gum or inhalers are the most common methods, administered in a course of reducing doses designed to wean you away from tobacco. They are not hugely successful, as they merely deal with the nicotine and not the fact that people actually like the whole business of smoking, and thus they don't stimulate any desire to give up.

Willpower

Whatever method you try – including hypnotherapy – you're going to need a fair amount of willpower to get out of the habit of how, where and why you smoke. Or you could do it old school, by willpower and nothing else.

F

Fact: Doctors in the UK are now allowed to write "smoking" on a death certificate as the cause of death.

When you stub that last one out:

Half an hour later
Reduced heart rate and blood pressure.

Eight hours later
The carbon monoxide in your bloodstream has been metabolized and not replaced, normalizing the levels of oxygen in it.

Twenty-four hours later
Your heart is no longer putting itself under added strain as your blood is thinning – odds on having a coronary have already lengthened.

Forty-eight hours later
Damaged nerve endings are regenerating meaning your skin will start to feel more sensitive.

Three days later
Your sense of smell, and therefore your sense of taste improves.

One week later
Your lung capacity will be noticeably improved.

One month later
Your sperm count has risen massively and your skin looks a lot healthier as the collagen is building up once more.

Six weeks later
You get terrible cravings, as the last vestiges of nicotine are leaving your body; it means you've successfully given up.

Three months later
Your circulation and immune system have improved to the degree you will feel much more energized and less susceptible to low-level infections.

Five years later
Your likelihood of heart disease or lung cancer is half what it was when you smoked.

Ten years later
Your system is now more or less the same as somebody who has never smoked.

The best of the web

britishlivertrust.org.uk
A charitable organization, whose site offers everything you need to know about looking after your liver, recognizing signs that something is wrong and seeking help if it is.

thamesvalley.police.uk/UNDERZONE
Aimed specifically at young people, by a particular police force, but full of good advice for everybody everywhere when it comes to keeping safe and on the right side of the law.

ezinearticles.com/?Herbal-Remedies-And-Drug-Addiction
A fascinating and useful collection of writings on addictions, how to break them and appropriate herbal remedies.

smokefree.nhs.uk
The health service's stopping smoking site, offering help, tips, advice and where to find local groups and clinics.

quit.org.uk
A charity set up to help people stop smoking, offering text message support, events, awards, and a telephone hotline: 0800 00 22 00.

bhf.org.uk/smoking
The British Heart Foundation site, offering detailed reasons why you should quit, plus support groups and a hotline: 0800 169 1900.

None of it's good

Although you might not inhale cigar or pipe smoke they're still not safe, as your mouth, throat and larynx will be exposed to smoke with some of it still seeping down to your lungs. Then the sheer scale of the task means one fat stogie or decent-sized pipe can produce as much smoke as a whole packet of cigarettes, meaning even the small percentage of it getting in your lungs is going to be considerable.

Also, this last point means there will be a great deal of smoke in the air around you. Secondary smoking can affect you as much as the people you are with as you will still be breathing it in.

Ten top tips if overindulging

▶ **Drink water alongside your alcoholic drinks** It will go a long way to cutting down on the dehydration that will make you feel miserable the next day.

▶ **Always have a "designated driver"** Even if you all went to town on the bus. You are much more likely to be a victim of violence if you are drunk, so make sure one of your group has their wits about them at all times.

▶ **Don't build your spliffs with tobacco** If you're going to smoke weed at least avoid the addictive qualities and added chemicals of cigarettes.

▶ **Watch that wineglass** Many UK pubs and bars have quietly got rid of 125ml wineglasses and replaced them with 175ml or 250ml glasses, meaning, if it's the latter, you'll have put away a whole bottle when you've only had three glasses.

▶ **Have a couple of nights off every week** This will allow your system to recover and prove you've not got an uncontrollable problem.

▶ **Don't do drugs in unsanitary surroundings** Chopping cocaine out on the cistern cover or the seat of a public toilet will never be the healthiest preparation for a substance you're about to hoover up into your lungs.

▶ **Beware the drunken words "don't worry about a condom"** The UK statistics for drink-related unplanned pregnancies and STDs are alarmingly high.

▶ **Don't tell people you're giving up smoking** It will seem like it's all they'll ever talk to you about.

▶ **Vodka will still give you a hangover** This is because it will still dehydrate you.

▶ **Make sure you know what you are taking** This is not always possible with unregulated illegal drugs, but don't trust strangers in clubs.

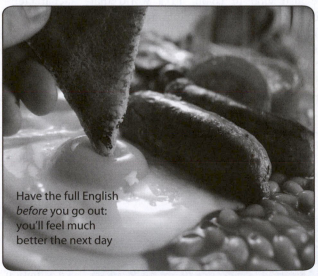

Have the full English *before* you go out: you'll feel much better the next day

In the head (11)

What's going on in your head is probably the most important aspect of your overall health, because it's what's in charge of everything else. However, as modern life increases the pressures on men, this headspace needs some maintenance of its own.

Emotionally speaking

For us human beings, emotions are among the most powerful and primal communication tools in our social toolbox – everybody the whole world over understands a smile and most of the other involuntary facial expressions. Emotions are also vital to colour in a world that would otherwise be horribly grey. If you didn't feel happy when you heard a certain piece of music or sad when your team lost or even jealous when your partner flirted with somebody at a party, our lives would be pretty boring ones.

As they are unconscious reactions and serve to put the rational brain on high alert, they are the first line of defence in awkward or harmful situations. Emotions also provide the glue that holds society together, inasmuch as it is the prompting of emotions in ourselves and others that governs how we behave to each other.

The key to self-awareness

It's through your emotional behaviour that those around you will identify your character – a happy person, a miserable sod, a soppy git, Mr Angry and so on – but, more importantly, it's also how you will define yourself. By being aware of your emotions, you will be provided with irrefutable proof of how you were affected by or behaved in certain situations, which will allow you to define your own personality.

Knowing this, and with your rational mind analysing each incident in its entirety, you will be able to better understand what constitutes acceptable social conduct and how you should behave to achieve it.

This is where it becomes apparent that behaving rationally and behaving emotionally are far from mutually exclusive. Emotions provide an instant, unfiltered assessment of a situation. The rational mind then almost immediately works out how to deal with that situation and files it in the memory for the next time you come up against something like that. It's actually very easy for the memory to store this information,

F

Fact: The cortex is one of the last areas of the brain to physically develop, which is why children and adolescents are far more prone to emotional outbursts than adults.

How it all works: the brain

The brain is made up of about 100 billion brain cells known as neurons, which are divided into about fifty different types, each variety dedicated to a different area of activity – balance, pleasure, speech, hearing, memory and so on. These groups of neurons function as individual units and in concert to coordinate thoughts, moods and actions – a relevant analogy is the sections of an orchestra working as entities within themselves and together to create a symphony.

Neurons process and store information, and transmit it by generating tiny electrical impulses to send a chemical along their tendril-like axons and across the gap (the synapse) to a neighbouring cell. The receiving neuron will absorb the information carried on the chemical. Throughout the brain these connections create intricate "road maps" to allow our thoughts to be so varied and precise, and to instruct the body to carry out physical action. These chemicals are known as neurotransmitters and they increase or alter the electrical signals to dictate brain activity and so control our bodies and minds. They apply to different aspects of the brain and among those discussed in this book are dopamine (emotion, movement, pleasure), serotonin (sleep, temperature regulation, appetite) and glutamate (memory and learning).

There are five main areas of the brain that operate different aspects of how we live our lives, and they are split into the categories of the "lower" and "higher" brain. The lowest of the low is the brainstem in which the body's most basic automatic functions are controlled – eating, breathing, the digestive process, heartbeat and so on. This is the first area of the brain to develop in babies. Next up is the limbic system, prompting impulses, instinctive behaviour and involuntary expression of emotion – actions like smiling, frowning, laughing or cussing. This will be the second area to develop, and the next, the cerebellum, is relatively small but contains around half of the brain's neurons. It is responsible for voluntary movement, balance and coordination. It processes information from the senses and translates it for the nervous system to be able to send signals to whatever parts of the body need to be manoeuvred.

All of the above are essentially instinctive, but the last two parts of the brain, the higher brain, are cognitive. They develop as we mature as adults and are the frontal cortex and the prefrontal cortex. The frontal cortex is where high-level thinking goes on, and an astonishing number of electrical impulses zip about between neurons at fantastic speeds to facilitate thoughts or ideas. These ideas can involve future planning, goal setting, or creativity; they can be abstract, or based on what is being received from the senses, or derived from information already taken in – memories; or they can simply set off voluntary movement of the body. The prefrontal cortex is the brain's executive decision maker. It simultaneously absorbs information from all the senses, the memory and our aims for the future, to make the choices we need. It will make judgements between right and wrong or when to take chances; it also governs our behaviour as social beings and exercises restraint as regards emotions or desires. It is the nearest tangible manifestation of a conscience, and is fundamental to what we call intelligence or character.

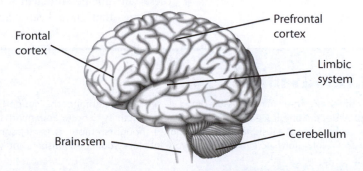

Frontal cortex

Prefrontal cortex

Limbic system

Brainstem

Cerebellum

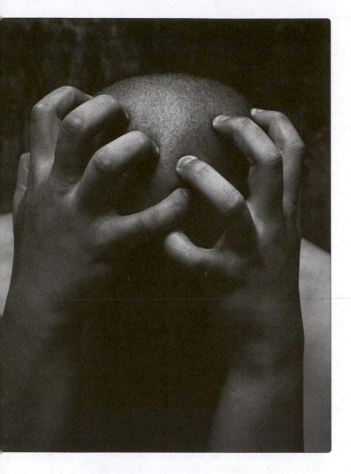

Keeping a lid on it

A certain amount of emotional behaviour is a huge advantage. It can sharpen your instincts and reactions, improve awareness of what is happening and introduce a necessary degree of creative – i.e. illogical – thinking. But giving emotions too free a rein can be just as damaging as totally suppressing them. Inappropriate behaviour, such as laughing during a funeral service or looking disgusted at what is put in front of you at a dinner party, will ultimately land you with few friends, while not being able to control anger or fear can put you at serious risk. Violent behaviour is usually a result of a lack of emotional control, and alcohol suppresses the ability to control emotions, hence the high incidences of late-night city-centre bloodshed.

The control of emotions happens in the secondary circuit of the brain's emotional response unit, in the pathway between the amygdala and the cortex, as the former feeds information to the latter to trigger a rational response. Everybody reacts to emotions in different ways because everybody's cortex will have different capabilities; therefore, the signals it sends out to calm the amygdala will be of varying strengths. In some cases these will not be sufficient to override the emotions that have been triggered. Also,

as emotionally charged situations are always more memorable than bland ones.

Where it can all go wrong, however, is when your conscious mind is either not reacting fast enough or with insufficient influence, and your emotions are getting the better of you on a regular basis.

Brain versus mind

Your brain is the spongy grey mass of tissue, blood vessels and membranes that supports the neurons; it provides the physical environment for electrical activity to occur. Your mind is what is created by that activity as a residual pool of memories, thoughts, emotions, perceptions, imagination and resolve, forming what becomes your intellect, your consciousness and your creativity.

the pathway that sends the signals between the two areas may not be strong enough to handle the signals needed to cope with very powerful emotional responses. However, it is very possible to influence how much you are able to regulate your reactions.

Because the degree to which we control emotions is learned behaviour – from when we are children we are taught, and in turn practise, self-control – this circuitry can be improved upon. The cortex is like any other part of your brain, and will get stronger the more you use it, thus working hard to control your emotions will make it easier the next time, and so on. Having a strengthened cortex will also improve the neurological

pathway between it and the amygdala, as the deeper these routes are worn the more efficiently they will carry signals. It's because emotional self-control quickly becomes habit-forming that it is rare to see people who blow up sometimes – usually they are reliably calm or predictably unpredictable.

Practising yoga and meditation will contribute to you being able to control

F

Fact: The human brain is capable of making some 100 trillion calculations per second.

Keep it real

A proportion of the apparent signs of depression, particularly among younger men in the Western world today, are down to the goalposts having been moved as regards expectations. Dr Sandra Scott believes that the celebrity lifestyles that dominate so many areas of the media have a great deal to answer for.

"Some of the problems regarding the stress and depressive symptoms which so many people are experiencing at the moment is that young people now have such high expectations of how they should be or what they should achieve. We live in a world in which we're surrounded by media telling us what our aspirations should be, that we can all have and should want these very wealthy lifestyles and we can all do anything we like. The media are good at what they do and the messages get through.

Unsurprisingly therefore, many people, again particularly young people, have these huge ideas about who they can be and what they can have. This is fine, up until a point, a realistic point. It is of course important for young people to dream and to want to push themselves to reach their full potential. However there can be a problem when there is a significant gap between the dream and their reality. Surveys repeatedly reveal huge aspirational gaps for today's youth, and not achieving unrealistic dreams can lead to unwarranted feelings of failure which can make people feel that they're not happy, and this is simply because they don't have what they think they ought to have.

Ultimately, if you continually feel that you can achieve these artificially high expectations and then you don't, you can end up with a sense of failure, which is entirely unwarranted. But it's dominant feelings of failure that are associated with depression.

It's as if an artificial pressure has been placed on people, and the first step as far as taking some of the pressure off is to take a good realistic look at what is really achievable for you with your unique set of skills or talents. And not what you just think you should be getting. A lot of people would be a lot happier if they just did that. Being more realistic and grounded will also help you deal or cope with disappointments and knock-backs when they come along – and they always will. It will be easier for you to put them in perspective, to accept that they are as much a part of life as the good stuff and to move on."

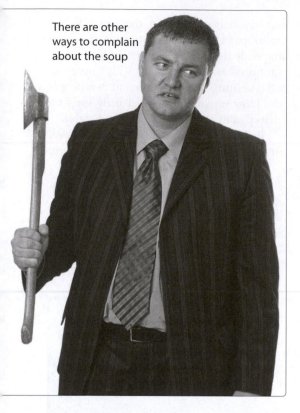

There are other ways to complain about the soup

your emotions in general, as they provide a far better understanding of the mind and how it works in conjunction with the body and its physiological responses. Breathing techniques will also help, as they will put you in a better position to control the changes the emotions are bringing to your body, and so not let them get out of control – the whole notion of taking a deep breath when entering an emotional situation is based on this and entirely valid.

Anger management

Counting to ten when you feel your anger is about to boil over is not only the most convenient diffusion technique, it's also one of the most effective. Primarily, it will divert your attention from whatever has set your anger off for at least ten seconds. This provides an important interval that will give you time to form rational thoughts

as a response to the situation, rather than react purely on emotion. Being able to think may well prove the difference between an impulsive action that may escalate the situation and a considered one that will calm it down.

As you count, take a deep breath on each number – exhaling in between, of course. Not only will this slow your counting down, but it will also relax you and offset the fight-or-flight stress triggers.

Just your imagination

Stress as a tangible condition, with identifiable outside causes, was dealt with in detail in Chapter 6. But equally important is internally produced stress and how it affects you. This can often be harder to handle and have a more serious impact, as there will be little apparent logic to how it can come about, and fewer external sources that can be addressed.

Your own worst enemy

As adults we are all going to worry at some points in our lives. It's an inherent cognitive activity that causes agitation within our

T

Tip: Although it's true that important decisions based purely on emotion will rarely be very good, it's just as correct that if you totally suppress your emotions the human decision-making process becomes seriously impaired, as there will be little room for creativity or flexible thinking.

F

Fact: To a large degree your mind tends to function "in the future". It will be anticipating things that are about to happen rather than reacting to what has already occurred.

brains and is usually related to something that might or might not happen in the future or that has happened in the past. As such, worry is a major precursor to stress and all that goes with it – sleep disorders, gastric problems and headaches. But also, as you'll have noticed from what it is you worry about most, it's more or less irrational – the past cannot be changed and any future we worry about is usually one we have no control over. Unfortunately though, this lack of logic as regards worrying often serves to become a worry in itself, making us feel worse and hugely increasing potential stress levels.

The good news is that we don't have to worry at all, or if we do at least we have control over how much, because worrying is a learned behaviour, not something that is hard-wired into our systems. It is believed that worrying is cultural in the West because from late childhood onwards,

we are subconsciously taught we need to prove we are taking our lives "seriously". The manifestation of this is that those who worry the most somehow have the most gravitas. This is borne out by the fact that the children of carefree parents tend to grow up into pretty chilled-out adults.

Worrying also can be a convenient barricade to hide behind. It can stop you having to make decisions, taking risks, making changes in your life or even doing anything at all. To keep worrying about the component parts of a situation allows you to ignore the big picture, and thus avoid actually advancing things. It can also easily become habit-forming, and as well as triggering stress in your system, it will prevent you from getting the most you can out of your life.

T

Tip: Concentrate on being who you are – trying to keep up with other people simply for the sake of it is one of the most stressful things you can do, as a) you will never be in control of your own destiny; and b) it probably won't be right for you.

Are you insane?

Periods of self-doubt among today's men are increasingly commonplace. This is because of the growing levels of expectations, the constantly changing environment and almost total lack of discernible guidelines. Depression is of growing concern in the twenty-first century, as are thoughts that life is sometimes overwhelming. This isn't madness though, and is relatively easy to treat. It is highly unlikely that you are actually suffering from a mental illness.

If you are worried about such feelings, however, it's always best to address them as early as possible, and you shouldn't feel any stigma about seeking professional help. Your first step should be to consult your GP, who may recommend therapy or even prescription drugs to address whatever is causing you problems. Signs of serious mental illness, such as delusional behaviour, schizophrenia or paranoia, will be very obvious to those around you, and, hopefully, they will have persuaded you to get help – or gone as far as they can to get it for you.

Don't worry, be happy

Having anxieties about major events in your life or a radically changed situation – a job interview, life after death of a spouse, an exam, moving house – is perfectly natural, as you will need to think things through as thoroughly as possible and try and consider every eventuality. Under these circumstances you are merely motivating yourself into analysing whatever it is facing you, which proves you are taking responsibility. Then if they become the trigger to take positive action, what you are doing is entirely healthy.

Problems occur when worrying becomes counterproductive. It settles in almost as a mental defence mechanism and thus can lead to problems with concentration, chronic indecisiveness, low self-confidence and, in severe cases, obsessive behaviour or panic attacks, as well as the physical manifestations of stress. This is known as mild anxiety, and around twelve percent of men in the UK suffer from it. If you recognize any of these symptoms in yourself it will be worth talking to your doctor about how you feel, which in itself will go a long way to stopping you worrying about worrying. There is also a range of self-help techniques:

T

Tip: If you are a worrier, avoid caffeine and alcohol as both will serve to raise anxiety levels.

Alternative approaches

Reflexology, aromatherapy, acupuncture and massage have all been cited as natural remedies for worry and anxiety, and while they might not work for everybody, one of them might be right for you. After all, because worry is all in your mind, if you think a therapy is doing you good it probably is. Yoga and meditation will help you relax, and assist in controlling your emotions, while breathing exercises help keep you calm in stressful situations.

Recommended complementary medicines for anxiety include celery juice, St John's Wort and kola nut, all of which lift the mood. Kava-kava root suppresses the nervous system to lessen feelings of anxiety – not unlike alcohol except not addictive; and ginkgo and vitamin B complex can sharpen brain activity to make decision-taking less of an overwhelming proposition.

There are also a number of herbal supplements you can take that may relieve conditions that can contribute to your low mood – don't forget, what might seem like depression may be due to an easily treatable set of symptoms. How you feel might be a result of hormonal imbalance, low blood sugar or simply not getting enough sunlight. A general lack of vitamins will contribute to a general mood-lowering, particularly the B vitamins as they are needed to efficiently metabolize the fats that will keep your brain and nervous system in tiptop condition. Omega-3 fatty acids will be vital for the same reason, as your brain is over fifty percent fats. Wholefoods containing complex carbohydrates will help regulate your blood sugar, and swapping to them from sugary food will revitalize you by giving you a much more even energy supply.

Getting out in the sunlight genuinely does lift a mood. It suppresses the production of melatonin in the pineal gland, which, as the hormone most associated with sleep, can lead to feelings of physical and mental lethargy if levels of it are high during the day. Excess melatonin secretions during the day will also cause the night's production to suffer and sleep will be disrupted. It is believed that sunlight boosts the brain's production of melatonin-inhibiting serotonin, and levels can also be raised by taking a herbal supplement called 5-hydroxy tryptophan. Likewise, the herb rhodiola will help the brain utilize serotonin and thus lift your mood.

Chill out (dude)

Telling people not to worry sounds almost as trite and as irritatingly pointless as telling them to "Cheer up, it might never happen!" However, in order to reduce your levels of self-generated stress, it helps to remind yourself of the futility of fretting about the following:

Yesterday
What is in the past has already happened and therefore cannot be changed. Worrying about it will not alter this fact, so concentrate on minimizing any prospective fallout or subsequent events.

Things you cannot control
The only excuse you have for worrying about the outcome of, say, a football match or board meeting would be if you were playing in it or sitting at it and, therefore, able to directly influence it.

Situations you have already made your contribution to
You've been for the job interview, sat the exam, put the bid in, or made the pitch: now forget about it. Remain secure in the fact you've done the absolute best you can and let the previous point come into play.

Stuff that has no immediate effect or purpose in your life
Although as good, humanitarian people it is natural to worry about things that are removed from our lives, sometimes it's stress we could really do without. Know where to draw a line as to feeling compassion for far-flung suffering.

Keep a diary

Writing down how you feel about various aspects of situations will allow you to more easily identify your own habits and so be careful of allowing them to apply to future events. Also, it will force you to analyse your reactions to things as they are occurring in fine detail and so reach a better understanding of what you need to address.

Talk about things

But only to people you are sure you a) trust; and b) respect the judgement of, as you do not want the additional worries of who they might tell or how they might spin your problems; also you need to be able to accept their opinions. Don't forget that the purpose of these discussions is your anxieties, so you need to be talking about your reaction to situations rather than the situations themselves – you are looking for

B

Best investment: ginkgo biloba

This plant that has been cultivated in China for thousands of years, and is starting to become recognized by conventional medicine as being an effective remedy for lethargy or low moods. It is taken as tablets made out of the extract from the leaves and improves blood circulation in even the smallest capillaries, meaning it increases blood flow to the brain and so aids memory and sharpens concentration.

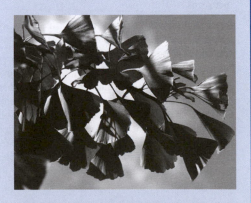

Tip: Going for a run or doing physical exercise that requires very little conscious thought can help you think clearly as it allows more connective pathways to be formed in the brain for creative thinking.

help with your worrying rather than career/marriage/whatever advice.

Don't talk about things

This might seem like perverse advice: you shouldn't bottle things up of course. But to talk to all and sundry means you will end up with too many conflicting opinions, which is even less help than none at all. Be just as careful about seeking advice purely from people you know will agree with you too. While this may temporarily boost your confidence, that will soon disappear and leave you equally anxious as you will have moved no further forward.

Confront your demons

Do it simply, in a way that gradually introduces you to this new, decisive you. Identify worries you have over seemingly less-than-crucial occurrences – will your team win, how many golf balls will you lose this afternoon, why didn't that woman on the train smile at you yesterday – take a deep breath and shrug them off. Start by willing yourself to go into situations like that without a care and it will spill into other, more important areas of your life.

Tip: When problem-solving, don't start from the obstacle and attempt to work forwards; think of the prospective goal and then work backwards.

Psychologists, psychiatrists & psychotherapy

Both psychologists and psychiatrists treat people with mental problems, and both treat problems that vary in seriousness from occasional anxiety attacks to full-blown schizophrenia, but surprisingly few people can differentiate between the two. The distinction between the professions is all in the suffix: "…iatry" means it is a branch of medicine, while an "…ology" is a science. Thus psychiatry will be the treatment of the mind – the psyche – and its disorders from a medical perspective, while psychology is the study of all aspects of it, not necessarily just the problems.

A psychiatrist will have gone to medical school and will have qualified as a doctor of medicine before specializing in psychiatry. A psychologist will have completed several years of academic training and their doctorate will be a PhD.

Clinical psychologists are those that treat people with mental disorders, but most psychologists doing practical work specialize in a field such as sports or education or occupation, and concentrate on improving performances. The largest proportion of those qualified in psychology work in research into the human mind and behaviour. Because of its medical background, the vast majority of mental problems will be managed by psychiatry, either with prescribed drugs – psychologists cannot prescribe as they have no medical credentials – or psychotherapy. This is the "talking therapy", in which behavioural problems, bad habits, fears, relationship or emotional issues and stress are overcome by talking through the patient's history to uncover and address the root causes of problems.

The man with a plan

Having clear long-term and short-term plans will always be preferable to drifting aimlessly through life, because knowing what you are going to do puts you in control. It is this being in control that is the key, but you have to be in control of your plan as well, which means it will have to be as fluid as your circumstances. Too often people vastly increase their stress levels and end up achieving far less than they set out to by bending their lives to accommodate a rigid plan.

When to bring in the professionals

If you have tried self-help, or applying the chill out checklist (see p.241) to individual situations and have made such lifestyle changes as eating healthily, exercising and getting plenty of sleep – all of which serve to make you feel less anxious in general – yet feel worry is still inhibiting your life, you should get help.

The first place to go is your family doctor. There is a chance they may prescribe tranquillizers or antidepressants, but in the first instance they are more likely to advise you to take up some form of talking therapy. This will probably take one of three forms: cognitive behavioural therapy, which examines the way you think and will look to alter it to confront and conquer your anxieties; counselling to assist your decision-making process so it is no longer overwhelmed; and psychodynamic psychotherapy, which delves into the psyche to uncover and confront whatever is at the root of your behaviour – it is like a milder version of psychoanalysis. In any of these events you may be referred back to your doctor for a prescription to alleviate your symptoms.

The most important thing to remember about mild anxiety is that it can be addressed, whether it is the result of a mental illness or not, and sufferers shouldn't be shy to talk to their doctor.

Perfection is overrated

This has been said elsewhere in this book, but it is particularly relevant here, as so much of the stress we put ourselves under when carrying out tasks at home or at work comes from what we tell ourselves is a search for perfection. Too often we are far harder on ourselves than we would be on anybody else, but while there is nothing wrong with setting

Five ways to fend off worry

1. Don't get overtired: it's much easier to get irrational about things if you're exhausted.

2. Stay busy: the more time you have on your hands, the more likely you are to think up things to worry about, and if you are actually contributing to something you'll worry about it less because you have a degree of control.

3. Learn to delegate: in spite of the previous point don't take on too much as you may feel overwhelmed, which will add to your anxiety levels, and you won't have time to assess situations properly.

4. Be enthusiastic: in all areas of your life, as it's a great deal harder to worry about something if you're excited about where it could be going.

5. Relax: beating yourself up about worrying too much creates a vicious circle that doesn't take long to bring on real stress.

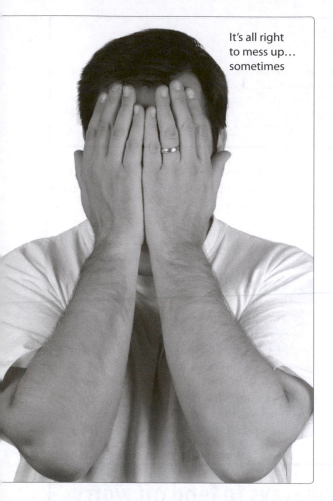

It's all right to mess up... sometimes

effort/reward ratio, but can also do you a great deal of damage. Not being able to leave something because you are perpetually dissatisfied with it is an incredibly stressful experience, as it means there is no closure and it will always be on your mind.

The chances are it will have a negative effect on those around you too. Quite the opposite from your so-called perfectionism bringing admiration or even appreciation from colleagues, there is a much greater chance it will irritate them enormously. You will probably be holding others up while you mess about with whatever it is, then at best they will think you are indecisive and at worst anally retentive. Either way it is unlikely to increase your chances of promotion.

Doing yourself more harm than good

The fundamental problem with endless tinkering is it says more about how you relate to what you have already done than it does about what you are trying to achieve, and your obvious dissatisfaction speaks of a lack of confidence. The chances are that these fine-tunings will not make or break the final result, if indeed anybody else notices, and a task that was finished earlier would still gain the same acceptance or acclaim. It will also do wonders for your confidence when this happens, as it will make you aware that you are intrinsically

our internal bars high, this can easily become counterproductive as it means we're either seldom satisfied with anything we achieve or are unable to finish a project.

Although doing a sloppy job will benefit nobody, least of all yourself, striving to achieve perfection – that is, perfection as you see it – not only seldom brings a worthwhile

Pick your battles

There are things worth getting stressed about, where the fight-or-flight syndrome will probably give you an edge, but there is also a huge amount of stuff that isn't worth worrying about. Be selective about what you are going to be bothered about, and make sure you don't expend mental energy on anything that doesn't merit it or will be taken care of anyway.

Are you paranoid?

Probably not, although if you are smoking massive amounts of weed or maintaining a serious cocaine habit then you're probably well on your way.

In psychiatric terminology, paranoia describes the condition in which somebody has delusions about being victimized by an individual or group intent on doing him harm; delusions of harm actually being inflicted on him by an individual, a group, a disease or a parasite; the belief that a person's actions are actually being controlled by a force greater than oneself; or that that person is an emissary for a higher, otherworldly power. An irrational fear of something such as water, flying or spiders or public speaking is a phobia rather than paranoia.

Although the term is commonly used to describe anybody with apparently exaggerated concerns about people around them – fellow board members, the police, your mother-in-law – doing them harm, it has applications in and outside of psychiatry. They all involve delusions of some sort, and need not be restricted to fear of harm: erotomania, for example, is the paranoid delusion that the sufferer has somebody sexually obsessed with them.

better at what you are doing than you might realize.

There's also the purely pragmatic aspect, inasmuch as fiddling and fiddling with something because you are not wholly satisfied with it will always come to a point, probably sooner than you think, at which

T

Tip: Don't always do the best job you can. Instead do the best job you can before six o'clock – it's important to have a life outside of work for no other reason than to be able to put your work in the context in which it will be received.

physical and mental fatigue means it starts to become self-defeating. Also, you will always find something else to change or fine-tune, so unless you're a mathematician, there will never be an automatic cut-off point.

Depression: a twenty-first-century condition

There are over 1.5 million men in the UK suffering from depression, and as many as ten percent admit to extended periods of feeling down. In the past these men were more likely to be older, as retirement, loss of partners, poor health and daily life becoming progressively more difficult contributed to

Brainstorming works

As the first stage of any problem-solving exercise, throwing out ideas, good and bad, with little or no restraint, has been proved to be one of the most successful methods of coming up with innovative or effective solutions. Brainstorming stimulates brain activity and encourages lateral thinking, and doesn't have to be carried out in a group. Individual brainstorming is equally valuable – just make sure you write down those ideas as soon as they pop into your head.

feelings of loneliness or frustration. These days, though, growing numbers of young men, from adolescents upwards, are being diagnosed with depression as modern life brings increased expectations and pressures.

There is, however, a world of difference between going through a bit of a bad patch and full-blown depression.

What is depression?

Chemical depression accounts for the vast majority of cases of depression. It occurs when the brain does not produce enough of the hormones which lift the mood – serotonin and norepinephrine – and because they work on the nervous system it can trigger any of the symptoms of depression (see box below) in any combination. It then quickly becomes a downward spiral of constantly bleak moods, and because the symptoms will make the sufferer feel worse, even the subconscious notion that it might be depression furthers the cycle.

Those suffering from chemical depression are far more susceptible to bad

The symptoms of depression

Perpetual feelings of sadness or emptiness
You will find very little pleasure in many of the things you used to enjoy, and will notice what is wrong with a situation before you spot the advantages or good points.

Feelings of hopelessness or worthlessness
A pessimistic mood affects your approach to just about everything in life – friends, family, work and so on. You will feel it is better to do nothing about things rather than face the inevitable disappointment of it going wrong.

Inability to concentrate or make decisions
This is linked to the above, as at the back of your mind you are thinking "What's the point?", and therefore not really putting any mental effort into anything. You will also find it difficult to remember details.

Irritability
Because, somewhere deep in your brain, your pre-depressed self knows this state of affairs isn't right, you are continually dissatisfied with how you are feeling and functioning. You just want to be left alone most of the time.

Disrupted sleep patterns
Depressives either can't sleep or sleep fitfully through anxiety, or they oversleep, thinking there is little worth getting up for – this is more common among younger men. Both symptoms contribute to the general fatigue that accompanies depression.

Eating disorders
Weight gain or loss may be noticeable as it's not unusual for a depressive to lose interest in food or to eat too much out of habit or restlessness.

Loss of energy and susceptibility to infection
Your whole system will be functioning well below its best, and therefore it won't be making full use of nutrients being absorbed even if you are eating properly, thereby compromising your metabolism and your immune system.

Thoughts of suicide
The two positive notes here are that it is only the severely depressed that think this way, and far fewer act on it than don't – according to Mental Health America less than fifteen percent of the severely depressed commit suicide, yet over seventy percent admit to thinking about it.

reactions to upsetting occurrences in their lives, but a traumatic event such as the death of a family member or a long-lasting stressful situation can set depression off in those with no hormonal imbalance. This is psychological depression, and more likely to be a temporary situation that is best treated with a talking therapy.

The term "clinical depression" refers to either sort of depression that is serious enough to be sustained and affect every aspect of your day-to-day life. It is not something that clears up in a few days.

What can you do about it?

If you feel you are suffering from any sort of lengthy depressive episode, i.e. you are showing the symptoms listed on p.220, you should seek professional help. Start at your doctor's surgery, where you will be given an initial diagnosis. That will determine what, if any, further action you should take – you may find it helps a huge amount just to talk to somebody about how you feel.

The prescribing of antidepressant drugs is a common option. These can become

B

Best investment: oily fish

Once again your mum knew what she was talking about when she told you to eat your fish because it would make you smarter: a good supply of omega-3 fatty acids is vital to maintain the brain cells' outer membranes and so assist nerve signals, memory and the ability to learn. Beyond that, though, whole grains, pulses, liver, poultry and eggs help

the mind to function, as the B vitamins – particularly 1, 3, 6 and 12 – aid the nervous system and mental performance, and work to stabilize emotions. The amino acids found in high-protein foods such as dairy, meat and fish help build neurotransmitters, and carbohydrates aid the absorption of tryptophan, which contributes to the brain's serotonin production.

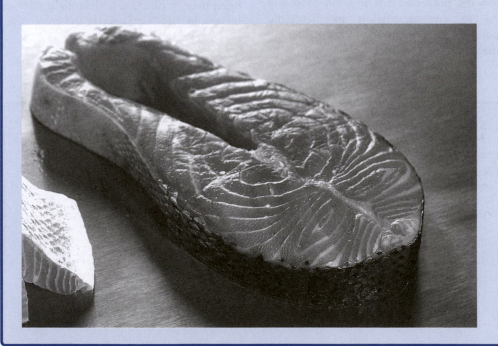

addictive, but they work to lift the internal mood, which will either become an end in itself or make the sufferer far more open to talking therapies. The majority of treatment for depression is a combination of drugs and talking therapies, but for anything to have the best chance of working you have to initiate it as soon as possible.

There are also a number of things you can do yourself, which will help alongside any medical treatment or will work to lift your mood if you are merely feeling down.

Stop drinking or taking drugs

Although alcohol may make you livelier in the pub, it's a depressant as it reduces your levels of serotonin so ultimately lowers your mood. The aftereffects of many recreational drugs will leave you feeling less positive than you were before you got high.

Eat right

Avoid refined sugars and binge eating, as these will send your blood sugar levels into wild fluctuation, and the crashes can have a seriously detrimental effect on your mood. Also the processed fats in junk food will add to any depression by depleting your body's stores of the mood-lightening vitamins B and C.

F

Fact: As well as the risk of suicide, depressives have a higher mortality rate, as their physical health and immune systems suffer due to disinterest in their own well-being.

Get some exercise

Walking or running or working out will help your system function properly, which will improve your health and will release endorphins, the "feel good hormone". Exercise helps you sleep better too, while from a psychological point of view, you'll have improved self-confidence and feelings of self-worth as you will look better and feel more vitalized.

Get some sun

If you can do that exercise outdoors it will be doubly beneficial: oxygenating your brain helps it function and sunlight releases melatonin, which makes you feel more alive.

Understanding antidepressants

Prescription antidepressants are contentious. Debate over prolonged use of them rages on: largely centred upon whether they are a cause of long-term damage. However, other discussions revolve around the relative effectiveness of treatments involving talking therapies that are popular in the UK, concerns about over-prescribing in general and the range of alternative treatments on offer. Drug therapy is still widespread, of course, and in around eighty percent of cases it is successful at rebalancing hormones and chemicals within the body to relieve feelings of depression. The two main types of antidepressant being prescribed are:

Selective serotonin reuptake inhibitors (SSRIs): the most widely used antidepressant, this has very few side effects and works by increasing the levels of serotonin in the brain. Prozac is an SSRI.

Serotonin-norepinephrine reuptake inhibitors (SNRIs): very similar to SSRIs, but as norepinephrine increases the heart rate and triggers glucose release within the muscles, it acts as a stimulant, and therefore is not good for those with insomnia.

Are you depressed?

Once again, probably not. The chances are you are experiencing a temporary depressed mood, rather than any sort of clinical disorder, and it will be the result of an external event or situation making you feel sad or miserable. When that changes or, with time, you come to terms with it, the chances are your mood will lift.

Have a laugh

Read a book or watch a film that you know will be funny, as not only will it serve as a handy distraction, but laughter reduces the levels of the stress hormones cortisol and adrenaline – the idea of laughter therapy as a bona fide treatment is currently gaining ground.

Don't suffer in silence

Nearly three-quarters of all adults suffering from depression are not getting treatment, a figure that is much higher for men than women, in spite of more women suffering from depression than men.

Dr Sandra Scott explains why this is and what should be done about it:

"Get help if you need help: if you really believe you've got something seriously wrong with you. One of the reasons we believe the rates of depression are lower for men than women is that many men are reluctant to talk about emotional problems, so their difficulties can go unnoticed by those who can help them. Sometimes it may be going against everything you believe in, but if you are unhappy and have been for some time and cannot shift it by yourself, then get help.

There is still a huge feeling among many men that it's not really appropriate to seek that sort of emotional help. Thus if they go to a GP they are much more likely to talk about the physical symptoms of depression rather than the psychological ones. They also

Talking about it

As you'd probably expect, talking therapies involve exactly that – talking. But talking to somebody who is trained in listening to people with anxieties or troubles, then helping them find the answers within themselves. These listeners could be psychiatrists, psychologists or counsellors, and there are a number of different talking therapies, but what they have in common is a much lower relapse rate than medication.

The main reason why talking therapies are more successful is because they do not simply treat the symptoms and chemically engineer a change of mood, but as the sessions progress will work on the cause of the depression. Some will seek to change patterns of behaviour, others will establish the root cause of your unhappiness and help you to confront and deal with it, and others will simply allow you to talk about stuff to somebody who will listen without judging and then support you as you look for a solution to whatever is troubling you.

Even if you're not depressed and are maybe just having a rough time in your life – jobwise, in your marriage, with your sexuality – just being able to talk honestly and openly with somebody can be a huge help.

Britain's Department of Health offers a comprehensive downloadable brochure on talking therapies that is equally relevant on either side of the Atlantic. Visit: dh.gov.uk/en/publicationsandstatistics.

The best of the web

bacp.co.uk
The British Association for Counselling and Psychotherapy offers a range of services that include finding an accredited psychotherapist, information about counselling and what you should expect from therapy.

nmha.org
Mental Health America (formerly the National Mental Health Association) offers information about care, medication and legal issues, plus a series of downloadable factsheets and easily understood answers to FAQs.

mentalhealth.org.uk
A charity that provides information about mental health, conducts research and campaigns to improve public services and spending in that area. The site features an A–Z of Mental Health, which explains just about any condition or term.

rcpsych.ac.uk
The Royal College of Psychiatrists offers a vast range of well-researched, up-to-date and readable information on mental health and its treatment, including ten downloadable leaflets on frequently enquired about subjects.

cmha.ca
The Canadian Mental Health Association offers a wide range of advice and information about all aspects of mental health, also a series of DIY tests designed to assess your state of mind.

mhfederation.org
The Mental Health, Addiction and Retardation Organizations of America raises money for the US's mental health charities and organizations, but also offers a vast range of help and information.

mind.org.uk
The UK's leading mental health charity, which works to ensure those with mental health problems are looked after properly and treated with equality and dignity.

can present things differently from women – they are more likely to try to hide sadness and present with aggression and frustration. Young men tend to deal with their symptoms differently – for example, by increases in reckless behaviour such as taking drugs and alcohol abuse, and their depression can go unrecognized or be labelled as something else.

It may be that you will be more comfortable going online at first to try to look up the symptoms of what you are feeling and to get more information about your condition. This is a very good first step, because if you don't understand what your issues are it is much harder to speak about them even if you want to – at least as articulately as you may need to in order to ensure you are understood.

Write things down too. Sometimes putting it down on paper or typing it onto a laptop simply helps you take it seriously, which may spur you on to do something about it. Also, it will help you accurately capture what you really feel, and what it felt like at the time. Because sometimes when you're caught up in whatever moment it was, when you come to recall it, you can actually have forgotten just how bad things were, or the important details, such as what triggered your downward spiral in the first place.

The most important thing is for men to realize that it's okay to ask for help, that depression is a biological illness, and that there are all sorts of ways they can get help. Clinical depression involves a chemical imbalance. If you had diabetes – another

Ten top tips for the best mental health

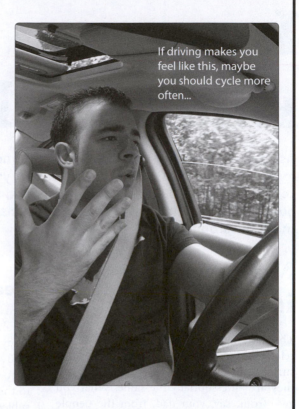

If driving makes you feel like this, maybe you should cycle more often...

▶ **Talk to somebody** Do so as soon as you feel you are becoming overwhelmed or that you might be becoming depressed. The earlier you get help the more effective it will be.

▶ **Eat plenty of fish** The omega-3 oils in such fish as salmon or mackerel will nourish your brain, which is over fifty percent fat.

▶ **Be aware of your emotions** Notice how they are making you behave, then practise keeping them under control – some emotional input is healthy, too much can be dangerous.

▶ **Get out more** Sunlight triggers the release of melatonin, which boosts feelings of well-being.

▶ **Know when to stop** Don't carry on with a project or a job imagining you are a perfectionist and everything has to be exactly right.

▶ **Find out your family history** Depression can be hereditary, and so you will be more susceptible to it if your father or grandfather suffered from it.

▶ **You probably aren't going mad** But it is very healthy to wonder about it from time to time.

▶ **Counting to ten really works** If you feel yourself starting to lose it, start counting and take deep breaths as you do so.

▶ **Don't drink if you feel depressed** It will only make you feel more so.

illness caused by a chemical imbalance – you'd obviously have it treated by a medical professional. Depression is no different."

In a relationship ⑫

As human beings we are social animals, and throughout your life you will form a series of relationships, which will let you know you are part of a larger community, that you are accepted, cared for, trusted and liked. All of which is hugely important in a man's measure of himself and how he is progressing in the world around him.

No man is an island

The remarkable thing about all the different relationships you have is that, while on the surface they may all be wildly different, they are all essentially the same. What you get from, say, your dad, from the people who work with you or from someone you fancy will (hopefully) be hugely varied. Yet each relationship will stand or fall on things such as consideration, mutual respect, a degree of tolerance, unselfishness and the ability to be able to trust within it. These lie at the base of every tangible reward that may result from a relationship; they form the foundation for whatever longevity it might assume.

But it is crucial they be balanced on both sides. So be prepared to learn to communicate. It's not something all men do naturally, but it will be the difference between relationships working or not; approach being communicative like learning any other skill. Consciously build on your experiences and don't dismiss anything as something that should happen by itself or not at all.

Keep your friends close

Men and women who have friends they are in regular communication with live longer and enjoy better mental and physical health. One study carried out by the Harvard Medical School likened the effects of not having friends to the dangers of obesity or smoking, as the subjects with no or few friends had higher cholesterol levels, less-efficient immune systems and greater rates of chronic stress. The study concluded that having people to share situations, ideas and circumstances with were happier, had a higher sense of self-esteem and were more likely to look after themselves. This reduced the likelihood of stress, which in turn lowered blood pressure, heart rates and cholesterol levels. It also lessened the likelihood of risky behaviour – to the degree that those with friends even drove more carefully.

Meeting new people is the gateway to new friendships. But while it might follow that the more people you meet, the more friendships you are likely to form and the greater support structure you are likely to enjoy, friendships are about quality rather than quantity, and a few good friends will be much more valuable than dozens of acquaintances.

How it all works: the perfect relationship

Respect works both ways

Treat others in relationships in exactly the same way as you want them to treat you – this applies to work, marriage, friendship, team-mates, or anything at all. If you treat others carelessly, then you have no right to complain if you are being given a hard time.

Take a hit for the team

What's worth more, your pride or your relationship? Sometimes it will be for the greater good to just live with something you might not be overly happy about – a healthy relationship will never be about winning.

Be honest

Don't bend the truth to try to get your own way as you'll either have to live that lie forever, or it will catch up with you and bite you on the arse.

Wrap things up

Look for closure in any dispute. If you let feuds or fights fester they will never "just go away". In a relationship, try not to go to sleep on an argument.

Give as much as you expect to take

If you are going to bend your friends' ears with your problems and get a considered, caring response, then be prepared to spend as much time playing agony uncle to them; likewise take your partner's problems as seriously as she or he takes yours.

Don't give up

Just because a relationship has got a little tricky there's no need to walk away from it. Always look to sort things out before you consider dumping somebody.

There is nothing you can't talk about

If you are keeping secrets then it is not a relationship founded on mutual trust, which means it will be doomed from the start. This isn't quite the same as the "Be honest" point: it's more serious.

Know when to call it a day

Trying to start again won't always work. Sometimes it'll be best for all concerned if you bring an unfulfilling relationship to an end.

Listen up

A dialogue is a two-way street, so if you are just using the periods when the other person is talking to think up what you are going to say next, your reactions won't have anything to do with their point of view.

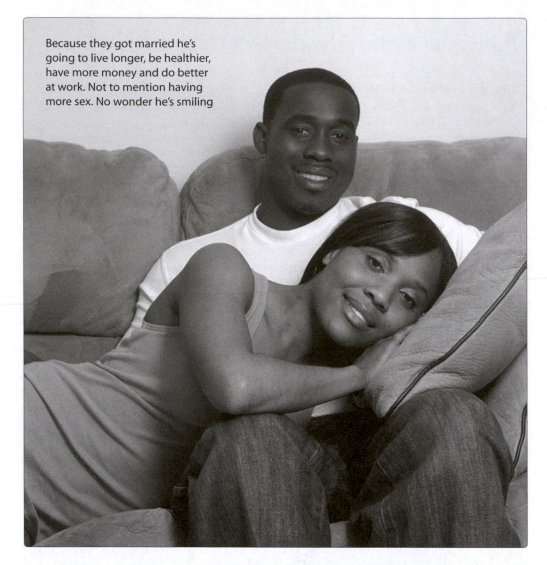

Because they got married he's going to live longer, be healthier, have more money and do better at work. Not to mention having more sex. No wonder he's smiling

Friends can lend a sympathetic ear when times are bad; they are also the people with whom you can enjoy sharing your successes. They will boost your confidence and provide moral support or physical back-up when you need it, and, perhaps most importantly, will not be slow in letting you know if you are acting like a jerk. And you will trust their judgements as much as you expect them to trust yours.

The coupling conundrum

The human race is genetically engineered to keep going. To ensure the best chance of survival, at some point most of us are going to form some sort of meaningful personal relationship, with a view to it lasting a long time. Because this is so fundamental to who we are, these relationships can bring the most joy and fulfilment to our lives. They can also cause enormous problems.

Step away from the lingerie department!

According to Sarah Hedley, the worst thing you can buy your wife or girlfriend is underwear.

"Don't buy her underwear. Imagine what it looks like from the other side – 'I bought you this underwear, now can we have sex? Oh yes, and can you put it on first?' You need to be a bit more sophisticated than that.

Don't buy her shoes either. Regardless of whether she likes the shoes or not, there will be a whole experience attached to shopping for them that you will just have stolen from her. Take her to lunch, go shopping with her for that pair of shoes, and she'll get the whole experience without having to foot the bill."

But remember that perfection is overrated. If you want to find that life partner before both of you are dead then let go of your checklist of what they need to be. Learn to see past their "flaws" – just as you'll hope they will accept yours.

Why get married?

For the last 40 years men have been getting married older. In 1972 the average age of a UK bridegroom was nearly 25; in 2009 it was just under 32. But, despite this fact, there is little in life that offers as much obvious benefit to a man as getting married (or being in a committed long-term union) – if the demographic research is to be believed. Married men live longer than their single counterparts; they are likely to earn more, be promoted at work earlier and receive more positive assessments; get ill less frequently; have more sex; suffer less depression and have far fewer problems with drink or drug addictions; manage their money better; suffer fewer stress-related complaints; and are nearly twice as likely as single men to say they are happy with their lives.

Incidentally, many similar things are statistically true of married women – the only negative point being reported is that married women tend to do more housework. However, even this can be ascribed more to having children than having a husband.

That said, if you think you aren't ready to settle down just yet, you probably aren't. Letting circumstances or other people try and convince you otherwise is never a good idea.

B

Best investment: a bunch of flowers

Flowers work. Practically everybody loves getting a bunch of flowers – men and women. And after they've been given, they'll cheer up a room to such a degree that everybody who comes into it will smile. Also, next time you buy a bunch for somebody check out the looks you're getting from women as you walk along carrying them.

Not just a knees-up

The reason why those in formal unions do so much better in general is because they satisfy us on both a deep-seated intuitive level and a practical one – both of which are pretty straightforward.

As we get older, we invest more in our friendships and so expect more in return. Thus loyalty, reliability, stability and so on, play as much of a part as the more immediate reasons to hang out with somebody. It's relevant that friendships made among older people tend to last longer, with a greater degree of trust involved. A good marriage satisfies so much of this innate need for dependable company, to leave us feeling fulfilled on a deep subconscious level. It's why the proportion of married men who claim to be happy with their lives is nearly twice what it is for single men, and why a married man's mental health is considerably better. This feeling of well-being is something they take with them into other aspects of their lives, notably the workplace, where it contributes to their greater success levels.

Of course, it also satisfies the "propagation of the species" aspect. Psychologically, this commitment to settling down with a permanent partner represents the successful negotiation of some sort of "growing up" watershed, and then becomes a precursor to having children.

A

Expert advice: "Massage is one of the best things you can do in a relationship – I know it's a cliché, but the reason it's a cliché is because it's true. With so many men, it's a bit of a foreplay tactic, with them just using it to try to get in some woman's pants. But if you appreciate it for what it is, as a way of helping your partner de-stress and having physical closeness of a non-sexual nature, then it really comes into its own. Massage classes for couples are really booming, because it gives people another way to be physical: I don't feel like sex tonight, but how about a massage?"
Sarah Hedley

On a far more prosaic level, sharing your life with somebody who cares about you as much as you care about them means you look after each other as a matter of course. And look out for each other – people in long-term relationships are much less likely to be victims of crime than single people. According to the surveys, married men have lower blood pressure and cholesterol levels. Much of this improved health is down to the "nag factor" of being married. In the nicest possible way, someone with a long-term partner is more likely to be prodded into watching their weight, getting their blood pressure and cholesterol checked, going to the dentist, getting that bad back looked at and so on.

Then, if they do get ill, it's far more likely to be dealt with at the early stages. All of which contributes as much to the low sick-day count as the frequent and scathing accusations of being a "bloody hypochondriac" with "man flu". It's so much harder for married men to shirk their responsibilities if they are hungover, no matter how truly awful they might feel.

In fact, it's also much less likely they're going to be hungover. Most men's rates of risky behaviour drop significantly once they tie the knot, simply because, according to surveys, they believe that "isn't what life's all about any more". They feel part of something bigger, and while most won't – and shouldn't – completely give up going on the lash, most simply won't want to nearly so much.

More than simply a piece of paper

The number of couples cohabiting before getting married has massively increased over the last sixty years: over half of married couples in the UK and US lived together first. Yet, interestingly, those couples that did are much more likely to eventually get divorced than those that didn't. It rather flies in the face of the modern belief that getting to know one another properly before tying the knot will build a stronger union.

A cynic might say that pre-marital cohabiting signifies an underlying selfishness on both sides – neither party is prepared to fully commit, creating an "if you pass this audition then maybe I'll marry you" state of affairs. Often there might be calculated pragmatic reasons for living together – it's cheaper, you get regular sex and you have somebody to talk to after a bad day at work – but none of these are exactly indicative of lasting commitment.

It seems as if, regardless of how un-twenty-first-century the institution of marriage may appear, the act of going through a formal wedding ceremony in front of your family and friends elevates the level of commitment to a degree that simply moving in together can't. Although, once again, there is no scientific evidence to support this, research has shown that, in spite of being outwardly dedicated to

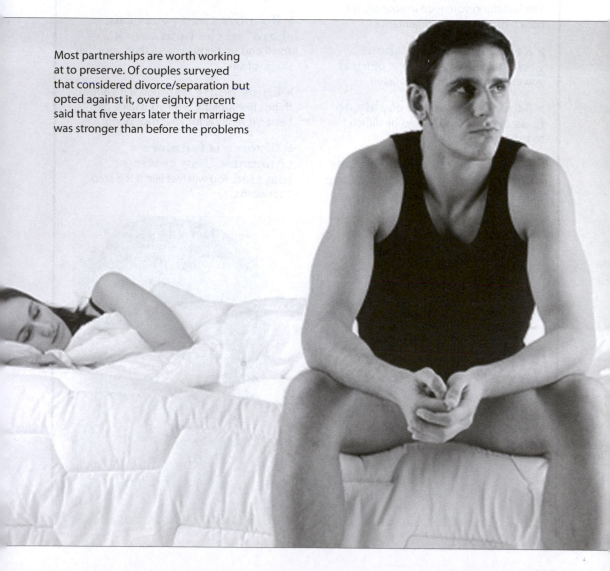

Most partnerships are worth working at to preserve. Of couples surveyed that considered divorce/separation but opted against it, over eighty percent said that five years later their marriage was stronger than before the problems

Ten top tips for good relationships

▶ **Getting married is good for your health** And your wallet. And your career.

▶ **Choose your friends for quality rather than quantity** The last thing you need in your life is a bunch of pointless acquaintances.

▶ **Relationships are about giving and taking** Treat others as you expect to be treated yourself.

▶ **Adulterers will probably do it again** They will always be difficult to trust.

▶ **Don't ever threaten to leave if you've no intention of going through with it** Not only is this wrong on so many levels but one day your partner may call your bluff.

▶ **Try not to tell too many lies** Unless they're little ones and you're doing it for the greater good and not just to save your own skin.

▶ **Relationship counselling works** It's successful in over three-quarters of cases.

▶ **Do more than your "fair share" of the housework** You'll end up getting more than your "fair share" of sex.

▶ **Enjoy being nagged** If it's about things like looking after yourself a bit better, it really is for your own good.

▶ **Divorce is far more traumatic than getting married** You will feel like it is a step backwards.

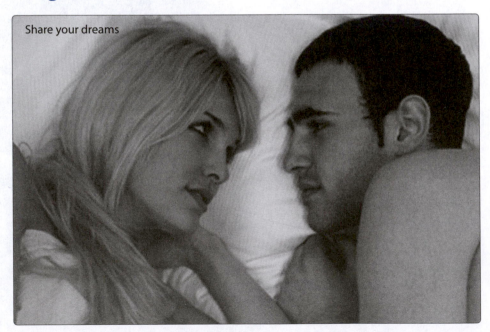

Share your dreams

Battered husbands: the reality

A recent American survey found that 27 percent of adult men had been the victims of domestic abuse, and that men in their twenties and thirties suffered far more than their older counterparts (which could suggest this might be an escalating trend). The health firm that conducted the survey also believed the actual figure was far higher, but that many men were too embarrassed to admit they were bullied.

The definition of abuse in the survey included physical assault (with or without weapons), sex against their will and "non-physical abuse" which covered threats, controlling or manipulating behaviour and persistent disparaging remarks.

the relationship, cohabitees set greater store on their independence. They are less likely to share finances and more likely to be unfaithful – both men and women are apt to carry on behaving like two single people instead of half of a couple.

Should you get counselling?

For many couples, relationship counselling is the absolute last resort. This is because, traditionally, outside help in something as personal as a marriage is seen as unnecessary intrusion. Yet the success rates are very high and over eighty percent of couples in Britain who have received counselling say it put their relationship back on track. Relate, the UK's biggest counselling service, believe this figure would be even higher if couples came to them earlier. Ideally, you should get help the minute you feel you need it, rather than when the sniping begins, otherwise you may both be too defensive to allow a solution to be found.

If you take counselling as an option, you should attend sessions together (although individuals may still find it helpful) and be prepared to tell the full story of your relationship. The counsellor will then help you both understand that story and pick out significant points and habits formed. As a result, the three of you will be able to identify the strengths and weaknesses of the relationship and start to redefine how it can go forward by emphasizing the former and accommodating the latter.

Usually the results of counselling are very straightforward, and the changes a counsellor will suggest should be easy to absorb into your lives. This is because those in the relationship are so often wrapped up in its minutiae they cannot see aspects that are very obvious to outsiders. Also,

Foreplay vs choreplay

Men who do housework get more sex, and not merely as a reward. Sarah Hedley explains:

"We are all very, very time poor at the moment and if you can give your partner back some time then they will have time to feel more free to relax and de-stress, to feel sexy. Because there are only so many hours in the day, if one person is left to take care of the responsibilities of running the house, then that person will run out of time and energy to do anything else. Do the hoovering, or whatever, then there will be more time left at the end of the day for you to be with each other. It's called choreplay, and it really works."

D.I.V.O.R.C.E.

Regardless of how much better it will be for most people to remain married or in a relationship, there will be many for whom getting out of it would be far better for their health. Because the home is traditionally a place of safety, away from the stresses of the world as well as the dangers, the effects of living in a relationship gone bad can be more damaging than having a miserable time at work. It will have a lower profile though, as the resulting senses of shame or failure or disappointment at a marriage going wrong are, for many men, far more difficult to talk about than problems at work.

In cases in which a single unforgivable act, such as infidelity or violence, has caused all vestiges of trust or respect to have disappeared, it will be clear cut. But in other instances, wherein the reasons for the breakdown are less easily identifiable, setting proceedings in motion will be far less straightforward. Because divorce is such a drastic step and rarely one that ends in happiness for both parties, before you reach for m'learned friends, ask yourself these six questions. And make sure you get well-considered, satisfactory answers.

Why do you want to get divorced?	If you are just having a row, then realize that is what it is and that as an isolated incident it can surely be resolved. However, if it's one more manifestation of deep-seated differences that you can no longer live with and you are certain can never be sorted out, that's a whole other matter.
Did you ever truly commit to start off with?	Are you together for the purely practical reasons of servicing the needs of two individuals – mortgage, bills, sex, company? Then you should probably call it a day without making yourselves miserable in the process. But if you're a genuine one-half-complements-the-other couple, think twice.
Are you simply bored?	The chances are your partner is too, therefore, if you sit down together and talk about it, it will be relatively easy to do something about. Be prepared to take a bit of stick though, and you might have to give up your right to the bacon always being on the left-hand side of the eggs.
Is it that the grass seems greener outside of your relationship?	If you're contemplating getting out of your marriage not because there's anything too wrong with it but because what's going on elsewhere seems so much more exciting, be warned – it rarely is. The chances are you will soon get tired of whatever it is you're coveting at the moment. (See previous point.)
Are you threatening divorce just to get your own way?	Ironically, if you have no intention of going through with it then you absolutely should. Any relationship that is being held together with that sort of threat is already finished.
Do you still love your partner?	If you do, then divorce is going to be doubly difficult.

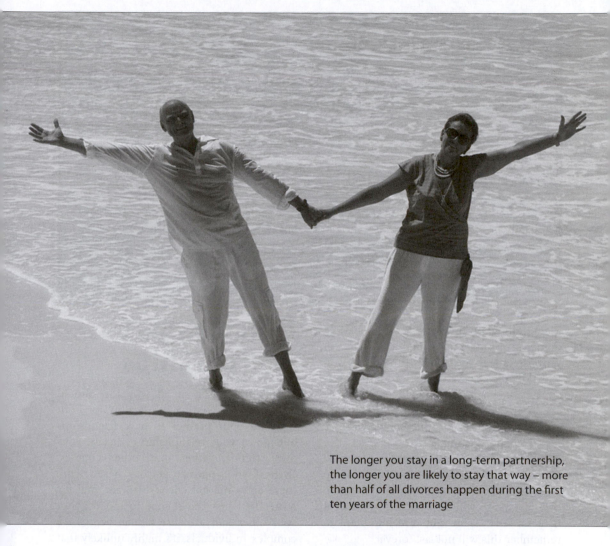

The longer you stay in a long-term partnership, the longer you are likely to stay that way – more than half of all divorces happen during the first ten years of the marriage

the chance for both parties to talk openly to somebody other than each other can bring to light things that have never been discussed before.

Fit for divorce

It's possible that if you're seriously contemplating divorce, it will be a liberating state of affairs and that becoming single once again will hugely enrich your life. But then again it might not. Like more or less everything else in this book, getting divorced will be a great deal easier if you are ready for it, although these preparations will be mental rather than physical. Initially you have to be steely enough to face the pain this divorce is going to cause to your partner, children, parents, in-laws and mutual friends. It's going to affect all of them, none of them well – and children particularly acutely.

It will mean a bigger disruption to your life than getting married or, if you have kids, having children did. Then you were eased into those situations with a great deal of positive preparation, and those experiences were adding to your life. Divorce will entail

261

a rethinking of finances, accommodation, domestic arrangements and habits. It will seriously affect your state of mind too; you will probably face a degree of loneliness as a result.

There will be the sheer stress brought on by all of the above, added to which there may well be the unpleasant prospect of a messy legal battle with somebody you used to share a bed with. The act of splitting up a partnership you have invested so much in over the years will also put a serious dent in your self-esteem. But it is important to remember this will not last forever.

It's not just about you

Then there's the collateral damage. Getting divorced will mean the world will look at you differently to when you were Mr Family Man. Just as married men tend to do better at work, divorced men's careers can slow down suddenly, and in social situations it might be the only thing that defines you to some people for a good while.

Friendships vs partnerships

There's no reason at all why this should be a cause of conflict. It's healthy for both you and your partner to have friendships outside of your relationship – that is, your own friends, rather than other couples. Even if your partner is your best friend, these extra-marital friendships are vital for more than just the chance to moan about your other half. Because human beings are complex individuals, it's highly unlikely that most of them are going to be satisfied with the relatively tunnel-visioned approach to existence that would be offered by no life outside a domestic relationship. Provided, of course, you remember what your priorities have to be and that they don't interfere with your life at home.

A wider view of life

Primarily, outside friendships bring an all-important different perspective on life, an angle other than that within the household. This can be a huge advantage when it comes to discussing problems, just as they can be an important pressure-release valve for thoughts you perhaps couldn't express at home. These friendships offer the chance to behave in ways that might not be entirely appropriate at home. They may allow the chance to pursue activities that do not interest your partner but which mean a great deal to you.

For men, these friendships will often mean people they were friends with before they met their partner. Be careful, however, that this doesn't lead to problems in itself. These will be people who will know you as well as your partner does, if not better, and such friendships can lead to jealousies or feelings of exclusion. Think about it very carefully if these long-standing friends are women. Ex-girlfriends are generally bad news as far as your present relationship goes. Even if you are very sure that they have been securely consigned to history, the chances are your other half won't see it that way.

T

Tip: Remain sensitive to whoever you are dealing with. There is nothing dishonest about presenting slightly different facets of yourself in different relationships, and it is vital not to treat everybody you deal with in exactly the same way – it's pretty much a given your partner won't appreciate being called "mate" as she or he gets punched on the shoulder.

On holiday

A good holiday a couple of times a year is one of the best remedies known to man for stress, boredom, overwork and feeling run-down. Two weeks away somewhere sunny or spectacular – or both – is as good for the body as it is for the soul. Provided you stay healthy while you're away.

The not-so-friendly skies

Quite apart from the stress caused by the seemingly compulsory delays, baggage surplus fees and often unhelpful staff, air travel can be physically bad for you. The main culprits are dehydration, poor air quality, reduced oxygen availability, immobility and bodily expansion.

Hydration, hydration, hydration (Part 1)

Humidity levels in the main cabins of commercial airliners will vary, but, uniformly, they will be lower than is good for you at take-off and will continue to fall as the flight progresses. Put simply, the longer the haul the drier the air around you. You are liable to dry out far quicker than on the ground and your equilibrium will suffer as:

Deep vein thrombosis

As the name suggests, this is a blood clot or thrombus that occurs in the large veins, such as the femoral, deep within your legs. Deep vein thrombosis has become associated with long-haul flying due to the extended stretches of inactivity in the constrictive position of aircraft seating: a situation that increases the likelihood of a blood clot. Large veins are more susceptible to sizeable blood clots, and while they may not do much damage in your legs, substantial pieces can break off and work their way up to the veins that feed into the heart and lungs, to cause serious problems. The effects of DVT may not be felt until some time after the flight, as the blood needs to flow freely once more for the clot to start moving through the veins.

The chances of a healthy person getting deep vein thrombosis are slim, but those odds increase greatly among smokers, the overweight or those with a family history of blood-clotting complaints. The same precautions for swollen feet should be taken to avoid possible DVT, but if you are susceptible to blood clots, it is recommended you wear calf-length compression socks to keep the blood flowing smoothly in your lower legs.

How it all works: ear popping

The ear is split up into three parts: the outer ear – the part you can see, which leads down to the eardrum; the middle ear – comprising the eardrum and the air-filled cavity behind it; and the inner ear – which contains the nerve endings that transmit signals for hearing and balance. Sound is processed as the sound waves come down the ear canal of the outer ear to vibrate the fan-like membrane of the eardrum in the middle ear, and register in the inner ear. For this to happen efficiently, the air pressure on both sides of the eardrum must remain the same, and it will be constantly readjusting itself in the middle ear with air brought in through the Eustachian tube, a tiny tube that connects the back of the nose with the middle ear. If changes in pressure on the outside of the eardrum are swift, the Eustachian tube cannot equalize it within the chamber behind the drum and a vacuum is caused. This will suck the eardrum inwards, stretching it and preventing it from vibrating properly, hence the muffled hearing and discomfort inside the ear when cabin pressure changes. The same state can occur if nasal blockages from a head cold prevent air from reaching the Eustachian tube.

Yawning and swallowing can relieve the situation, as it activates the muscles that open the Eustachian tube and pushes a small bubble of air into it from the nose. You may need to do it several times though. If that doesn't work, increase the pressure through the Eustachian tube by taking in a mouthful of air, holding your nose shut and trying to push the air out through your blocked nose. Do this gently, because blowing too hard without clearing the blockage could damage your inner ear.

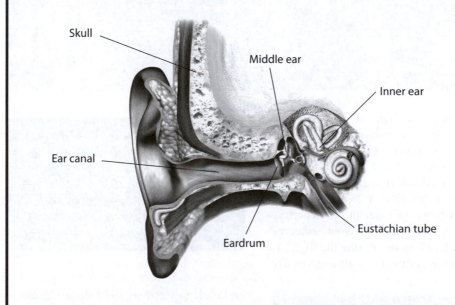

Skull

Middle ear

Inner ear

Ear canal

Eustachian tube

Eardrum

a) oxygen levels in cabin air are lower than air you'd normally breathe; and b) cabin pressure reduces oxygen saturation in the bloodstream. Should you start to dehydrate, your blood will thicken, thus transporting oxygen around the body and brain with less efficiency. And with less oxygen to utilize, an uncomfortable fatigue and drowsiness can result, which could also increase stress levels. (Interestingly, the air quality on the flight decks of most commercial airliners will be of a much better quality than in the main cabin, as higher oxygen levels serve to keep the pilots sharp.)

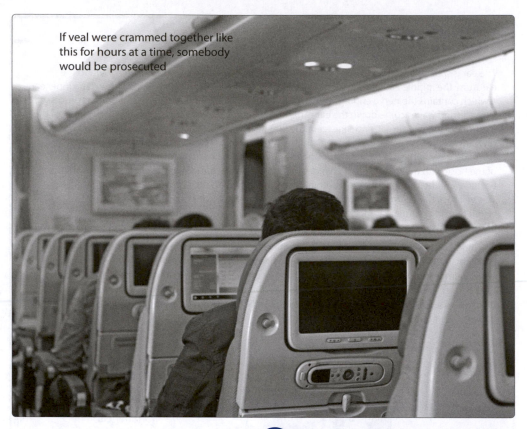

If veal were crammed together like this for hours at a time, somebody would be prosecuted

Approach any flight of over a couple of hours like a marathon runner: begin your hydration process beforehand. During those two or three hours between check-in and boarding, drink at least 500ml of water, topping up with a further 250ml before the gate; buy a bottle of water in the departure lounge to take on board. Avoid coffee or alcohol both before and during the flight, as they will serve as diuretics – although you're

T

Tip: As soon as possible after landing immerse yourself in water – in a bath, in the swimming pool, or in the sea – as this will assist the rehydration process and help you to relax.

T

Tip: No matter how thirsty you are, never drink tap water on aircraft, as there are no set standards for in-flight water purity, and also you will have no idea in which country the tanks were filled.

on holiday, of course, and rules are made to be broken.

Once in flight, you need to be drinking 250ml of water each hour to stay hydrated and if you experience a dry mouth, itchy eyes, dull headache or general discomfort, you are on the way to dehydration. Wetting your face with a spray or a dampened handkerchief can help, and you should continue to rehydrate for a couple of hours after the flight has landed.

Have a good flight

• Make sure you've informed the airline in advance about any dietary or health requirements, then, when you check in, make sure these requests have been registered.

• Don't let airline staff stress you out, no matter how awkward they are appearing to be – console yourself by remembering you're going somewhere exciting and they're not.

• Be prepared for delays: carry any medicine you may need along with an MP3 player, reading material, carbohydrate snacks and plenty of water.

• If you are delayed and it can affect a condition you suffer with, make sure you inform airline staff at the earliest opportunity.

• Don't get drunk; relax with a drink or two, but don't overdo it as alcohol will have a more acute effect when you are in the air and will serve to dehydrate you more quickly.

• Remember to avoid excess tea and coffee as these are also diuretics.

• Move around the cabin if you can (without getting on fellow travellers' nerves, obviously).

Pressure situation

At cruising altitude the air pressure in commercial airliners' cabins will be lower than on the ground, meaning your blood oxygen saturation will be lower than normal, by as much as ten percent. This shouldn't affect anyone in good health – although it may contribute to drowsiness or lack of concentration – but if you have cardiovascular problems or are very overweight, seek advice before you fly.

During your flight, cabin pressure will cause the gases in your stomach to expand by as much as twenty percent, therefore avoid gas-producing foods such as cabbage or broccoli, or beer or fizzy drinks. Wear trousers that can be discreetly expanded and be thoughtful of fellow passengers should internal pressures get too much to bear.

If you experience aching lungs, clammy skin, dull headache, nausea, lack of focus or impaired vision, the chances are you're becoming oxygen deprived. Explain to the cabin crew that you are having difficulty breathing and ask if the oxygen can be turned up; this should get you back on course.

Air quality in aeroplanes is a questionable issue. Airlines maintain it is perfectly adequate – better than most office blocks, they claim – while so much anecdotal evidence suggests otherwise. It's no coincidence that a fair few people pick up a low-level bug on a long-haul flight.

Don't sit still

For most of us, air travel means being squashed into a confined space in an uncomfortable position, unless you can afford to fly business class. As seat pitch – the distance between the front of your seat and the back of the one in front – seems to be getting shorter, this situation isn't liable to improve. Such constriction of movement and pressure on parts of the body can cause a serious restriction in blood flow, which brings on big problems.

The most immediate effect is a swelling of the feet and ankles. This is commonly assumed to be down to cabin pressure, but it's simply a gravitational pooling of blood in the veins in those areas due to sitting with your feet on the floor for a long period of time. The dispersal of blood from these areas will also be hindered by pressure on the legs and waist from sitting, which constricts veins.

As elevating your feet will not always be practical, sit with your legs out as straight as

For the frequent flyer

If regular business trips are playing havoc with your fitness regime, follow these guidelines:

• Carry your own snacks, so that the two hours between check-in and flight time isn't spent grazing high-carb convenience food.

• Air travel causes fatigue through dehydration and poor air quality, which leads to feelings of hunger, so drink plenty of water and carry your own healthy food.

• Stay away from the room service menu, especially outside of restaurant hours. It's too easy to be tempted and the chances are it will offer quick-fix calorific stodge.

• Two or three extra beers a day will soon make themselves known on your waistline, so don't drink either for business bonding or out of sheer boredom.

• Set a time to work out or run and stick to it, either getting up early or blocking out an hour of your schedule.

possible, rotate your ankles frequently and stretch your calf muscles every half hour or so by drawing your feet up and pointing your toes. Get up and walk about at least once every hour, as the contraction and expansion of the muscles in your lower legs will pump the blood away from where it is collecting. This exercise will also ease constriction all over your body and stimulate your heart rate to assist blood flow.

Jet lag

There is not much that can be done about the discomfort and tiredness that can be brought on by crossing into different time zones and having to readjust your body clock. The best you can do is prepare by being rested, well nourished and properly hydrated before you travel. Then, when you arrive, set your watch to the local time immediately and throw yourself into the new schedule. Avoid big, carbohydrate-heavy, drowsiness-inducing meals, drink lots of water and carry on as normally as possible for the time zone you are in. If you feel you will be too tired to make it through the evening, have a short nap during the afternoon, but keep to local hours.

Keep healthy and fit on holiday

The best way to keep fit on holiday is swimming. However, it's a good idea to pack a pair of running shoes in case the weather's terrible or swimming isn't an option. Getting out on the road for a jog on a few early mornings will keep things ticking over. It can benefit more than your health, as being out and about in the area you're staying when it's waking up is a great way to discover some of its true character. You'll see views that go unnoticed and spot landmarks or sites that may be worth going back to when you've got more time.

Watch what you're eating – especially if you're drinking a great deal – as it's easy to pile on the weight in just two weeks of eating rich hotel or restaurant food. Don't neglect breakfast, but don't turn it into a bagel and croissant-heavy carb-fest. Instead opt for cereals, fresh fruit and yoghurt and don't overdo that caffeine if you're going out in the sun, as it will speed dehydration. Go for fruit or fruit juice at lunchtime to keep your blood sugar levels up, and visit a local supermarket, street or farmers market to stock up on fruit, nuts or other healthy

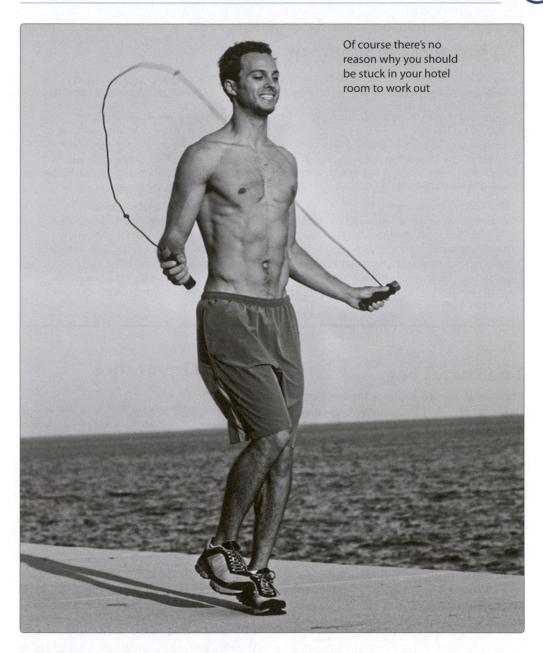

Of course there's no reason why you should be stuck in your hotel room to work out

snacks. Treat yourself to a decent dinner, as if you've eaten healthily all day you deserve it – you are on holiday, after all – and it's important to get something in your stomach before a night on the town.

Really, all healthy eating abroad requires is to bear in mind any rules you stick to at home, and not go overboard. If you find the restaurant gives you a huge portion, don't be shy about asking for a doggy bag – it could take care of your next meal. If your holiday offers the bonuses of really fresh fish and poultry or locally grown fruit and vegetables, take full advantage of them.

A hotel room workout

If your hotel doesn't have a gym, the following routine works most of your major muscles and should help keep you trim until you get home. Do as many reps (repeats) as you feel are beneficial.

Press ups – work those arms, shoulders and upper back
Employing a selection of different approaches to your press-ups, such as clapping, spreading your arms wider, raising your feet off the floor, will utilize different muscles.

The lunge – quadriceps
Stand with your feet slightly apart and hands on hips; step forward with your right leg, until your right knee is bent at right angles and your left knee is almost touching the floor, while your back remains straight. Step back with you right leg to starting position. Repeat with your left leg.

Donkey kicks – hamstrings and hips
Get down on your hands and knees; lift left leg up to bring the knee to the chest; then kick back with it as far and as high as you can. Bring it back to your chest and return it to the floor. Repeat with the right leg.

The crunch – abdominal muscles
Lie with your back flat on the floor and your feet raised so your knees are at right angles, your shins are parallel with the floor and your arms are crossed over your chest. Raise your upper body to crunch your ribcage towards the pelvis. Lower your shoulders back to the floor and repeat.

The travel bug

Millions of Britons contract food poisoning abroad every year, and although most of it isn't life-threatening, it's more than enough to ruin a holiday. The most likely complaints are described on p.107, and in hotter countries such things as dairy products and seafood will be particularly susceptible to spoiling if not kept properly, as will cooked food that is not refrigerated as soon as possible.

Be well prepared for an increased likelihood of bacterial infections by getting as fit and healthy as possible beforehand – if you're in tip-top gastric health you'll be less vulnerable. If you take on as many nutrients as you can in the lead-up to your holiday, your immune system will be as ready as it can be to ward off attack. Likewise, if you are going to a very high-risk area, a course of probiotics (see p.105) in the weeks before you fly out will make sure the good bacteria will be prevalent in your gut, no matter what.

Health insurance

Many budget tour operators make more money selling travel insurance than they do selling holidays; hence the pressure on you to buy it. But while you should definitely have medical and/or travel insurance before you fly, make sure it's got what you need. A general rule of thumb with insurance policies is that you get what you pay for, and the less expensive the policy, the flimsier your coverage.

Make sure yours not only covers you for having to go to hospital, but will pay all medical bills abroad – this is because items like ambulances, drugs, surgery, convalescence, meals in hospital and follow-up visits to outpatient clinics or doctors may all be billed as separate items. Also, if it covers getting flown home, check that it includes your partner or family.

The European Health Insurance card

This UK government-issue card entitles the bearer to access to whatever state-provided medical care is available in whatever European Union country they

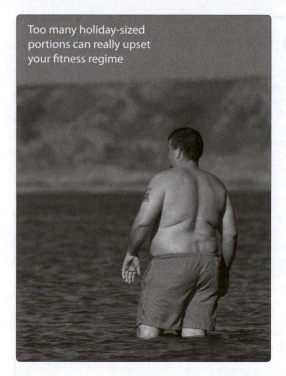

Too many holiday-sized portions can really upset your fitness regime

are visiting, and is also valid in Iceland, Liechtenstein, Norway and Switzerland. Many travel insurances will be invalid if you are not carrying one of these cards, but they are not a substitute for health insurance when away as there could be many expenses incurred that are not covered by that country's state healthcare.

No such service exists for Europeans travelling to the US, or for Americans travelling anywhere in the world, and private travel health insurance should be purchased. European Union citizens in the UK can apply for a European Health Insurance card in any post office, or online at ehic.org.uk.

Water, water, everywhere

Just because you see local people drinking the water, don't assume it will be safe; for you, they may well have built up immunity to bacteria contained within. And it's not just drinking the water: in many countries a common cause of water-related food poisoning is ice. Tempting as it may seem, if you are not sure it has been made with sterilized or chlorinated water, don't load that rum and Coke with ice; make do with chilled mixers instead. Also, salad items that have been washed in tap-water could be contaminated – and this applies to all food items that will not be cooked. Remember to peel all fruit before you eat it.

Most of the larger hotels practically anywhere in the world will be safe in this regard. Water will be treated to make sure it is good for use in the kitchen or ice machine, but it's still not advisable to drink it as it won't be quite what you are used to and may cause stomach upsets. In all cases it's best to steer clear of roadside food vendors, unless what you're about to eat is well cooked and still sizzling hot. It might even be worth investing in a small, inexpensive cool box; it will keep fruit fresh and drinks cold on the go or in your hotel room and you can donate it to the

B

Best investment: a box of drinking straws

Carry it with you at all times, as it will allow you to buy drinks from street vendors and enjoy them without the risk of picking up any bacteria: your mouth won't have to touch the bottle or can.

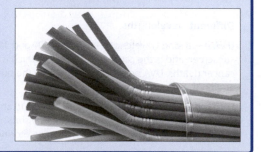

How it all works: tanning and burning

A suntan is the darkening of the skin through exposure to the UVA and UVB waves of the sun's ultraviolet rays. It occurs because the melanocyte cells in the epidermis, or outer layer of the skin, are stimulated into producing extra melanin to protect against potential DNA damage by the ultraviolet rays. Melanin is the pigment that provides the skin with colour and protects against the sun by dissipating UV rays as harmless heat. This is why people from hotter climates have dark skin, as large amounts of natural melanin are protecting them from the sun, and why suntans fade after a holiday when protection is no longer required. During the protection process, UVA radiation produces an oxidizing effect in the melanocytes, darkening both the pre-formed and existing melanin, while the UVB rays cause the increase in production. The initial effects of the darkening will be immediate, increasing in intensity – the deep tan – after a couple of days.

Sunburn happens when living tissue is overexposed to UV rays (both UVA and UVB radiation) and the production of extra melanin either isn't sufficient or hasn't happened quickly enough to prevent some DNA damage occurring. Once this happens, the body sets off a series of defence mechanisms, depending on how serious the sunburn is. The painful redness and inflammation is a result of the epidermis releasing protective chemicals, which trigger a swelling of the blood vessels nearest the skin surface. If the burn is more serious, blisters form as the blood vessels leak a fluid that protects the skin as it recovers, and they shouldn't be burst. Peeling occurs when the damaged skin cells are jettisoned en masse, because their DNA make-up is no longer what it should be, the brain has deemed them "out of control", presenting a big risk of turning cancerous. However, it is very important to remember that just because you've peeled, the risk of skin cancer hasn't gone away – there is a high chance the UV rays have penetrated deeper, causing problems that will reveal themselves at some time in the future.

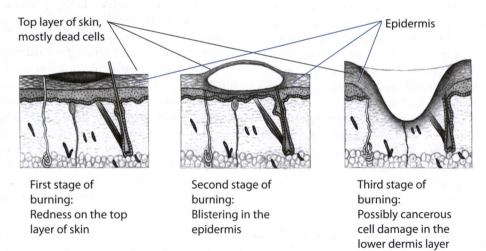

Top layer of skin, mostly dead cells

Epidermis

First stage of burning: Redness on the top layer of skin

Second stage of burning: Blistering in the epidermis

Third stage of burning: Possibly cancerous cell damage in the lower dermis layer

Different wavelengths

UVA has a long wavelength – between 400 and 315 nanometres – is less easily blocked by sunscreen and is the cause of melanoma, which is the starting point of 75 percent of all skin cancer deaths. UVA penetrates deeper into the skin, adversely affecting collagen and elastin, thus ageing the skin.

UVB has a medium wavelength – between 315 and 280 nanometres – is more likely to cause sunburn but more efficiently filtered out by sunscreen. It is believed to cause moles and some skin cancers, but UVB contact with skin also can produce beneficial vitamin D in the body.

room's next visitor when you go home.

Be careful of swimming in contaminated water too – raw sewage is the most common pollutant and, however careful you think you are being, some of it will enter your system and it can bring on extreme forms of gastroenteritis. Dirty water can cause rashes and infections in your bodily orifices as it seeps into ears, nose, eyes and the penis.

This was a very real problem in the waters around the UK, back in 2007, when floods led to overflowing sewers and long-term contamination of many parts of the coastline. Never swim in water where a dead animal or bird has been found; this will be a breeding ground for botulism, especially if the water temperature is very warm.

Pollution aside, before swimming in the sea, you might like to check what time the tides are; if it turns while you are out and you don't notice you could get into serious trouble.

A place in the sun

A bit of heat and a suntan are reasons many people go on holiday, yet it is also the reason why there are currently so many cases of skin cancer being diagnosed: an amount that has quadrupled among UK citizens over the last forty years. Although exposure to sunlight stimulates vitamin D production in the body, it only takes twenty minutes or so, a couple of times a week, of going about your regular business in the sun to get the maximum effect from this. A longer period, or increased intensity, will not add any more vitamin D but will leave you open to all the risks of UV radiation.

But, in spite of it being widely accepted that the notion of a "healthy tan" is an oxymoron, you can still get away with doing it in the traditional manner… as long as you're never less than very careful. If your shadow is shorter than you are, the sun's rays will be dangerously intense and extra care needs to be taken.

Tanning types

Because tanning is a reaction to damage already being inflicted, how well you will tan depends on your skin's ability to produce enough melanin to protect you from being burned (see box overleaf). In this respect, everybody's skin will respond differently, depending on how much melanin a person has to start with. There are a number of categories of skin type that need to be considered.

Very fair
This is a skin type that will burn very quickly, probably not tanning at all. Exposure should only be for very limited periods – the incidents of skin cancer in Scandinavia are nearly twice the EU average. This group should apply sunscreen of Factor 30 and upward.

Freckles or numerous moles
Those with this type of skin have a much greater likelihood of skin cancer, thus should also use above Factor 30.

Fair
Will burn easily, thus only a light, golden brownish tan will be possible. Sunscreen should be between Factor 15 and 30.

Light
As burning will take a while to happen, a mid-brown tan is possible, provided it's achieved gradually. Sunscreen Factor 8 to 15.

Dark or olive
Thanks to a large degree of inherent melanin, this skin type will not readily burn and so will tan profusely. Sunscreen Factor between 4 and 8.

Very dark
Although black people can sunburn, it is rare and takes a long time. UV rays can still be harmful, so a Factor 1 to 4 is still

recommended for entire days in the sun, especially for those not used to it.

A sunscreen summary

The SPF rating of sunscreen is the degree of protection it offers the user – it stands for Sun Protection Factor – and the higher the number the longer, not the stronger, the protection offered. What the number signifies is a multiplication factor of the amount of time you can spend in the sun before you'll burn: if, with no protection, it takes you twenty minutes to burn, then applying Factor 5 will extend that to one hundred minutes, while Factor 2 would mean you could stay out in the sun merely twice as long than you could without protection.

However, these timings are rough guidelines that don't take into account the intensity of the sun you'll be under. Also, be wary of those offering all-day protection – Factor 50 and upwards – as they will still need regular re-application: they will wear off, or sweat off, or wash off while you are swimming.

Remember to reapply sunscreen every couple of hours, regardless of what

Sun safety

The sun will be at its most intense between 10am and 2pm
Restrict your sunbathing to much shorter stretches during this period.

Just because you're not hot, it doesn't mean you're not burning
Out on a boat or on the golf course, for instance, the wind may well be keeping you cool, but the UV rays will still be getting through.

Check your sunscreen is of the "broad spectrum" variety and filters out both UVA and UVB radiation
It is not unusual for less expensive sunscreens to only block UVB rays, leading the user to believe they are better protected than they are: although UVB rays cause proportionately more damage, the UVA rays will still burn you if you are overexposed to them.

Make sure you apply enough sunscreen
It's not at all uncommon for people to under-apply sunscreen and thus compromise its protection capabilities. If you don't want to put on a great deal then switch to a higher SPF, but remember to reduce the time limit accordingly.

Reflective surfaces like sand, water or snow will intensify the sun's rays
This not only increases the amount of UV radiation hitting the skin, but also means it will be coming at you from a different direction as well – whitewashed walls or pale patios will have the same effect.

Be careful of those bits of you not used to the sun
Areas of your body usually exposed will have a more protective level of melanin than the bits that only see the light of day on holiday or when sunbathing.

The sun's rays will be more intense the higher up you are
And not just because you're closer to it either, but because the thinner air provides less resistance to UV radiation.

Wear a hat – even if you've got a full head of hair
The head is particularly sensitive to heat, thus leaving it uncovered greatly increases the risk of sunstroke. Opt for one with a wide, all-round brim, as that will provide sunburn protection for the nose, ears and neck.

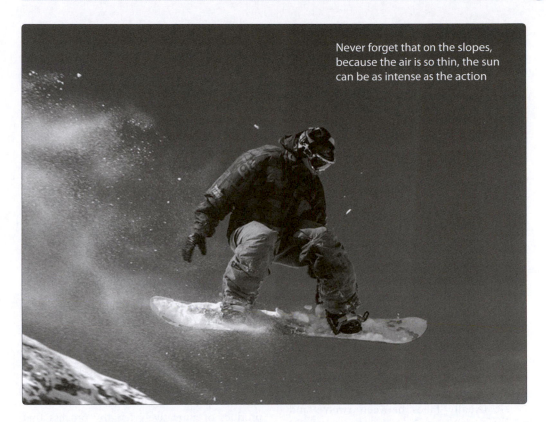

Never forget that on the slopes, because the air is so thin, the sun can be as intense as the action

time limit the Factor calculation gives you. This is because that time represents how long your skin will be safe in the sun with sufficient application, not how long each application lasts. Sweating, moving about, lying down, putting on and taking off clothes all contribute to it wearing too thin to be of any use after a couple of hours. Always reapply after swimming, even if yours is of a waterproof variety, and if playing sports make sure it is one of the specially formulated sweatproof, performance types.

If you've still managed to get burned

There is no "cure" for sunburn, and the best you can hope for is to manage the symptoms with a minimum of discomfort and without increasing the damage already done.

The first thing to do is get out of the sun immediately – this is important because in some cases sunburn may not become apparent for several hours, meaning significant damage has already occurred. Sunburn symptoms are partially the result of the body trying to cool itself down, so help it by applying cooling gel or after-sun lotion. Compresses made from towels soaked in iced water can be particularly effective, but avoid thick creams as they may prevent the skin from dissipating the heat and so intensify your condition.

Anti-inflammatory medicine – a brand containing aspirin or ibuprofen – will help ease the pain and bring the swelling down. After that, apply a moisturizing cream, something with aloe will soothe, or a cream containing between 0.5 and 1 percent hydrocortisone will boost the healing process. The aloe plant grows abundantly in tropical climes: it is recognizable by thick, spiky, fleshy leaves and tubular flower shafts rising from their centre. Cut one of the leaves open to release a thick liquid that will cool, soothe and moisturize irritated skin.

Don't burst any blisters as these will be protecting the new skin that is forming, and drink plenty of water as it's likely you'll be dehydrated from your time in the sun.

It usually takes between twelve and twenty-four hours from the time it started for sunburn to peak, therefore it is important you stay out of the sun, or keep the burned area covered, for the next two days. Seek professional help if the symptoms persist after two days, if you are feverish, or if over half your body is covered with blisters.

Keep your cool

Heat stroke, or sunstroke, is the name given to the extreme end of a condition called hyperthermia, during which the body is absorbing, or producing, more heat than it can dissipate. It's the opposite of hypothermia, when the body is losing more heat than it can produce or absorb.

If you have reached the point of heat stroke, your body temperature will be dangerously elevated as your internal thermostat will have been overloaded and can no longer function properly. This occurs because the cooling mechanisms have been overwhelmed by any of the following: high external temperature, intense or prolonged physical exertion or dehydration. As a result the body's temperature rises from between 36 and 37°C to 40°C or above, at which heat exhaustion causes collapse, and any further rise becomes potentially life-threatening as systems shut down. This, however, is the end product of a relatively lengthy process that will give plenty of warning signs that you are overheating or dehydrating.

Hydration, hydration, hydration (Part 2)

Starting to sweat when you get hot is perfectly normal, as the droplets of perspiration draw heat from inside the body to deposit it on the outside of the skin, where it dissipates through evaporation. However, the body needs to be sufficiently hydrated to allow it to sweat enough to keep cool under intense conditions, so it is vital to drink more water as the mercury rises.

Dehydration comes on very quickly – if you feel thirsty, it's already started because your body is letting you know – and once you've lost up to five percent of your body weight through fluid depletion you will experience all-over discomfort, muscle cramps and headaches. While this would impair an athlete's performance, it won't, at that point, be too dangerous. Any further loss of fluid though, and sweating will become so difficult that the body's internal temperature starts to rise drastically. If physical effort or high external temperature are continued it will increase massively, bringing progressively dangerous warning signs.

First, breathing becomes difficult as the heart beats faster to try to get enough oxygen around the system via the bloodstream. The skin reddens because blood vessels dilate to assist this movement of oxygen, but that causes blood pressure to fall and dizziness can result, often accompanied by nausea and headaches. Reacting to this drop in blood pressure, the blood vessels close up, often giving the skin a bluish tint, and lack of oxygen to the brain can contribute to loss of balance and impaired concentration. By now the blood is thickening through lack of oxygen and the rising core temperature brings on hot flushes, counteracted by chills.

If lack of water continues to allow the body to get hotter, breathing will become very shallow and confusion, impaired vision and overall weakness will set in. Then you will pass out. Worryingly, among older people fainting can be the first obvious sign of heat stroke, as other symptoms may not appear too unusual or will pass quickly.

If heat stroke strikes

Heat stroke can be avoided by keeping hydrated and not getting too hot – wearing a hat is vital as, just as your head loses heat easily in the cold, so it absorbs heat if exposed to the sun. If you feel any of the symptoms leading up to heat stroke, get out of the sun straight away, preferably into an air-conditioned environment to speed up the cooling down. Start drinking water, but don't gulp it down: take it on board gently.

If the situation advanced to the stage of feeling weak and disoriented and air-conditioning is inaccessible, assist the cooling down by fanning the body and head, and covering them with a sheet or towel soaked in cold water. Once anybody has reached the point of heat exhaustion, they should be moved out of the sun and an ambulance called immediately.

Your traveller's first aid kit

It should be kept in a cool place and contain:

A variety of plasters
Antiseptic wipes
Antiseptic cream
Various-sized gauze dressings
Rolled crepe bandage and safety pins
Disposable sterile gloves
Scissors
Tweezers
Painkillers
Insect bite cream/spray
Digital thermometer
Distilled water for cleaning wounds or eyes

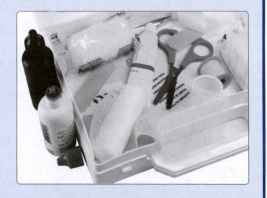

Skin cancer's spreading

Although the fatality rates for skin cancer are relatively low, it is the fastest rising form of cancer with the number of new cases having tripled during the last twenty years. And the reason the percentage of people dying from it in the US is so much smaller than in the UK is because they are a great deal better educated about its dangers.

What is skin cancer?

The vast majority of skin cancer is caused by cumulative overexposure to UV radiation over a period of time, which is why skin cancers are more prevalent among older people and usually appear on exposed areas of skin such as hands, forearms, necks and faces. In these cases, it is due to DNA damage to the epidermis cells, which start growing outside the control of the usual cell construction instructions and can become cancerous. The risk of contracting skin cancer increases hugely if you have suffered bad sunburn – sufficient to blister – at any time in your life, as this may have caused DNA damage.

Skin cancer falls into two main categories, non-melanoma and malignant melanoma, with the former being the less serious and easiest to treat, and the latter the cause of the majority of all skin cancer deaths. Non-melanoma skin cancer comes in two varieties. Basal cell carcinoma (BCC) is the most common form of skin cancer, the easiest treated and the least likely to spread.

What happens in Ibiza stays in Ibiza

Although losing a few inhibitions and carrying on in ways you wouldn't dream of at home is often the whole point of going on holiday, it's important to bear in mind that risky behaviour abroad could always be that bit more hazardous.

Drinking

Lower duty means cheaper prices and, as is very often the case abroad, the measures will be larger and the beer stronger, making it possible to drink much more than you are used to or indeed meant to. (Though, of course, if you're actually in Ibiza, you may well find the bar prices cripplingly expensive.) You could unwittingly become perilously drunk, affecting not only your health but also your personal safety and that of those around you. Never forget all the same dangers discussed in Chapter 9 will still apply, but problems can increase exponentially in an unfamiliar environment and with a police force who might not be sympathetic to hordes of rowdy tourists.

Sex

With a drunken situation comes the same likelihood of unprotected sex that there could be at home. Pack more condoms than you think you are likely to need, as you don't know how easily obtainable they will be where you are going. Make sure you carry them on a night out.

And while partying with the locals, be aware of the increased rates of STDs and HIV in some parts of the world. Be reminded that going with a prostitute abroad is no less seedy, and no more of a good idea, than doing so at home.

Drugs

Don't take anything if you're not sure what it is and be aware that local varieties may be much stronger than you are used to. Also, just because drugs appear to be "part of the culture" – i.e. seemingly sold and used openly – this doesn't mean the local police and judiciary will be in any way tolerant if they choose to haul you in. Find out about the local laws and do not flout them.

F

Fact: Sunbed tans contribute to skin cancer as much as the sun's rays, as in both cases UV radiation is involved.

Warning signs are small waxy nodules on your face, ears or neck, or flat, scar-like growths on your chest or back. The other type is squamous cell carcinoma (SCC), which is more likely to spread, but is just as easily treated if detected early. Symptoms are small, hard red bumps, or red, scaly, scab-like patches or crusty sores that refuse to heal on skin usually exposed to the sun.

Melanoma is the most dangerous form of skin cancer, with malignant melanomas accounting for around three-quarters of all skin cancer fatalities. Although the risks increase with age, this is one of the few cancers that can affect young people – melanoma is not uncommon in the 15-to-40-year-old age group. It is highly noticeable and if caught early is 99 percent curable; visible warning signs are new moles (dark or black spots or patches on the

AIDS/HIV around the world

Sub-Saharan Africa	5.0 percent of population living with AIDS/HIV	22.5 million people living with AIDS/HIV
Caribbean	0.9 percent of population	212,000 people
Eastern Europe & Central Asia	0.9 percent of population	1.6 million people
USA & Canada	0.6 percent of population	1.3 million people
South America	0.4 percent of population	1.5 million people
Australasia	0.4 percent of population	75,000 people
South & Southeast Asia	0.3 percent of population	4 million people
Western & Central Europe	0.3 percent of population	760,000 people
North Africa & Middle East	0.2 percent of population	350,000 people
East Asia	0.1 percent of population	800,000 people
Globally	0.8 percent of population	33.2 million people

Source: UNAIDS/WHO, 2011

skin) appearing, existing moles changing colour or shape, a mole that suddenly starts persistently itching or hurting, or a mole that starts bleeding or seeping.

The highest rates of melanoma are among white men over the age of fifty. This is believed to be linked to findings that men in their forties spend more time outdoors than any other demographic, and therefore have the greatest exposure to UV radiation.

Skin cancer is a big medical problem for New Zealand, Australia and South Africa, countries with high levels of sunshine and large Caucasian populations. Those of African or African-Caribbean descent or from the Indian subcontinent should also check regularly for skin blemishes that could be cancerous. While the melanoma rate amongst Caucasians is twenty-two percent compared with one percent among black people, the fatality rates are considerably higher among the latter because, frequently, tumours will be allowed to progress further without being noticed for what they are.

A suitable case for treatment

Any of the warning signs should prompt a visit to the healthcare professionals, at which point you will either be referred to a specialist or told it is nothing to worry about. If it does need treatment, there are several different choices and the success rate is high – provided it is diagnosed early enough. It is impossible to overstress that anything on your skin you suspect might be cancerous should be properly

T

Tip: Between dusk and dawn it is even more important to wear plenty of insect repellent, or to cover up, as during this time the malarial mosquitoes will be feeding.

investigated at the first viable opportunity.

Get the needle

The majority of holiday-makers will not need to get vaccinated before they travel, but as destinations become ever more far-flung, so the diseases on offer will be equally exotic, and need to be protected against.

Although requirements and advice can alter as health concerns change within different countries, a general principle is that anywhere outside of Northern and Western Europe, North America, Australia and New Zealand can pose a health risk, so seek advice from your travel agent or doctor or check the NHS Direct website (nhsdirect.nhs.uk).

In high-risk countries, the need for vaccination will be far less pressing if you are merely going away on a brief business trip, during which your time will be spent in air-conditioned, five-star luxury with minimal contact with the country you are visiting. Even then, however, you should take advice before deciding whether or not to get vaccinated, and whether or not those rules will apply if you are vacationing at even the highest end holiday resort. You will still be spending time in the open air, the sea, the swimming pool or on the beach, leaving you susceptible to a range of viruses. Also, bear in mind that some tropical countries will ask for evidence of certain immunizations as an entry requirement

It will also be vital to make sure your childhood vaccinations – diphtheria, tetanus, whooping cough, polio, Hib (influenzae type B), meningitis C, MMR and pneumococcal – are up to date, and this may mean a booster shot. Your doctor will advise on this, and arrange for the jabs should you need them.

If your travel agent tells you vaccinations are not required for a certain destination, make sure they are not merely referring to a vaccination certificate – inoculations themselves may still be appropriate and recommended.

> **T**
>
> *Tip: Apply insect repellent over your sunscreen to ensure effectiveness, and reapply after every reapplication of sunscreen, or after every couple of hours.*

From whom and for what?

If you believe you may need vaccinations, the first place you should go is to your doctor – this is vital if you are already on medication, as you will need to make sure the vaccine you are about to take will not have any adverse effects. At the surgery you may be able to get the immunization you require on the spot, especially if it is merely boosters to the British childhood schedule. However, many surgeries will not keep stocks of the less commonly called for vaccines, and you may be asked to come back at a later date or referred to a specialist holiday health centre, which are usually situated in larger branches of pharmacy chains.

You will be charged by the surgery both for the vaccine and the act of

Treatable STDs around the world

Sub-Saharan Africa	11.9 percent of adult population infected	53.5 million people infected at any one time
Caribbean	7.1 percent	1.63 million
South & Southeast Asia	5.0 percent	6.6 million
Eastern Europe & Central Asia	2.9 percent	5.13 million
Australasia	2.7 percent	506,250
USA & Canada	2.4 percent	5.19 million
North Africa & Middle East	2.1 percent	2.6 million
Western & Central Europe	2.0 percent	5.06 million
South America	1.9 percent	6.08 million
Globally	3.8 percent	82.296 million

Source: UNAIDS/WHO 2011

How it all works: vaccinations

Inoculations against specific diseases stimulate the body's immune system into producing the required antibodies by introducing controlled doses of the disease to be protected against into the system. When the body is attacked by hostile or unknown viruses or bacteria, the system produces the relevant protective antibodies to fight it off, and in the case of a genuine infection often the infection takes hold due to lack of antibodies. Vaccination brings in a small quantity of potentially hostile bacteria or viruses, causing the system to produce the right antibodies, but the biologically altered invaders will not actually inflict the diseases themselves. Once these antibodies have been produced, they remain in the body for years, allowing the immune system to recognise the disease in its real form and to wipe it out before it takes hold. Each separate vaccinable disease requires its own individual injection.

injecting it because vaccinations for travel are not provided for on the NHS – it is to specifically protect against disease you won't get in Britain, so why should they? The cost of holiday vaccinations is generally inexpensive.

Timing your jabs

Don't leave it too late to find out if you need vaccinations. Many take time to produce antibodies so six weeks before you travel should be the minimum. Be mindful that vaccines can require two or more shots

The best of the web

mcsuk.org
The website of the Marine Conservation Society, where you can find up-to-the-minute information about the levels of pollution on beaches around the UK.

fitfortravel.scot.nhs.uk
Part of NHS Scotland and a comprehensive advice site for travellers' health, it has up-to-date details of which countries require what immunization.

masta.org
The Medical Advisory Service for Travellers Abroad, was founded by the London School of Hygiene and Tropical Medicine. It has a network of travel clinics all over the country and much useful advice on immunization.

traveldoctor.co.uk
How to prepare before going abroad, what to do if you become ill and many useful travel tips.

skincancer.org
Comprehensive American site, dedicated to advice about all aspects of skin cancer from clear explanations of what it is to facts and figures to precautions to be taken if heading for the sun.

airlinequality.com
An impartial guide to the world's major airlines, including those all-important leg room and seat pitch surveys.

who.int
The World Health Organization has all the facts and figures about the state of health or risk of disease all over the world.

given with an interval of at least four weeks in between each one. Also, in the case of some multiple inoculations, while they can all be administered at the same time to different parts of the body, if that is not possible there must be a gap of three weeks between shots.

Ten top tips for travelling healthily

▶ **Pack more condoms than you think you'll need** Then make sure you've got a couple with you when you go out.

▶ **Never drink water in an aircraft bathroom** Quite literally, you don't know where it's been.

▶ **Double your regular water intake when flying** Then make sure you are properly hydrated before boarding, as cabin humidity and lower oxygen levels will dry you out much faster.

▶ **Get out of your seat and move around** Do so for a minute at least once an hour on a long haul flight, and rotate your feet at the ankles as often as you remember.

▶ **Make the most of local cuisine** Provided it includes locally grown fruit and vegetables and genuinely fresh meat and fish, but not if you're in Las Vegas, obviously.

▶ **Any sort of risky behaviour you indulge in at home will be even riskier abroad** You won't know what the local attitude is, you may not be able to speak the language and, surprisingly, people might be all too willing to take advantage of tourists.

▶ **Get vaccinated early** Many vaccinations will take a few weeks to become fully effective.

▶ **The sand, snow or sea will intensify the sun's rays** Take extra care when out in it under these conditions.

▶ **Don't turn breakfast into a carb fest** Followed by a morning of inactivity it will send you home considerably wider around the waist.

▶ **Hangovers are always worse in a hot country** This is because of the ease of dehydration.

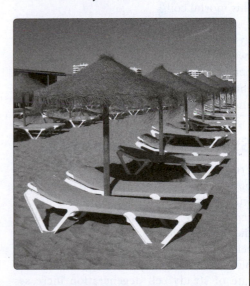

In later life (14)

According to medical science, on the physical side it's downhill for us from our mid-twenties onwards. Worst of all, although we get smarter, we get progressively less able to do anything about all these good ideas we might have. While this book won't make you live forever, it can help you put off the effects of ageing until the last possible moment.

Youth is wasted on the young

As the years pass by your body will unfortunately start to wear out, much like most things in life. Alarmingly, if you are a man living in the developed world you are liable to reach your peak physical condition a full fifty years before you finally shuffle off this mortal coil.

Which means, because you are likely to live for seventy years or more, for at least two-thirds of your life it will never get any better than it is right now. This is a great shame because with age comes experience and increased mental powers.

Structural alterations

From the moment you are born your body is in a constant state of regeneration, with cells dying all the time and getting replaced by new ones. As you get older, the rate at which you can manufacture new cells slows and eventually they begin to die out faster than they can be restored. This rate of steady cell degeneration increases with each passing summer, and will affect different aspects of your body in different ways.

Osteoporosis, as the result of a reduction in bone density, is probably the most common effect of ageing, and affects as many as one in ten men over the age of sixty. It occurs gradually, and comes about when the bones are not getting enough calcium and phosphate to keep rebuilding themselves. This means they are brittle and increasingly prone to fracture. Dietary intake of these minerals may need to be stepped up, because, as you age, your body will actually start reabsorbing them from your bones back into your system. It may be necessary to take calcium supplements, especially if you are lactose intolerant and don't drink milk. Regular exercise – running and walking, in particular – will also help preserve bone density, as the system adapts to cope with the rigours of impact and retains more minerals in the bones.

The tissues connecting the bones will suffer too, as the body's cell production starts to slow down. Joints become less flexible, and this can result in a painful stiffening. Time-induced wear and tear is also a big factor, and the cartilage that sits in between the joints' moving parts will wear thin over time, meaning it provides less protection from friction and impact. This can lead to inflammation and stiffness and can be further aggravated by a reduction in synovial fluid – the joint's internal lubrication. Stretching exercises will help keep joints mobile, while you can also help maintain fluid levels by taking fish oil supplements. Due to changes in posture, compression of vertebrae and shrinkage of connective tissue, a man can lose up to two inches in height between the ages of forty and seventy.

Loss of muscle tissue can start occurring naturally as early as your thirties, and exercise will become increasingly important to maintain bodily mass and strength. Muscles may also lose density as their regeneration slows and the body deposits fat within them. They might also stiffen as the regenerated tissue is tough and stringy due to larger cells. Maintaining muscles to provide support and protection as bones degenerate is essential, just as strength will be needed for balance, mobility and coordination.

As you age your body gets worse at regulating its internal temperature, thus you need to be much more careful about exposure to extreme temperatures.

Age and the organs

The vital organs start to decrease in efficiency as they get older, but this is gradual and in the cases of a healthy liver and kidneys, not really dangerous. They are rarely used to maximum capacity, thus any decline will be taken up by their natural reserves.

Ageing affects the heart in a number of ways. The muscles within it decline and the walls become less elastic, meaning it beats slower, with a shorter pumping stroke, and calcification can occur in heart valves, as the body absorbs calcium from the bones (see above). These factors restrict blood flow, as does the hardening of artery walls in and outside the heart. This increases the chances of congestive heart failure, heart attacks or strokes, and raises blood pressure to put more strain on your pump. Reduced blood

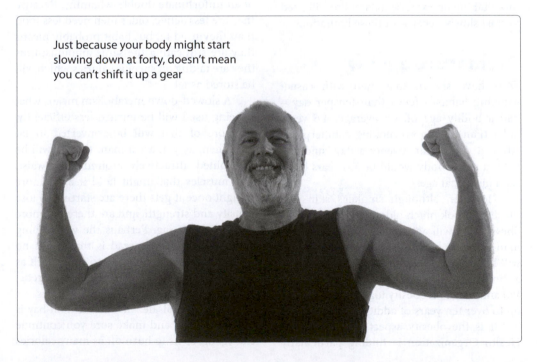

Just because your body might start slowing down at forty, doesn't mean you can't shift it up a gear

T

Tip: As you age your body will not be able to regulate its internal temperature so efficiently, thus you will need to be much more careful about exposure to extreme temperatures.

flow will slow the response to stress or danger and impede healing abilities, while decreased oxygen to the muscles adds to fatigue.

This reduced oxygen delivery will not be helped by your lung capacity getting smaller as you get older, because the muscles that control breathing are weaker and the ribcage becomes stiffer and less able to expand and contract. This means more air remains in the lungs after exhaling, leaving less space for what the next breath ought to be bringing in.

Men who have exercised throughout their lives will reach their senior years with much stronger cardiovascular systems, but those taking up exercise in later life will need to start slowly because of these limitations.

Premature ageing

Tests have shown that men with casual smoking habits – fewer than ten per day – had a bodily age of, on average, 4.6 years older than their non-smoking counterparts. After a forty-year twenty-a-day smoking habit a man's body would be 7.6 years older than his actual age.

However, although smoker's skin will make you look much older than you are, it is obesity that will actually age you quicker. A man who has been obese for over ten years will have a bodily age of 8.8 years older than a slim fellow who was born in the same year. Put smoking and obesity together and it adds up to over ten years of additional ageing.

It is the obesity aspect that the World Health Organization is finding particularly worrying as, while smoking figures have gone up and down over the years, obesity is increasing relentlessly, especially among young people. There is a growing number of overweight children and adolescents who are experiencing adult-related conditions such as heart disease and type 2 diabetes much earlier than previous generations. This is being perceived in medical circles as a dangerous "advanced ageing", leading to fears that, as their conditions put greater strains on their systems for longer, their life spans will be reduced.

It is accepted that while advances in modern medicine are already reducing the impact of obesity and associated conditions, nobody is yet sure what knock-on effect such childhood ill health will have in later life.

Middle-aged spread

How did that get there? That spare tyre suddenly appearing around the midriff seems almost inescapable to most men in their forties and comes about as the result of an unfortunate double-whammy. Because they are less active, older men need less food than they used to, but habit probably means they are still eating the same amounts; thus they are taking on surplus calories which will be stored as fat.

A slowed-down metabolism means what is being used will be burned less efficiently, so more of that will be converted to fat too. Then, as you are a man, this fat will be distributed attractively around your waist. The muscles that might hold it a bit more upright once it gets there are starting to lose density and strength, and are therefore more likely to let it sag. Perhaps the worst thing about middle-aged spread is that it has no respect for age – it can start to show itself as soon as your lifestyle becomes less energetic, which might be as early as your twenties.

The only failsafe way to keep it at bay is to eat healthily and make sure you continue exercising, so as to burn off as many calories

Are you getting enough?

It may not be possible to get enough nutrients from your diet – especially as you will naturally be eating less, so these supplements will be particularly important:

What it is	What it does	What you need
Calcium & vitamin D	Maintains bone strength and density; vitamin D allows the calcium to be absorbed efficiently; aids the nervous system	800 milligrams & 5.0 micrograms
Beta-carotene (vitamin A)	Helps build bones; prevents eyes drying out	1000 milligrams
Vitamins C & E	Prevents lipid oxidation, thus aids blood flow and reduces plaque formation and blood pressure	60 milligrams & 10 micrograms
Folic acid	Promotes alertness	400 micrograms
Vitamin B complex	Assists cell growth; aids the nervous system; helps guard against macular degeneration (age-related blindness)	B1 1.2 milligrams B2 1.4 milligrams B3 16 milligrams B12 3.0 micrograms
Zinc	Boosts the immune system	10 milligrams

as you take in. A combined schedule of strength and aerobic training should see some reduction (see Chapter 4), but don't be fooled into thinking endless repetitions of sit-ups or crunches will get rid of it. Although firmer abs will help your posture as your gut will be less able to drag you down, and that will save your lower back, you can't spot reduce through targeted exercise. If you start to lose weight all over, eventually that spare tyre will start to deflate.

The eyes have it... or perhaps not

Sight generally begins to worsen after the age of forty because the cornea and the lens of the eye start to become opaque and the pupil gets smaller, contracting the field of vision. The most obvious effect is an almost universal problem with reading: a need for either magnification or more light to cope with small text. (This is one of the reasons that electronic reading devices are proving so popular among older generations: the option of altering text-size being a distinct plus.) Also, shifting focus from one object to another will take longer and some green/blue colour blindness may occur.

As far as your ears go, it's not great news either. Although your hearing will worsen, your ears will keep getting bigger – men's ears continue to grow at approximately 0.22mm per year for their entire lives.

Snow on the roof but a fire in the hearth

Although the numbers of living sperm per emission go down with the passing of time, there will be very little change in a man's fertility as he gets older; indeed it is not uncommon for men above the age of sixty to father children. Sex drive can decrease slightly, as some testicular mass may be lost, meaning testosterone levels can decline, and it might take more to get you aroused, as responses will be slower. Repeat performances could be confined to memory too, as it will take longer to replenish seminal fluid reservoirs and to get another erection.

In spite of erectile dysfunction being more common among older men, this is not inevitable. It comes about because of other medical conditions that are more prevalent among this age group, such as diabetes and high blood pressure. Older men get fewer erections than their youthful counterparts, though, and that's just a fact of life.

Eating late

Because very little will change as regards your digestive system as you get older, other than a slowing down of your metabolism,

dietary requirements for a healthy later life aren't actually that much different from what you've always been eating. To achieve the necessary nutrition you'll need to maintain a good balance of fresh fruit and vegetables, protein, fibre and carbohydrate, but there will be certain things you should avoid. Foods high in cholesterol should be given the swerve; no more than 25 percent of your calorific intake should come from fats and as little of that as possible should be saturated; and sugar needs to be limited, because of the increased risk of diabetes.

It will benefit you to eat less more often – five or six small meals a day – and to make sure you keep up your water intake, even if it does mean visiting the gents more often than you might like.

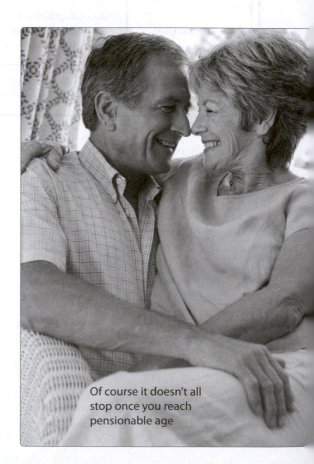

Of course it doesn't all stop once you reach pensionable age

How long can you go on?

It is believed that the upper age limit for the human body is around 120 years, and to get there you will need an ongoing lifestyle that promotes health, fitness, low levels of stress and strong emotional support. It is far from unusual for the people of the islands of Okinawa in Japan to live past one hundred years old, and their lifestyle couldn't be further removed from so much of the Western world. Their diet is low in fat, refined sugar and processed foods, yet high in fibre through fresh fruit and vegetables. Everybody exercises, regardless of age, and a strong sense of spirituality, family and community eases stress levels. The rates of prostate and colon cancer in that region are eighty percent lower than in the US.

Don't stop now

As middle-aged spread starts to creep up on you, it's easy just to surrender and watch it accelerate. But you could do something about it. Even if you've never exercised before it's never too late to start with this relatively easy programme – you don't even need any special equipment. Do as many repetitions of each exercise as you feel is giving you a good workout.

Sit and stand

Exactly what it says on the tin: sit on a straight-backed chair with feet flat on the floor and knees bent at right angles; with your hands dangling loose by your sides, stand up straight; sit down again, slowly; repeat. To make it a little more difficult, hold your arms straight out in front of you.

Standing press-ups

Stand about one metre away from a wall, and put your hands flat on it, each about 20cm outside your shoulders, with your arms straight; keeping body and legs rigid, bend your elbows so your face is brought towards the wall; stop when your elbows are bent at right angles; press back until your arms are once again straight; repeat.

Step-ups

Stand at the bottom of a flight of stairs or in front of something that is at least 25cm high and will support your weight; step up on to the first step with your left foot then bring your right foot up alongside it; step down with left foot then bring right foot down next to it; to complete one exercise, repeat movement starting with right foot; repeat for each foot.

Hamstring curls

Stand straight with your feet about 30cm apart, holding the back of a chair if you need it for balance; bring left heel up towards left buttock by bending knee; slowly lower foot back to the floor; bring right heel up to right buttock; slowly lower foot back to the floor; repeat with each foot.

Reverse crunches

Lie on your back with hands by your sides or behind your head; bend knees to right angles and lift feet 15cm off the floor; keeping knees bent at right angles and using abdominal muscles, lift feet until shins are parallel with the floor; lower slowly to 15cm above the floor; repeat.

Knee lifts

Stand straight with feet about 30cm apart, holding the back of a chair to the side of you if you need it for balance; lift left knee straight up in front of you, until it is bent at right angles with thigh parallel with floor; lower foot slowly to the floor; lift right knee to right angles; lower slowly to floor; repeat with each leg.

Age and IQ

Although it is a long-standing comedy notion that old people are unable to come to grips with anything that hasn't been made out of wood, there is actually no natural decrease in mental capacity as you get older. The number of nerve cells in the brain (neurons) do not go into decline with age, and they continue to make the new connections needed for learning and memory.

Any reductions in brain power as you get older will be the result of a disease rather than an inevitable occurrence. In 1998, Professor Whalley, head of mental health at Aberdeen University, was able to prove the theory. The exam papers from an IQ test, sat by some 100,000 11-year-olds in 1932, was discovered in a cellar. Whalley and his research team then gave the same test to 125 volunteers he tracked down from that same group, carried out under exactly the same conditions. The 77-year-olds fared considerably better than they did aged 11. The most interesting finding was that the levels of improvement were more or less the same across the whole group, meaning everybody seemed to have acquired more intelligence. The IQ levels had remained constant over that time too, and the brighter-than-their-peers kids were still the sharpest tools in the box as pensioners.

Sorry, I've forgotten your name

Researchers at the University of Toronto recently found that older people have difficulty

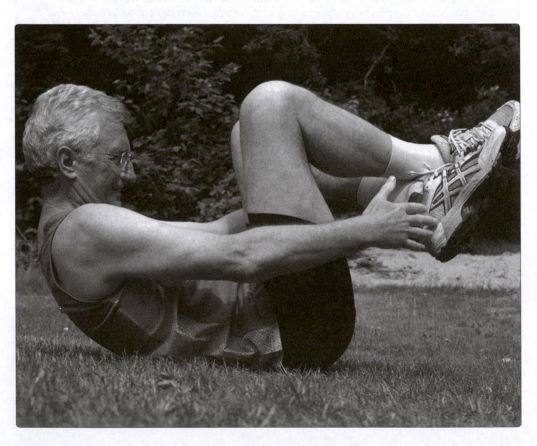

remembering isolated facts like names or telephone numbers because the older brain has a wider focus. This means when being introduced to somebody in a room full of people, rather than concentrate on a single fact – the name, for instance – they will be taking in the wider aspect and will have to sort through a jumble of information in order to immediately retrieve that one name.

While this may lead to what appears to be slowness of thought and distractibility, it is why the tests proved older people to be better at analysing situations, making broader-based judgements and being more mentally flexible if circumstances change. This happens because the extraneous information the older mind has been absorbing will be processed and sorted, allowing for a wider spectrum of knowledge to be called upon when considering the situation at a later date. Although much of the information absorbed appears trivial when taken as individual aspects, it meant the older people knew more about every situation than their more tightly focused younger counterparts, thus were better equipped to work out what needed to be done.

The downside was that this was thought to be why older people seemed to have problems making instant decisions or thinking on the hoof – fluid intelligence. Interestingly, though, they were far more likely to say they didn't feel ready to make a decision, rather than take a guess and try and pass it off as "gut reaction" like many of the younger test subjects did.

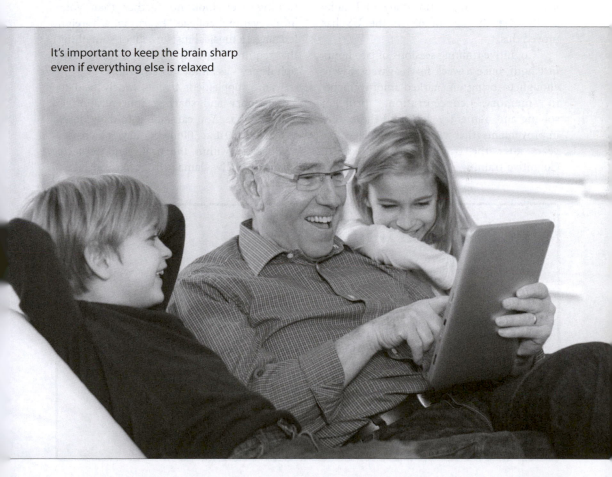

It's important to keep the brain sharp even if everything else is relaxed

> Tip: The older you are, the longer vaccinations will need in the body before they become effective, so be sure to leave plenty of time if getting jabs to travel abroad.

Staying sharp

The notion of the brain as some sort of muscle that will function much better if it is regularly exercised has been gaining credence for some time now, as older people with smart spouses or intellectually challenging working environments tend to stay sharper later in life. A long-term study of healthy adults over the age of 65 in the US has proved this.

Cognitive training sessions of two hours in length, once a week for five weeks, were enough to bring on marked improvements in memory, concentration, problem solving and numeracy skills and these were improvements that remained in place five years after the training sessions ended. Cognitive training is anything that stretches the brain by pushing it to solve puzzles or problems on the hoof – sudoku, crosswords, Rubiks cubes, word searches and mental arithmetic are all cognitive exercises.

The conclusion of the experiments was that if people regularly challenge themselves with short bursts of mental workouts, their brains' abilities will develop to maximum potential. "Tapping in to your cognitive reserve" is how scientists are describing it.

Don't wait until you're over sixty either. The younger you start these exercises the more benefit they will have and the same research showed the importance of entering those twilight years with the sharpest faculties possible.

If you have time on your hands and you want to keep the old grey matter turning over, look no further than your local evening college. Learning a foreign language, a musical instrument or something that requires dexterity – pottery, woodwork, upholstery – is an ideal brain trainer.

One supplement that is widely held to aid memory and sharpen concentration is ginkgo biloba. You can take it in daily doses of between 50 and 500mg per day. It increases blood flow within the brain and protects against oxidative damage from free radicals.

The dementia time bomb

There are now more sixty-year-olds alive in the UK than there are sixteen-year-olds. This is symptomatic of an expected average life span that has nearly doubled since 1900. While this represents a huge achievement for medicine and science, it also begs the question: is this curve heading further than is actually good for the human body?

Although keeping healthy and active can offset the physical demands of ageing, it seems less can be done to reduce the likelihood of Alzheimer's and other forms of senile dementia. Because the percentage of Alzheimer's sufferers rises so steeply as people get into their eighties – there are over 700,000 sufferers in the UK – with people living longer this figure is expected to more than double in the next twenty years, then double again in the following twenty. This is leading to concerns over the growth of a large number of people with a very low quality of life, who will be in need of constant care.

At the moment, this situation is not helped by the fact the levels of spending on research into Alzheimer's is less than ten percent of that spent on finding cures for cancer.

The best of the web

alzheimers.org.uk
The website of the Alzheimer's Society, a charity dedicated to raising awareness and funds for the fight against the disease. The first stop for anybody who wants to find out more about Alzheimer's or make a donation.

laterlife.com
Health, travel, fitness, relationships, courses, insurance, health farms… in fact all human life is covered here with the older person in mind.

healthscotland.com
From Scotland's NHS website, pages that deal comprehensively with all health-related aspects of getting old.

senior.com
Where the US senior community find out about health, travel, the law, care-giving, stay in touch or just hang out.

runningforfitness.org/faq/agegrading.php
Where to go to calculate how your running times compare with world records, as relative to your age.

50plus.org
The home of the Lifelong Fitness Alliance, an American organization dedicated to seniors' health and fitness, offering advice, tips and events listings.

Fading to grey

Alzheimer's disease is the leading cause of senile dementia in the developed world, and around three percent of those over sixty-five and forty percent of those over eighty will be sufferers. It is a progressive degenerative condition that attacks the cells in all areas of the brain to destroy the memory, the ability to function and emotional control. Symptoms include forgetfulness, loss of memory, mood swings, confusion and a noticeable lack of purpose in speech and action.

At the time of writing Alzheimer's is incurable, with very little evidence as to what might help prevent it. Very little is known as to whether it is caused by anything other than old age too, although there is evidence that it is hereditary, with children of sufferers having a fifteen percent chance of getting it themselves.

Age and immunity

The immune system will also function progressively less efficiently as the years roll by, and when you reach your sixties it won't be much more than forty percent of what it was in your thirties. This will happen on two different levels. Initially the central nervous system reacts more slowly and less sensitively to signals that infections are invading the body, and secondly the cells that will then be produced to fight infection will be less dynamic than they would have been when you were younger. This means older people are far more prone to viral and bacterial infections and need to take extra precautions.

Remaining well nourished is key to keeping your immune system working as well as possible, although staying fit is also important as it will help those nutrients

Ten top tips for growing old gracefully

▶ **Eat more smaller meals per day** Your digestive system may be functioning less efficiently and should not be over worked.

▶ **Make sure you get enough nutrients** You should be eating less than you did as a young man but you will still need the same vitamin and mineral intake.

▶ **Go swimming instead of running** It is a non-impact exercise, therefore, it will put no undue strain on your joints.

▶ **Get vaccinated earlier** Especially if it's for foreign travel as it will take longer for the vaccine to become absorbed into your system.

▶ **Just about everybody needs reading glasses by the age of fifty** Don't be shy about whipping yours out.

▶ **Don't be scared of keeping fit** It will actually get easier as you get older because your muscles start to function more efficiently.

▶ **Drink plenty of water** This is particularly important as older men are more prone to constipation, which can lead to hernias.

▶ **Stay sharp with some form of brain activity on a daily basis** Do sudoku or crosswords for instance, as this will keep the old grey matter functioning as well as it ever did.

▶ **Dress your age** Mutton dressed as lamb will rarely look any more impressive than mutton dressed as mutton.

▶ **Don't believe the hype** When you were a young person, you may have been brainwashed into thinking there's no fun to be had once you get past forty – this simply isn't true.

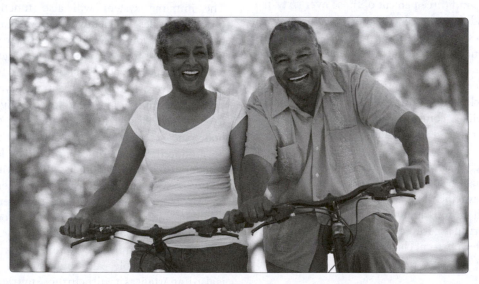

get metabolized. Healthy eating will become far more significant at this stage in your life, as you will be eating less but will still require more or less the same amount of nutrients as when you were younger. So you will need to make sure you are getting everything possible from the food. You may need to add to what you are getting from your food with supplements. B vitamins are imperative as they boost the immune system and maintain the nervous system; and make sure you are eating plenty of whole grains, pulses, nuts, eggs and dairy.

Any inherent inefficiency of the immune system means that vaccinations will be less effective, but they are still vital. Inoculations against flu, streptococcal pneumonia, tuberculosis and hepatitis B should be obtained, and the UK vaccination schedule should be maintained with whatever booster shots are necessary – at the very least, you will need to be vaccinated against tetanus and diphtheria.

Once the body passes the age of seventy it is likely to produce something called autoantibodies, which can attack the system to trigger rheumatoid arthritis and a hardening of the arteries (atherosclerosis). Making sure you are getting enough vitamins B3 and C will help fight against this.

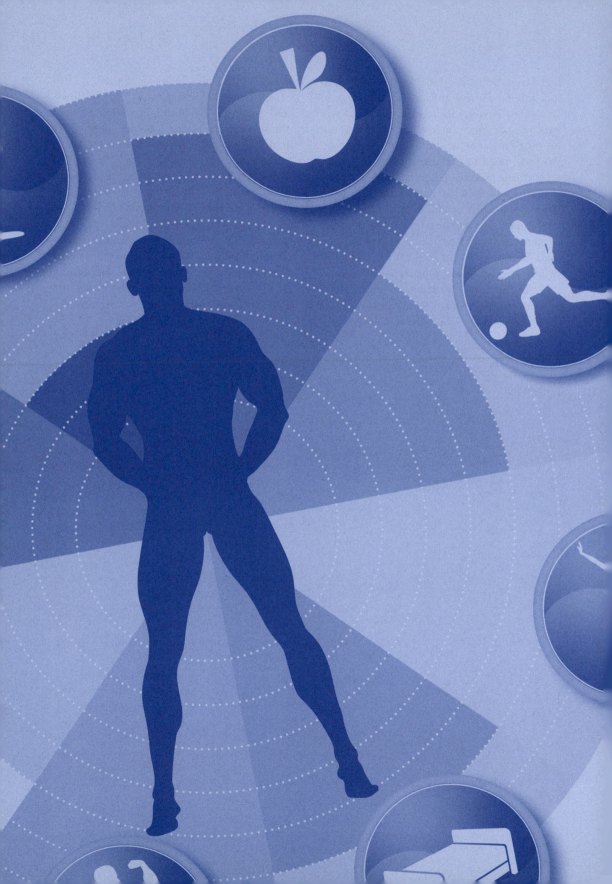

PART 2
FIT FOR LIFE

A man for all seasons

As you go through life, what is "normal" for you – as regards your health and fitness – will change. From decade to decade your requirements, your risks and how you need to handle things will be very different. But it's far from downhill all the way: each period has at least as many plus points as it does negatives.

Man in his twenties

It is at this point that a man can expect to have the most fun. A lack of familial responsibilities, the anticipation of possibilities, loads of energy and peak levels of testosterone turn life into an exhilarating experience. But it can also be the most potentially damaging time too. Male suicide rates are high among this age group; depression is a common problem and often undiagnosed; and young men in their late teens and twenties are the most likely to be victims of violence. Beyond that, this time of life is made even more confusing and contradictory by the continually teetering balance between what you and the people around you feel you should be doing, and what your capabilities and experience actually allow.

However, the advantages of being twentysomething vastly outweigh the downsides. At this point you should be at your naturally healthiest and fittest, as so much of your system peaks during these years. Your metabolism will be operating at its most efficient level. Thus in spite of you

eating so much because you are still growing, there is relatively little danger of you getting fat; also you should have masses of energy. This doesn't mean you shouldn't watch what you eat though, and your need for almost constant feeding ought to be sated with complex carbohydrates (whole grains, fruit and vegetables), rather than fat and sugar.

Technically you will be at your "manliest", as testosterone levels and sperm counts will be at their all-time high. This means not only are men of this age at their most sexually potent but macho-type behaviour among them is most widespread – hence the disproportionate statistics for violence. It might surprise you to learn that the biggest cause of death among men aged between seventeen and thirty in the UK is road accidents: the majority of all road accident fatalities are within this age group. It is also the age group that has the highest proportion of smokers, and it is now that a lifetime habit is most likely to start.

Any feelings of invulnerability will be further increased by the fact that your immune system is working better than it ever has, or will do so again, so fighting off infection will be relatively straightforward. But don't let feeling good lead you into complacency. It won't hurt you to have an all-over medical checkup (heart, lungs, blood pressure, cholesterol, diabetes, liver, kidneys and overall fitness) every two years. And if you wear glasses, get your sight tested every six months, as your eyes and their capabilities will still be changing.

Mind games

Apart from the fighting and the predisposition for STDs, the biggest problems of being in your twenties will be psychological, as in spite of the testosterone surge it is unlikely your self-confidence is keeping up with the macho public face.

What will seem to be expected of you by family, friends, bosses, teachers or yourself, as you start out in the world, can often put undue pressure on a young man, while decision-making will not be easy due to the limited amount of worldly experience you have. Confusion about sexuality is most common at this time, and love lives will be further complicated by what young men perceive they should be doing. Hormone levels and the rest of the world in general – websites, lads' mags, music videos, TV – will be telling you that you should either be coupled up or out sowing abundant amounts of wild oats, yet a genuine lack of self-confidence about appearance, sophistication and all-round manliness makes this a huge task.

It all amounts to the difficulties men have in passing from childhood into adulthood without the support system that women seem to have. Women are far more likely to talk about things among themselves or

What's good about being twentysomething	What sucks about being twentysomething
Your high testosterone levels mean you will be full of confidence	The amount of new life experiences you will encounter will often cause self-doubt
Suicide rates among this age group are falling	Incidents of self-harm are rising
Your muscles are at their strongest; your potency is at its highest; you have the least chance of putting on weight	You are the most confused about your appearance, your sexuality and your attractiveness
You will be meeting new people all the time	There is relatively little emotional connection between men of this age, thus loneliness can be a problem
Your metabolism is so fast you can eat what you like without putting on weight	You will need almost twice as many calories as your dad does, thus will need to be eating fairly constantly
Apparent lack of responsibilities	Pressure to get started on "life's ladder"
Your system will best be able to cope with the excesses of drink and drugs	You are far more likely to dangerously overdo it with drink and drugs
Your immune system will be operating at its peak and you will feel invincible	Because you feel invincible you are less likely to look after your health, thus serious conditions are often allowed to develop unchecked

Be careful of:

STDs and AIDS
Not because your system is any more susceptible, but simply because statistics say your behaviour is likely to put you at much greater risk.

Testicular cancer
Monthly self-examination is recommended; it is the type of cancer most likely to affect you at this age.

Weight gain
You are still growing and you will need to eat heartily, but be careful of getting fat at this point as it could become a habit. Now is the time to get into an exercise routine.

Anaemia
Iron deficiency, causing general fatigue, isn't uncommon in men of this age. So eat plenty of leafy green vegetables.

Acts of violence
The vast majority of assaults in the UK are committed by young men aged between fifteen and thirty on other young men aged between fifteen and thirty.

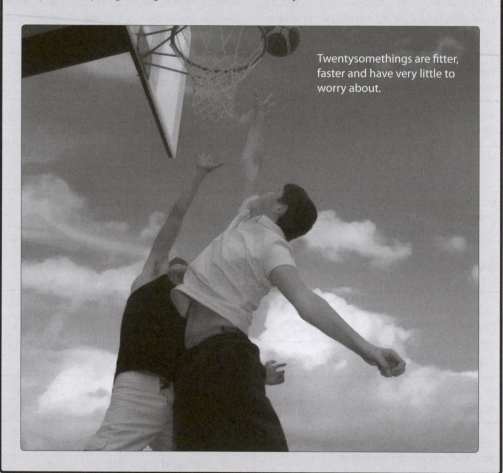

Twentysomethings are fitter, faster and have very little to worry about.

with their mothers, and have all manner of media offering them advice. Men could get through this difficult period more easily if they talked about what was going on in their lives and admitted to fears and insecurities, to each other, to their dads, to teachers or – before things get really bleak – counsellors. If they did more of that their biggest worries would be exactly how much fun to have that particular night.

Man in his thirties

By now, if you've made it out of your twenties without being stabbed to death or getting killed in a car accident, you should be a much more stable individual. Statistically you are likely to be either settled down in a relationship and starting a family or, at the very least, aware of the value of doing so. This is a completely natural result of a man's inherent programming for procreation and you are following through now because you have become self-confident enough to form close personal relationships. Also, you are grown up enough to be far less selfish than you were ten years ago.

This is a serious change of lifestyle that will allow you to get something a bit more meaningful from your leisure time than a skinful and a bit of a scrap, and many men will be rather grateful for this. But although the risky behaviour of your previous decade will be far less frequent it's unlikely such shenanigans have been consigned completely to history. It will still be necessary and not altogether unhealthy for you to prove

What's good about being thirtysomething	What sucks about being thirtysomething
You are much more confident than when you were in your twenties	Dissatisfaction is replacing insecurity and male suicides peak during this decade
You will probably be married or in a stable relationship	You'll have to adjust to a whole new way of life as half of a couple
Your propensity for risky behaviour will have decreased massively	You will be a trifle envious of your single friends still whooping it up
Your immune system will still be working well but less efficiently than when you were in your twenties	Your metabolism will have slowed noticeably, so it will suddenly become much easier to put on weight
Your earnings will have increased	Your financial commitments will have multiplied
You will be much better equipped to make big decisions	You will have many, many more big decisions to make
You are still young enough and by now experienced enough to get a huge amount out of your life	Trying to do too much, career-wise, leisure-wise and family-wise is a major cause of frustration

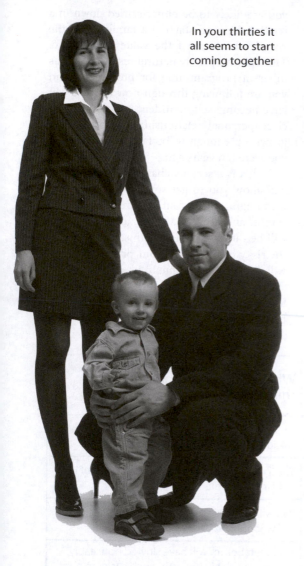

In your thirties it all seems to start coming together

having the energy of a young man, but with enough experience gained to know how to channel it. Also you are unlikely to have grown too cynical about the more humdrum things, so will still have a huge enthusiasm for life. However, while your potential for earnings and promotion prospects are looking healthy, your work-related stress levels will be increasing, added to which may well be the pressures of a newly growing family. It's little wonder the male suicide rate peaks among thirtysomethings and incidences of impotence are higher than at any age below eighty.

In spite of it being a period of high pressure, as a great deal will be expected of you by a growing number of people, you are actually far better equipped to deal with whatever life throws at you.

Stress and the thirtysomething man

It is now being recognized that men are suffering from stress at a much younger age, and it is over the past couple of decades that potential triggers for it have increased dramatically. A fundamental cause is the changes in social convention that have happened since their fathers were their age and for which so few contemporary life models exist. A generation ago a man lived with his mum until he got married, then he lived with his wife until one of them died. Nowadays the wealth of choice of domestic arrangements means there are so many that haven't existed long enough to have rules,

there's occasional life in the old dog. The big difference about going on the town at this age, though, is that you will exercise more restraint as you have more to lose. Now, if you do get into trouble, your life experience is far more likely to get you out of it without a trip to casualty. An all-over medical checkup (heart, lungs, blood pressure, cholesterol, diabetes, liver, kidneys and overall fitness) is recommended annually.

Career-wise, things should be taking off for you. You'll be in that unique position of

F

Fact: If you are still smoking at this age, you are probably smoking a great deal more than you were when you were in your twenties.

302

Be careful of:

STDs and AIDS
Although you are not at as high a risk as you were ten years ago, this is still a dangerous time for the many single thirtysomething men.

Drink and drug addictions
This is when habits start to gain a hold, as you are less likely to binge drink but more likely to drink every night, and will have more money to afford more and better substances.

Prostate problems
This is when you should consider getting examined every year for trouble with your prostate gland – not necessarily for cancer, but for lower-level infections and inflammations such as prostatitis.

Weight gain
Be warned, middle-aged spread starts now. Especially if you've recently achieved the enviable domestic situation of having at least two meals a day cooked for you.

and many require a great deal more effort to make them work.

Likewise men "growing up" later and later and often persisting with the carefree behaviour of their twenties well into their thirties and forties – adultescence, anybody? – conflicts with genetics and many of those around him will be urging him to settle down, start a family and get on at work. Once again this leads to stress because there are no cut and dried ways of doing things, and the more decisions that need to be made, the greater the pressure on the man making them.

Work and financial pressures have increased too, as, once again, the world they are making their way in will be very different to their father's. There is no such thing as a job for life any more; employment laws have been eroded to the degree that you may not be particularly well looked after if you do

keep your job; and international outsourcing means there is always somebody in a far-flung country who will do your job for less. Yet the financial pressures of this life stage remain at least as heavy as they always were, and your inherent need to be working will be unchanged.

It is vital that men of this age talk to people, to ease whatever pressure they might be feeling. If that stress is domestic-related, then you have to share it with your partner. Even if the problem is your partner.

Man in his forties

Astonishingly, forty is the cut-off age at which young people (those under thirty) think you become officially "old", a fact which seems to say more about the youngsters than their grizzled counterparts. Furthermore, in recent studies the most popular reason young people gave for their hedonistic behaviour was that they believed they had to whoop it up to the absolute max at that age because there is no fun to be had later. They also believed that not being "young" any more makes people inherently miserable and perpetually resentful of those who still have their youth.

Little do they know. Whoever thought up the title of that old Will Rogers movie, *Life Begins at Forty*, had it exactly right: as you ease into your fourth decade your quality of life is set to drastically improve. You will have developed enough understanding of the world and the people in it to be scared of nothing, and this self-confidence will help you get the best out of whatever you are doing because people will see the best side of you.

At work, you should be able to cope with increased responsibility without your stress levels rising, and you should be earning enough to have eased any financial worries you might have had during the previous decade. Many men are starting to reach their

Be careful of:

Failing eyesight
It's around now you will need reading glasses, even if you've had perfect eyesight up until now.

Weight gain
Your metabolism is performing less efficiently than it has been, yet you are probably still eating as much as you were ten years ago.

Blood sugar levels
Although it is being increasingly diagnosed among younger men, the most likely time for type 2 or adult onset diabetes to appear is in your forties. Men of Indian, African or African-Caribbean heritage need to be particularly vigilant.

Skin cancer
Because it can be a cumulative condition, it is much more prevalent among men of forty and above.

What's good about being fortysomething	What sucks about being fortysomething
You accept the fact you're not indestructible and take your health far more seriously	There are many more potential problems to be aware of
You are more likely now to want to get fit than at any other time	The highest number of exercise-related injuries is among this age group
Your earnings will be high	Your expenditure will be peaking as your family grows
You will rarely indulge in risky behaviour, and you will have considered the consequences	You may be tempted to buy a big motorbike or a sports car
Your family should have settled into a tight, trusted unit with children that no longer need constant attention	Single men in their forties are a notoriously broody bunch
You could well be achieving your career goals	If you haven't, work-related frustration may be starting to boil over
You will be starting to enjoy the good life	You will be much more susceptible to gastric disorders and peptic ulcers
You will be much more confident about discussing feelings and problems with other people – notably your partner	Because your responsibilities have increased – both at work and at home – you will have more potential problems to talk about

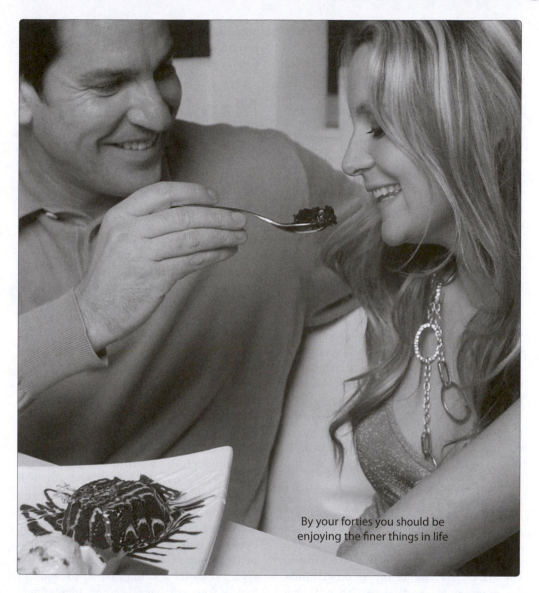

By your forties you should be enjoying the finer things in life

career goals at this time of life, which can be very fulfilling.

However, although most men will have settled on their career by this time, it is never too late to change tack – just make sure any life changes don't have an adverse effect on those around you.

Fortysomething men have become more health conscious than at any previous time in their lives – maybe this is a result of being nagged by their partners, but at least they are doing something about their well-being. Worries about cholesterol levels, heart disease and middle-aged spread mean that, at this age, men are very likely to start a keep-fit programme and begin watching what they eat. Also, it's far from unusual for fortysomething men to quit smoking and cut back a bit on the drink. Not a moment too soon, either. Make sure you are drinking enough water, as it's now your face will start to show wrinkles.

Your family life should, with any luck, be everything you hoped for by now. Time will have developed a relationship between you and your partner that thrives on trust and closeness, while, if you have children, they could be developing into people that you can actually have a conversation with, although you will still be very much in charge of them. You should have more leisure time, and either taking up hobbies or sports or just chilling out will help keep you healthy as it keeps your brain active and lowers your stress levels.

Really, the only downside of being fortysomething is you will start to notice you're not as young as you used to be, and the physical decline that started ten years ago is gathering pace. However, with your new fitness regime you'll easily be able to slow it back down again. Still, it's worth dressing your age. Although you may look in the mirror and see the same lithe twentysomething looking back at you, the chances are the rest of the world sees a middle-aged bloke who for some reason is wearing his son's clothes.

Getting fit at forty

It is at this point in their lives that men start worrying about their fitness levels and weight gain, and more men in their forties embark on exercise-for-fitness programmes (as opposed to sport-related) than at any other age. And they will need to be very careful about it.

Warming up will be even more important for them, as the unexercised cardiovascular system needs to be eased into it gradually to avoid harmful stress, and a heart rate monitor will be money well spent. Stretching and ballistic joint looseners are also necessary, as your tendons and ligaments will be tight and more prone to sprains and strains. An unbreakable rule must be to stop if you feel pain, and don't push yourself too hard in the beginning of your programme.

Man in his fifties

The main thing about your fifties is that, if you're in good shape, they won't be very different from your forties. The kids will be a bit older, your home life will still be steady, you will be safer than you have ever been – you are very likely to be buying sensible, safety-oriented cars and will generally take less risks. You'll also be at low risk of being a victim of assault. The career path will probably have started to flatten out, but you will have a bit more spare cash in your pocket – if the mortgage isn't paid off there can't be much left of it – which is just as well as there are few things in life more expensive than teenage children. But the good side of your kids growing up is that, unless they need money, you'll hardly ever see them, which can be very liberating inasmuch as it allows you and your partner far more time to have fun. Together.

Although you won't be as strong as you once were – muscle density and size will have been in decline for a while now – if you started an exercise regime in your forties this will have minimal detrimental effect. Also, being very fit will mean you have a much better chance of staving off the heart disease, type 2 diabetes and high blood pressure to which you will have become increasingly prone. It will help you keep your weight in check as well, which takes more effort now as your metabolism continues to slow down. It may be advisable for runners to alternate their runs with non-impact exercise, such as swimming. An all-over medical checkup (heart, lungs, blood pressure, cholesterol, diabetes, liver, kidneys and overall fitness): is recommended bi-annually.

You are starting to wear out by now, and your declining immune system means you

Be careful of:

Weight gain
Your metabolism has slowed considerably.

Type 2 diabetes
Statistically, you are more likely to be at risk, so watch your diet and get your blood sugar and cholesterol levels checked at least once a year.

Cancers
Skin, bowel, stomach and lung. If any moles start changing appearance, get them looked at immediately, and if you are a smoker get checked at least four times a year. Or better still, give up.

Declining eyesight
You may need stronger reading glasses.

Stress fractures or joint damage
This particularly applies to those who do impact exercise, like runners.

Digestive complaints
Your system will have got even less efficient as your production of stomach acid will have slowed.

What's good about being fiftysomething	What sucks about being fiftysomething
You are very chilled out about things in general	You've got the highest chance of being laid off at work
You will have more money and an appreciation for the finer things in life	Susceptibility to type 2 diabetes and noticeable weight gain
The likelihood of testicular cancer is by now very low	Cancers of the bowel, skin, stomach and prostate are most likely now
You are less likely to smoke	If you have been smoking all your adult life it is now that it will be doing you obvious and possibly fatal damage
You are in the decade when you are least likely to get injured in a road accident	You are three times as likely to suffer cardiovascular disease than you were a decade ago
The health and fitness regime you adopted ten years ago is really starting to pay off	Your muscles will be naturally much less strong than in the previous decade
You probably spend less time and money in the barbers	Greying male pattern baldness

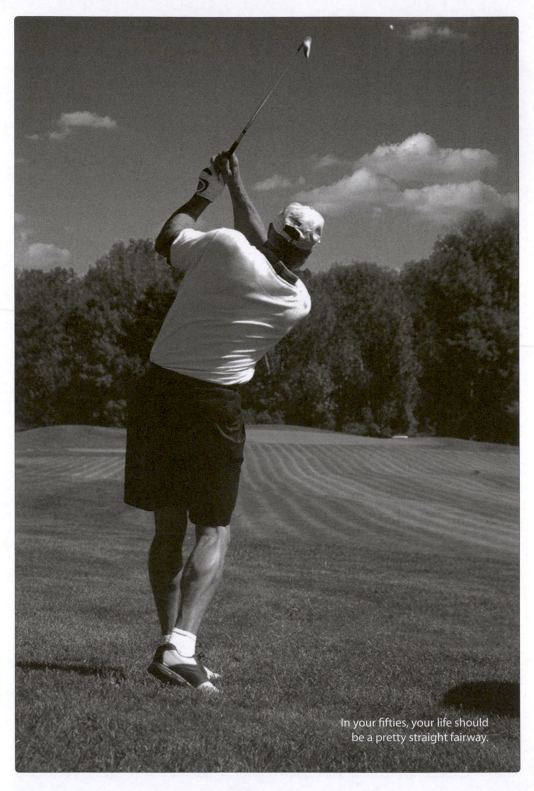

In your fifties, your life should be a pretty straight fairway.

are more susceptible to infection. If you eat right, stay fit and put a bit more effort into looking after yourself though, there's no reason why your fifties should hold you back from anything.

The hangovers don't get worse, but…

The actual dehydration and depletion of nutrients will hit you in more or less the same way it always has and you will have the same wretched morning after. Why it will seem progressively worse as you get older is because the disrupted sleep patterns will have a greater effect – although you will actually need less sleep, what you should be getting is more crucial and missing it far more noticeable. Not that you've got any business being out on the lash.

Man in his sixties (and beyond)

The chances are that as you celebrate your sixtieth, you'll have another twenty birthdays still to come, and that those coming decades can be pretty much pure unadulterated "me time". Welcome to the world of retirement and the chance to take a crack at pretty much anything you've ever had a hankering for. Within reason, of course. Provided you've kept yourself in reasonable shape, you will still be able to do pretty much everything you

Be careful of:

Rapidly declining eyesight
A hardening of the eye's lens and a weakening of the muscles behind it will mean focusing becomes progressively more difficult, starting with the closest field of vision.

Cancers
Get checked regularly for bowel, stomach and lung cancer (especially if you are still smoking) and keep a close lookout for signs of skin cancer.

Low-level infections
Your immune system becomes increasingly less efficient as you get older, meaning you have to make sure you keep it well nourished.

Boredom
Now you've got all this time on your hands there are loads of things you can be getting on with. Have a look online or in your local library to find out what's on offer.

Osteoporosis
Your bones will become progressively less dense than they were, so you need to make sure you keep your calcium intake up – but don't overdo it as that could cause constipation.

What you eat
Your system will be able to cope with junk food less easily, and because you will be naturally eating less you have to make sure your food is as nutrient-loaded as possible.

It's never too late

Four months after a double heart bypass and at the age of 59, Sir Ranulph Fiennes completed the Land Rover 7x7x7 Challenge, and between 26 October and 1 November 2003 he ran seven marathons on seven continents in seven days. Two years later he climbed 8690 metres (28,500 feet) up Mount Everest, then in 2007 scaled the notorious north face of Switzerland's 3970-metre (13,025-feet) Mount Eiger.

What's good about being sixtysomething	What sucks about being sixtysomething
People expect less of you	You will find yourself being patronized
You will be smarter than your younger counterparts thanks to greater experience and a "big picture" way of assessing situations	Your chances of Alzheimer's increases rapidly once you pass 65
Less stress in your life because, once you retire, you have far fewer schedules to keep	Higher potential for boredom and inactivity
Unexpected weight gain or loss will be a reliable early indicator that something is wrong	You will have to work harder to control your weight as your metabolism is still getting slower
You should be free from such money worries as a big mortgage or school fees	Living on a fixed income can cause financial problems
You become less susceptible to heart disease once you get past seventy	Your sixties are the decade in which you are most likely to suffer a heart attack or a stroke
Keeping fit becomes easier because your muscles will work more efficiently	Your muscles are decreasing in mass, density and strength
You understand life to a much better degree and therefore still have an enormous amount to contribute	Ageism from all those young whippersnappers

did before, albeit a bit more carefully.

The biggest barrier to a full and active life as a senior is that senior himself – if you think you're too old to partake in what's going on around you then you probably will be. Follow the example of places like Florida or continental Europe where being old simply means you've lived a little bit longer, and it's no reason not to get involved in anything. People there are fit, sharp and often difficult to keep up with, and quality of life is something of a self-maintaining spiral – because the demand for activities is there, the range on offer is enormous.

Don't be shy about checking out activities or even holidays specifically aimed at the over-sixties. They are often far more exciting than what's on offer in general and will also cater to the standards of comfort you need and expect.

Of course everything will be a bit more of an effort, and your declining hearing and eyesight will be testament to your noticeably wearing out. However, if you are keeping fit then although your muscles are naturally losing density and strength, you will be able to maintain them more efficiently at this age to retain strength.

You should be continuing to work out too, because at this age you will also be susceptible to high blood pressure, strokes and heart attacks. However, it may be easier for you to switch to a non-impact exercise such as cycling or swimming to reduce stress on your bones and joints. A good level of nutrition is vital too, as you will need to work that bit more to maintain your immune system. An all-over medical checkup (heart, lungs, blood pressure, cholesterol, diabetes, liver, kidneys and overall fitness) is recommended every three to six months.

Mentally you will be as sharp as you ever were, with greater analytical abilities, but again this will be down to you as you'll need to give your brain daily workouts to keep it fit. A downside of this, though, is that Alzheimer's and senile dementia become a very real prospect after the age of 65.

It really is still all there for you in your last two or three decades, provided you're willing to put a bit of effort in – both physically and mentally.

Looking after Number One

You could exercise, eat nutritiously, avoid risky situations, get and stay married, do everything within your power to keep yourself fit and healthy, but the chances are, at some time in your life, you are going to have to get professional healthcare. Whatever the reason, and whatever aspect of the service you will be dealing with, it will help if you know how to get the absolute best out of it.

Don't be afraid of the doc

Although this book can give you some good advice on staying healthy, it can't do everything. No matter how well you're taking care of yourself, the law of averages dictates that at some point in your life you're going to have to visit your doctor or go to hospital. And, as you are a man, it's statistically likely that you should have done it a while ago.

The vast majority of men only go so far as to visit the doctor when they feel they are so sick they can no longer do all the things they usually do – work, sport, socializing – without actually collapsing or throwing up, by which time this condition will have had to have persisted for several days. Which means there is virtually no chance of preventative healthcare or regular check-ups.

"Men do not go to the doctor's early enough," maintains our resident family doctor Liliana Risi. "They tend to let a complaint fester until it starts to actually stop them from doing something. It is almost becoming accepted among men that modern life puts so many time pressures on them, it is precluding something as good for them as looking after their health, but it has definitely slipped down the list of priorities.

"That said, no doctor wants people to turn up at the surgery every time they cough. There has to be a balance, and at the moment that balance has shifted away from looking after themselves."

According to the American Academy of Family Physicians, women visit healthcare facilities 2.5 times more often than men, and the reason behind this imbalance was found to be lack of habit-forming education – as girls, women are taught the importance of good personal health and it becomes ingrained. Boys rarely receive such teaching and as a result, from an early age, men believe healthcare is something that isn't for them. Although this credo is usually explained away as the stoicism inherent in "being a man", part of which dictates there will be something honourable in "not making a fuss", underneath it all is a mixture of embarrassment, machismo and fear – mostly fear. Widespread anecdotal evidence among British healthcare professionals suggests that there are several different types of fear involved.

Fear of the unknown is the biggest, as the doctor's surgery or a medical centre is a world that is totally alien to most people, like nothing else they are likely to come into contact with – it even has its own language. This means a feeling of being out of control of the situation, which makes many men very uncomfortable. Indeed even the anticipation of such a state of affairs can be intimidating. Then there is the likelihood that you are going to be told something you won't be overly happy about, which is never a situation most men rush to embrace. Ironically, the mere fact your complaint *might* be serious should give you far greater impetus to get it looked at sooner rather than later.

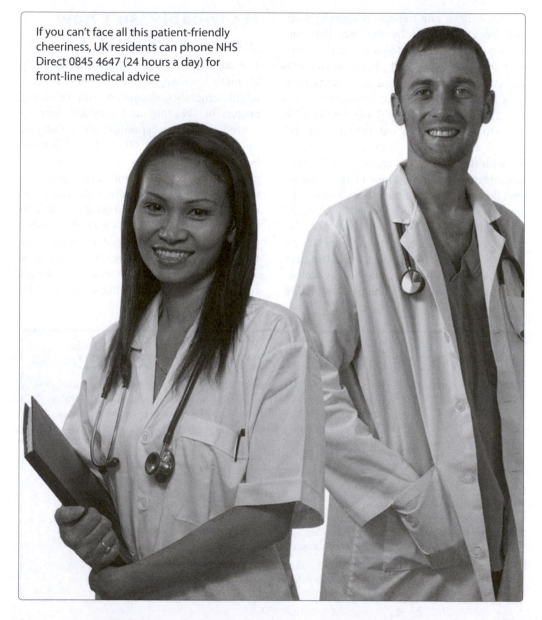

If you can't face all this patient-friendly cheeriness, UK residents can phone NHS Direct 0845 4647 (24 hours a day) for front-line medical advice

F

Fact: Unsurprisingly, married men are far more likely to go to the doctor earlier than single men, as their wives tend to take their health more seriously than they do.

Of course, any feelings of apprehension will be exacerbated by the fact that the reason you've decided to go to the doctor is that you aren't very well, therefore you will feel even more vulnerable. Thus, it takes even greater effort to make that appointment.

This last point deftly illustrates the self-perpetuating cycle of not getting yourself looked at when you should, and there is a widespread view among healthcare organizations on both sides of the Atlantic that this reluctance is contributing to so many men feeling stressed or chronically fatigued.

Again, it's not without irony that the aspects of their lives that get taken much more seriously – work, sport, socializing etc – would be much more enjoyable, effective or efficient if they kept themselves in tip-top condition. But on a more serious level, considering the current widespread levels of diabetes, obesity and sub-optimal nutrition, there is a worry that dangerous conditions are being allowed to develop unchecked.

Although it will take some mental effort on your part to initially break what has probably become a habit, there are a number of steps you can take to make your visit to the doctor easier and far more satisfying.

It probably isn't how you remember it

The days of the depressing-smelling, badly lit doctor's waiting room that some readers might remember, decorated with yellowing posters of skeletons and presided over by a fire-breathing receptionist are a thing of the past. In both the UK and the US there has been a revolution in how healthcare presents itself. Clinics and larger practices increasingly have purpose-built reception areas, designed to put patients at ease and to be as inviting as possible – even the smaller operations have been urged to make their premises more welcoming. Also, now it is accepted that it may take some time to get seen, waiting areas are being designed to be as soothing as possible.

Healthcare facilities aren't just for women

There has been a growing feeling among men that they have been marginalized by modern healthcare organizations, as many believe the services on offer have become increasingly female-centric. This view is particularly prevalent in the US, where a survey conducted by the *American Journal of Public Health* found that nearly one-third of men surveyed claimed they were put off seeking help because they thought health services had become "feminized" in terms of decor, presentation, reading materials and information on offer. The remarkable thing is this apparent gender bias came as the result of campaigns, on both sides of the Atlantic, to make hospital and health centre reception areas more welcoming and patient-friendly across the board.

However, this might just be an excuse. In 2000, in Seattle, to widespread media fanfare, a specifically men-oriented healthcare centre opened under the name The Garage, using motoring metaphors for different areas of healthcare – "fuel injection" (prostate), "tune-ups" (check-ups), "spark plugs" (Viagra) and so on. After six months and only seven patients, it shut down.

Meanwhile, Dr Risi assures us that healthcare facilities are *not* designed to be appealing to women and that men will receive equally thorough and sympathetic treatment.

Why men put off going to the doctor

Reason/excuse	The professionals say	How to get over it
Embarrassment	Doctors and health centre staff now have a much higher level of training as regards communication, discretion and putting patients at ease	Take your partner with you, and remember there is very little a twenty-first-century doctor won't have seen before
It's some sort of reflection on their masculinity	Everybody gets sick, regardless of how macho they are and no doctor would assume there is any shame attached to it	Bear in mind that looking after yourself will help maintain your manliness for longer
Don't have the time	Most health centres and surgeries now have opening hours extended beyond the traditional working day	Find a practice that offers a greater choice of access
Don't want to bother the doctor	That's what doctors are there for, and you will be a great deal more "bother" if you allow yourself to get very sick	Don't worry about imposing on a doctor's time – they haven't got anything else to do during surgery hours
Whinging is generally frowned upon	Looking after yourself is common sense, and would be applauded by a doctor, never thought of as whinging	Don't whinge; conduct a grown-up discussion with the doctor about what might be wrong
Not in men's nature to discuss problems	This is a big hurdle for a lot of men, and it often helps if they take somebody else with them	Take your partner, who may be able to explain your symptoms better than you can
Whatever is wrong will probably go away by itself	Although nobody wants to run to the doctor every time they sneeze, it is always best to go sooner rather than later	In the long term, be more aware of your own body so you can tell the difference between something minor and a potentially serious complaint
Scared of what they might be told	Whatever you are going to discover will definitely not be any less worrying if you find out about it in a month's time	If this is the case, you must be thinking something could be wrong: therefore it is best to get it checked out as soon as possible
Don't like being out of control of the situation	Healthcare professionals are now encouraged to involve the patient as much as possible, because it is vital they feel involved in their consultation and any resultant treatment	Prepare yourself as well as you can before you go, so you can hold a conversation with your doctor

Theses overhauls have increased the functionality of health centre reception areas, inasmuch as the use of space will be designed around patients' needs. Designs take into account patients' desires to move quickly from the entrance to a point at which they can be spoken to, as early contact with a healthcare professional puts a nervous visitor

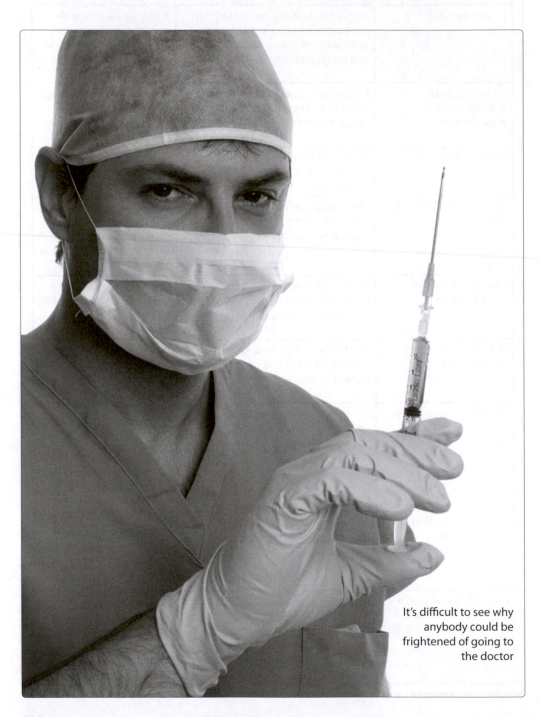

It's difficult to see why anybody could be frightened of going to the doctor

There's no need to go it alone

If you are particularly nervous, or you think it might help you better understand what you are being told, take somebody with you when you visit your healthcare professional. If it is your partner who knows your state of health as well as you do, this could be particularly useful as he/she may be able to bring up points you have forgotten or even be aware of some things you are not. Also, it will make it much easier to discuss and analyse what you were told when you get home. There is no reason whatsoever why a doctor should object to you bringing somebody else to a consultation, but it is always good manners to ask before you do.

at ease. Receptions are now being designed to respect a patient's privacy and wherever possible reception desks are positioned in such a way that conversations cannot be overheard in the waiting area. Also, private reception rooms are becoming standard in larger operations, so visitors can discuss their conditions with far less likelihood of embarrassment.

These improvements shouldn't really come as a surprise, because, as Dr Risi reminds us, "Doctors want to help people too!" She continues: "There has been a great deal of effort put into doctors' waiting areas and the reception areas of larger practices, because it was realized they had to work a bit harder to allow us to give the best healthcare we can. It was realized that if the patient feels alienated at the point of entry to a healthcare facility then that feeling won't get any better while they are waiting, and the consultancy is far less likely to be a satisfactory one.

"Reception staff are being purpose-trained too, to respond to people sympathetically and discreetly and to be aware that they could be putting people off. The addition of private areas at reception is making a difference, because people are finding out they can discuss sensitive or potentially embarrassing issues with total discretion."

Time for health

Three of the biggest barriers standing in between men and their pursuit of good health involve time: they haven't got enough

to be able to go to the doctor; health centre opening hours are inconvenient; the doctor has such a limited amount of time with each consultation, would-be patients don't feel like they are getting anything done. In today's healthcare climate, these are far from insurmountable.

As regards the first point, it comes down to time management and priorities. If you're thinking you don't have time to keep fit, it's a matter of sitting down and plotting how you actually spend the hours in your week – you'd be surprised at how much spare time you actually have. Or if you are really doing things every waking minute of your day, then it's all about weighing up the importance of keeping yourself well against other activities you might be pursuing. According to Dr Risi, men need to move "keeping healthy" much higher up the list of things they could not see themselves doing without. "So many men simply don't take looking after themselves seriously enough – it's why married men tend to have much better health," she says.

Health-centre opening hours, on both sides of the Atlantic, have taken into account the pressures on people's time during working hours and made moves to facilitate appointments. Many establishments now operate shift systems so people can be seen in the evening or early in the morning, or they are as flexible as possible within limited opening times.

The amount of time a doctor will have to see you is a problem that, unfortunately, has not got any better recently. But this isn't his

What you should get checked for and how often

Age	Checkup should include	Frequency
Twenty-something	Heart, lungs, blood pressure, cholesterol, testicular cancer, liver function, kidneys, blood sugar levels, weight/fat, overall fitness	Every two years
Thirty-something	Heart, lungs, blood pressure, cholesterol, prostate problems, testicular cancer, liver function, kidneys, blood sugar levels, weight/fat, overall fitness	Annually
Forty-something	Heart, lungs, blood pressure, cholesterol, blood sugar levels, skin cancer, liver function, kidneys, weight/fat, overall fitness	Annually
Fifty-something	Heart, lungs, blood pressure, cholesterol, blood sugar levels, skin cancer, thyroid problems, liver function, kidneys, weight/fat, overall fitness	Twice a year
Sixty-something and beyond	Heart, lungs, blood pressure, cholesterol, blood sugar levels, skin cancer, thyroid problems, liver function, kidneys, weight/fat, overall fitness	Every three months

or her fault and they will still try to do their very best in the limited time they have – in the UK, among GPs, the average time for a consultation is down to six minutes. In fact, the most common reason people in the UK have given for switching to private healthcare is that they feel the doctor has much more time for them.

But there is no point in putting off a visit or getting frustrated because of this. It is an unfortunate fact of life and the best thing you can do is follow the guidelines below and be as well prepared as possible before you get there.

Help them help you

When you go to visit a doctor, you know they won't have much time and you will want to get the best possible result from your consultation – the latter point is equally important to lengthier private consultations, as you don't want to waste money or need to go back for more repeat visits than you might have to.

Before you go

Make up your mind what it is you are going to see your doctor about – it may help to write it down – and be sure of what it is you are going to tell them. As Dr Risi says, "Take a checklist with you of things you want answered. Don't allow yourself to get

ر der3

knocked off focus and make sure you get across the point that you came there for in the first place. Otherwise you'll have to go back and that won't be the best use of your time or the doctor's."

This may involve a bit of self-diagnosis yourself at home first, and, contrary to popular wisdom, doctors are not averse to this. Dr Risi's view on this, which she believes is prevalent among the medical profession, is that with access to so much health information available online it would be odd if somebody didn't try and find out what was wrong with himself first.

Especially if he is of a group that is reluctant to seek professional help in the first place. It shows you are taking responsibility for your health, therefore taking it seriously. Then on a far more immediate level, any information you can provide about your condition, or the more specific symptoms you can describe, will help them reach a judgement in a shorter space of time.

When you are at the surgery

As well as taking a list of points you want answered, take a list of points you want asked. This may seem a little odd, but what will help your doctor more than anything is knowing everything he/she can about you. "We need," explains Dr Risi, "as complete a picture as we can get of a patient – are you married, what sort of job do you do and so on. This will all help to assess your state of mind, which will have a bearing on your state of health and what, if any, remedies should be prescribed to you."

This will mean that you will need to be prepared to give all sorts of information you might not have considered relevant, and if not asked for a rounded description of your

> # Get the most from your doctor
>
> Prepare well beforehand, so you are sure what your symptoms are.
>
> Write a list of what you want to ask and what you expect to be asked.
>
> Take somebody with you, if it makes you feel more confident.
>
> Volunteer information and hold a conversation with your doctor.
>
> Listen to what he or she is saying.
>
> Write things down.
>
> Don't be afraid to admit you didn't understand something or need it explained again.
>
> Try not to be rushed, but appreciate your doctor has time pressures too.
>
> Follow the advice given and courses of medicine prescribed.

life you should volunteer one. As Dr Risi stresses, a consultation should be more like a conversation and not simply a matter of you sitting down and having somebody with a stethoscope around his/her neck talking at you, and this will go a long way towards alleviating feelings of powerlessness the situation might be causing.

Take notes during your appointment, if you want to. This will have a twofold advantage: it will help you remember points you want to bring up for further clarification and it will help you remember things when you get home.

However, you need to listen. When you are nervous to start off with, and dealing with things you are unfamiliar with, it is very easy to fixate on ticking off the points on your list to such a degree you forget to listen to the answers you are getting.

GP's surgery vs Accident & Emergency

According to Dr Risi, going to A&E will not only put extra strain on an already stretched system, but will not do you the most good either.

"Don't go to casualty with anything other than an emergency or unless you've had an accident. This is very important, because those departments have a role to play, which is to patch up casualties and deal with accidents and emergencies – hence the name. They don't need their premises cluttered up with people who just aren't feeling very well.

Also, they don't specialize in that sort of stuff – illnesses – so if there is anything seriously wrong with you they will have to pass you on to somebody else. That means your treatment will then involve a lot more people and mean coming back for all sorts of appointments. If you're not feeling well, go and see your own doctor!"

At the end of your consultation

Although your time with the doctor will be limited – and he/she will have an internal clock that will wind things up at a certain point – try not to allow yourself to feel rushed. When you are asked if there is anything you didn't understand or anything that wasn't covered, consult your notes and make sure they go over anything you are not clear about or didn't get answered. It will save time for both of you in the long run if you get everything sorted out now.

Once you get out of there

Get any prescriptions filled as soon as possible, complete any courses of medication and make sure you follow any instructions you have been given.

While the modern healthcare professional may be keener on you playing doctor and self-diagnosing, he/she will not be so happy if you start making unilateral decisions as regards your treatment.

A feeling of false security

According to recent surveys in both the UK and the US, there is a wide gap between how men feel about their own health and what their state of health actually is – far wider than it is with women, who tend to have a far more realistic idea of how healthy they actually are. The vast majority of men said they felt their general health was either good or very good, regardless of their weight or eating habits or exercise regimes. What is worrying healthcare professionals is that these feelings of well-being are based on little other than there not seeming to be anything wrong, and this could be storing up serious problems for the future.

Many chronic or creeping conditions such as coronary artery disease, high cholesterol levels or vitamin or mineral deficiency do not necessarily involve feeling bad – or simply get adapted to as a new norm by men who are prepared to put up with them. Left unchecked, potential problems will not be addressed until they make a drastic or life-threatening impact. Far too many men are blasé about their state of health and, while not necessarily assuming something is wrong, be very aware that everything might not be as it should. You

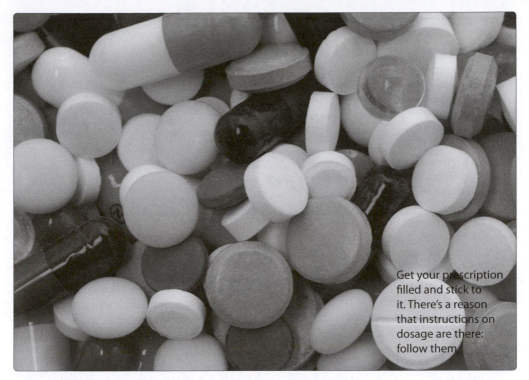

Get your prescription filled and stick to it. There's a reason that instructions on dosage are there: follow them

ought to get checked over by your doctor on a regular basis. At the risk of sounding like a failed Seattle healthcare practice with a motoring gimmick (see box on p.314), it's kind of like an MOT.

Natural alternatives

Currently, all across the Western world people are turning away from conventional healthcare and opting for an alternative approach. According to the World Health Organization, over fifty percent of the populations of Europe and North America have tried complementary or alternative medicines at least once, and in the UK and the US the annual spend on them is £120 million and $17 billion.

But are they any good?

Debate rages as to the value of alternative remedies, and as their effectiveness isn't backed up by the sort of clinical trials that would surround a pharmaceutical development, there is very little hard evidence to say whether they work or not. Although in many examples, there is a logic to some of these cures and it's possible to make sense of how they might work, people tend to arrive at them with a pre-formed viewpoint and are either very black or very white about the whole issue.

Some people will always try something natural first and will only "go chemical" if it doesn't seem to be having any effect. Others wouldn't touch iridology or acupuncture or suchlike with a pole. It is also believed there is a considerable psychological aspect to this and if patients believe whatever they are trying is doing them good, it will be. And there isn't anything wrong with that, either.

Alternative healthcare on the web

nccam.nih.gov
The National Center for Complementary and Alternative Medicine in the US will help you find a local practitioner.

icnm.org.uk
The Institute for Complementary Medicine will do much the same job in the UK, as they keep registers of approved healers.

who.int/mediacentre
The World Health Organization has general background and factsheets on alternative medicine at its media centre.

Although it might not seem like too much help, the best advice you can get as regards alternative or complementary medicine is to suck it and see. Talk to an established complementary medicine practitioner (see box above) as to what might be most suitable for you, then give it a go. Although it might not do you much good, it's unlikely to do you any harm.

Tablets of stone?

When you are given a prescription by your healthcare professional, it's highly unlikely you're going to be able to read what it says, and no more probable that you would know what it meant anyway. But it will always be in your interest to know what it is you are being expected to take and how you should be taking it. Follow this easy checklist and you won't get it far wrong.

1. Ask what you are taking. Not just the type of drugs, but the specific medication. Find out what brand name you are likely to be given by the pharmacist and if any should be avoided.

2. Find out what these pills will do and how they should make you feel. You want to be able to tell if they are working or not, and if there are liable to be any unpleasant side effects. You can always do this online, provided you know exactly what it is you are researching.

3. Make sure there is nothing you shouldn't be doing while taking them, such as driving or drinking.

Private vs public (in the UK)

According to Dr Risi, there are very few reasons for Brits to go private when it comes to healthcare.

"Unless you have a comprehensive private healthcare plan – which will be very costly in itself if you want to be covered for everything – then you are better off with the National Health Service. It does practically everything very, very well, and while it might take a little while longer than in the private sector, the job that gets done will be of the highest standard.

The only time I would recommend somebody to go private is if they have muscular-skeletal problems: the NHS doesn't do them very well. So if you need a long course of physiotherapy for something like a sports injury, you might be better looked after outside the Health Service. Bear in mind it will be expensive."

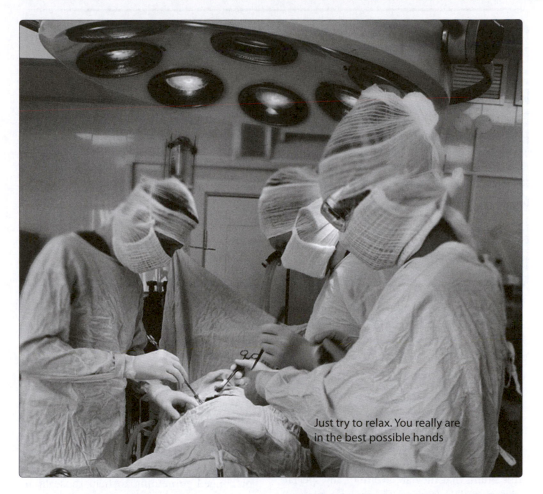

Just try to relax. You really are in the best possible hands

4. Get clear details of the course. This should include how long you need to take them for, how many per day and when they should be taken, for example, after meals or before you go to bed. The pharmacist should supply all this information, but you can never be too prepared.

5. Establish what you should do if you miss a dose. This is important, as there probably will be times when you don't take one, and you need to know what to do to make sure they remain effective without putting yourself in danger.

Going into hospital

In the weeks beforehand

You should have already received an admission letter, stating the time and date of your admission, the name of the ward you will be on and the name of your consultant. Get this photocopied so you can leave a copy with somebody responsible and you can take the original with you when you go.

If you change your mind about going into hospital for any reason, or want to change the date, use the contact number on your admission letter to let them know as soon as possible. That way you stand

If you're not happy with how you've been treated

In the UK, the first action you should take is to write to the doctor concerned and clearly and rationally express your dissatisfaction. Dr Risi says, "Write a constructive letter explaining what was wrong to the doctor concerned. They will welcome such communication as it helps them to help a patient further and to address something they might have been doing wrong. It shouldn't be assumed that if you complain about a doctor then you will get bad treatment in the future."

Beyond that, in the UK, the Patient and Advice Liaison Services, which will be based in your local Hospital Trust or Primary Care Trust, exists for more serious grievances. Then if you still do not get satisfaction from them, the General Medical Council, the British medical profession's governing body, has a complaints procedure that is outlined on their website gmc-uk.org.

In the US, you should start by writing to the doctor concerned, for the same reasons as in the UK, and they should accept it in the same spirit. If that doesn't work, complain in writing to the facility where the doctor practises, and as a final step, contact the relevant state's medical board.

---

the best chance of getting the alternative date you want or a convenient outpatient appointment, and it will allow the hospital the most time to reallocate your bed.

Two days before

Check the time and date you are due in, and call the contact number on your letter to confirm you are coming in. Make sure, at this point, that they are aware of any special dietary, religious or other requirements you might have.

Read the letter to see if the hospital has given any special instructions, such as not eating or drinking for a certain period or not taking medication.

24 hours before

Prepare what you will need to take with you:
1. **Clean pyjamas.** If you don't usually wear them, buy a pair. You may well be spending all day in them and most hospitals don't take kindly to patients kitted out in their underpants or, worse still, even less than that.

2. **Dressing gown and slippers.**
3. **Any medication you are taking.**
4. **Regular clothes.** Under some circumstances you might not have to stay in your pyjamas, and you will need something to wear when you go home.
5. **Washing and shaving kit, including a towel.** Unless you're in a very swanky private set-up, you will hugely appreciate the relative fluffiness of your own towel.
6. **Books and magazines.** Or iPad or Kindle: you'll need something to help those hours pass by.
7. **MP3 player.** If you're not a regular MP3 user, buy an inexpensive one specially and load it up with your favourite tunes. It will greatly lift your spirits and block out the general commotion of the ward.
8. **Tissues and wet wipes.** These will allow you much more independence if you are unable to get out of bed for a bit.
9. **A few quid, some of it in change.** Don't take too much money with you – it's pointless and big hospitals are far from free from petty crime – but you will need something for purchases from the trolley or shop.

On the day

1. Leave time. Leave more time than you think you are going to need to get there by your appointed admission time.

2. Don't drive yourself. There probably won't be anywhere for you to leave your car and you may not be in a fit state to drive when you are discharged.

3. Take a friend or your partner with you. It will be a pretty stressful experience and a reassuring presence will be valuable.

4. Take water. Buy a two-litre bottle of mineral water to take in with you. It will taste better than hospital water and save you having to keep asking for a drink. Unless, of course, you've been instructed not to eat and drink.

On your arrival

1. At the ward's reception make sure the staff are aware of any special requirements you might have.

2. If you have any medication, give it to the staff at this point, with instructions on how you should be taking it.

3. Establish visiting hours and whether there are any restrictions attached. Make a note of them for whoever you are with – many hospitals provide a booklet for patients' friends and relatives.

4. If you are proposing to bring any electrical items in with you, check at this point that it will be permitted.

5. Make sure you wear your identification wristband at all times.

On your discharge

1. Have somebody come and meet you – even if you are going home in a cab.

2. Make sure you fully understand any instructions, medication courses or further treatment schedule you have been given – don't be shy about asking questions or taking notes.

3. Take all your belongings with you from the ward.

4. If you have to pick up a prescription from the hospital pharmacy be prepared to wait a while, so try and time it so you don't keep a cab waiting or make somebody have to find somewhere to park.

Improve your performance

If you've got this far with this book, then you'll be very aware of two basic things: getting fit and improving how your body functions are going to vastly improve your quality of life in every respect; and doing them isn't exactly rocket science. So why are we in the grip of an obesity crisis, with heart disease and type 2 diabetes so sharply on the rise? Because even when faced with so many overwhelming positives, a vast number of people just can't be arsed.

Think fit

Picture yourself, but a more fit and healthy version. Better looking, with more energy. Sharper thinking, better-tempered, perhaps even more popular – certainly more attractive. A different you that gets more out of practically every aspect of your life; a version of you that enjoys sex more, and has more of it. While getting fit involves more than merely thinking about it, to get fit you have to think fit – it is the first step anybody has to take, whatever level of fitness they're starting from, or hope to reach. And it's often the biggest stumbling block.

T

Tip: Keep a bowl of fresh fruit at your workstation. It will be on hand for when you do require a snack, and you will be amazed at how popular you suddenly become, especially with your female co-workers.

Habitually healthy

One of the recurring themes of this book, both in the text and from the panel of experts, has been how changing your habits will be the foundation of getting fit and healthy. This is because to adopt any sort of healthy eating plan or exercise regime on a superficial level – i.e. to do it when you remember, or just when you fancy it – won't in the long term do you any good, as it won't be coming naturally to you. Which means, on a psychological level, it will remain something you don't really want to do and see as an imposition on your life. If you change your habits, then it actually *becomes* your life and anything else will be what you have to go out of your way to do.

The first thing you have to do is break the old habits. Chances are these habits were essentially self-destructive, as they got you into such a state to start off with. Eating badly is the most prevalent bad habit. As Dr Sarah Schenker explained back in Chapter 4, the fast-food industry is such a powerfully marketed affair it's impossible to avoid

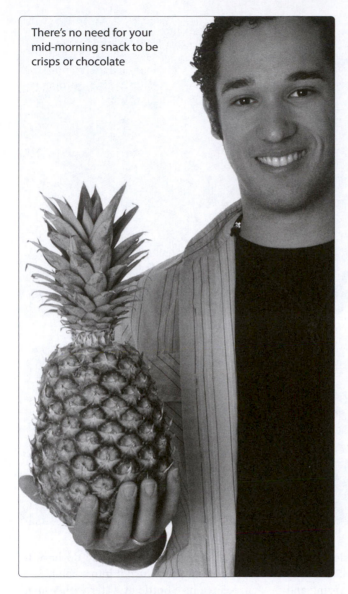

There's no need for your mid-morning snack to be crisps or chocolate

Don't go down to the shop when you have a break; get out of the office rather than sit at your desk with a sandwich; change your walk home from the pub so you no longer pass that kebab shop where they know you by name; hang with a different lunchtime crowd so you're no longer in that pattern of pub on Monday, McDonald's on Tuesday, fish and chips on Friday and so on. The time when you'll have to steel yourself the most is when you put your head down and ignore that very attractive display of Danish pastries when you get your early morning coffee in Starbucks – if you can't think yourself past it then get your coffee elsewhere, preferably an establishment where the staff aren't trained to try and sell you cakes. If you've ever smoked, and given up by going totally cold turkey, you might like to try the same approach to giving up junk food or habitually grazing. Stop dead; don't try to cut down gradually.

It's once you've broken these bad habits that you can start replacing them with good ones. As you remove the nutrient-free snacks you will still need to fuel your body, but now you can replace them with healthy food. Fruit, salads or yoghurt make convenient snack food, and get into the habit of drinking water, as not only will this keep your stomach full and remove the temptation to pop a can of soda, you really do have to work to keep yourself properly hydrated.

unhealthy eating opportunities: what were once called meals, of which we had three square ones a day, have now been relegated to "eating opportunities".

It's this widespread habit of grazing and snacking throughout the day that should be where you start. While you will need to think yourself out of reaching for the crisps or the chocolate bar or the fizzy drink, you can make it easier on yourself by avoiding certain situations that encourage bad eating.

Then, if you start to regulate the chaos out of our eating opportunities and turn them back into "proper" meals at "proper"

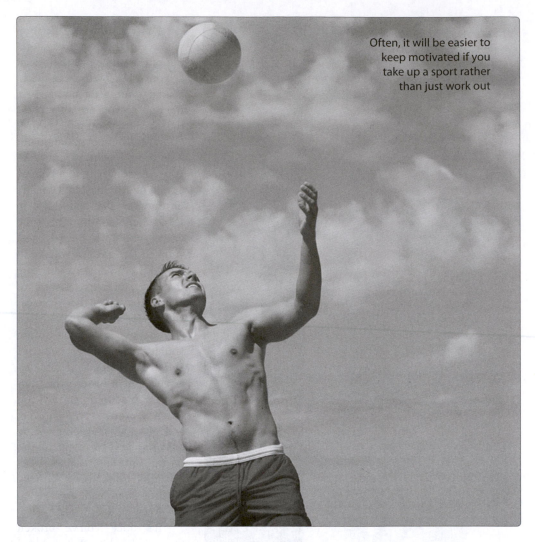

Often, it will be easier to keep motivated if you take up a sport rather than just work out

mealtimes, you will feel physically less inclined to snack. After this, it could only be force of habit that keeps you grazing and you'll just have to think yourself through it.

Get a drink habit

It's not just about what you eat, of course. Keeping lubricated helps keeps you fit. If you measure your water consumption over the course of, say, a week, you'll be surprised at how little you do in fact drink. To actually take on board the required two to three litres of water a day, you really do have to consciously work to turn it into a habit.

Keep a litre bottle of water with you all of the time, and perpetually swig from it in idle moments or while you are thinking about something. Eventually this will become like a nervous tic, in the same way as a smoker might spark up under the same circumstances, and that will be how you will genuinely keep yourself properly hydrated. Also, getting through a bottle with a predetermined amount in it will allow you to judge what you are drinking far more accurately than by filling glasses.

Supermarket sweep

You will need to change your shopping habits too. To get your new routine off to a good start, avoid big supermarkets, as they spend fortunes on creating environments in which you will buy pretty much what they want you to buy, rather than what is actually good for you. Until you are sure about your new shopping list, don't let them manipulate you into going astray. This may initially be slightly inconvenient, but you will thank yourself for it in the long run and you can always go back once you're confident about what you want.

Start at small shops – butcher, greengrocer, fishmonger – or market stalls, where the choice will be much greater and whoever is serving you will be able to give you advice on storing, preparing and cooking what you are about to buy. Just try to avoid their very busy periods and you will be surprised at how much benefit there is to be had from striking up a relationship with a shopkeeper or stallholder.

Routine fitness

As regards getting fit and staying fit, it is equally important that this becomes a habit; in fact your exercise routine needs to become as much a part of your regular routine as brushing your teeth or putting your phone in your pocket before you leave the house. If you can find just half an hour three times a week to get fit, it will pay genuine dividends if it becomes a habit.

Rather than look for random thirty-minute periods during your week, set aside specific times and adhere to them rigidly. Then make yourself stick to them in exactly the same way as you wouldn't miss the kick-off of a match, or not bother to turn up to a university lecture or forget to go to work.

In the beginning this may take some mental effort, especially if it involves getting out of a warm bed an hour or so earlier, but if you carry on then very soon it will become simply something you do, rather than something you have to go out of your way to do. You'll know when you've hit that level, because you will be adjusting other stuff in your life – like not staying out

---

Six quick fixes to get you off your sofa

Treat yourself to some brand new, hi-tech exercise kit You won't want to feel you've wasted the money, and if you look like somebody who ought to be working out, you'll feel much more like somebody who ought to be working out.

Get changed into those same hi-tech exercise clothes Eventually you'll get fed up with people asking you, "Are you going for a workout then?"

Have your gym buddy come and call for you If you can't nag yourself into getting started, then arrange for somebody else to do it.

Have a stretch You'll release endorphins, and immediately feel so much livelier, and your loosened, increased-blood-flowing-through-them muscles will start urging you to use them.

Tell yourself you're not going to do too much Opt for your most basic workout, then once you get started it's pretty much guaranteed you'll want to increase it.

Check out the TV schedules Repeats, reality and rubbish: there is probably no better motivation for getting out of the house.

late or on the lash – to fit around what has become an immovable fixture.

Fairly soon after that, you will get to a point where if you do skip a session your body lets you know because it's so used to expending increased energy at a particular time it was looking forward to it. This might mean that you will become a bit restless or feel frustrated, but it also means that, because you now truly have the exercise habit, unless you are physically laid up you will definitely not miss the next session. Of course, changing your life isn't all about beating yourself around the head with health and fitness. Be sure to take the odd weekend off and revisit some of your

How to keep going once you've started

Keep a record While this is an incredibly obvious thing to point out, you would be surprised at how many people don't keep a long-term training log of what they have been doing. There are numerous fitness websites that will offer an interactive log. The majority are dedicated to running or triathlon, but progresslog.com and activelog.com are good for all-round fitness records – or you could just do it the old-school way, with an exercise book and a pen. Either way, looking back at how much progress you have made is a powerful force to make sure you carry on.

Keep a record in photographs Everybody's got some sort of digital camera, so keep a week-by-week series of snapshots of yourself and how your body shape and general appearance have been changing since you started your regime. A good idea with this is to store it on your computer as a slide show. You could use it as your screensaver as a reminder of what you have achieved.

Set a target Having a tangible goal to reach in a certain amount of time is as vital as keeping a record. Moving steadily towards a specific target is the best way for many people to keep motivated; however be aware of the next point.

Don't set the wrong target For some people, overambitious targets can become a massive de-motivator, as they put an unnecessary stress on your exercise/healthy eating plan and turn it into a chore rather than something you should look forward to. Targets that are unreachable can have the same effect, while if you set your bar too low you won't get any benefit, thus won't see any improvement and will be much less inclined to continue.

Reward yourself Put a pre-decided amount of money in a jar for every inch you lose around the middle or put on around your chest, or kilogram you drop on the scales, and then after a couple of months use that cash to treat yourself. Ideally to something not very good for you (see next point).

Enjoy a blowout: a few drinks or a fine cigar There's no reason at all why you shouldn't do this every so often, because you will be able to do so without feeling guilty, while secure in the knowledge that your newly tuned body can handle it. Being able to cut loose occasionally will stop your fitness regime turning into a prison sentence – or at least make sure it's one with time off for good behaviour.

Put on a suit you haven't worn since last year This will make you feel doubly good about yourself – for losing the inches off your gut and cancelling out one of the most miserable things about putting on weight, that clothes you really like no longer fit you.

Buy some new clothes This will help you see yet another benefit to your newly toned body, and if you take your other half with you to help you choose, you'll be doing yourself another favour.

Go and see somebody you haven't seen for ages Because you've been getting in shape gradually, people around you won't really have noticed, but to look up somebody who hasn't seen any of it should really ramp up your compliment intake.

old haunts and bad habits. Everything in moderation; even moderation.

Motivational difficulties

One of the reasons getting started can be a problem is that you might be unsure why you want to do it in the first place. This isn't as straightforward as it might seem. One of the problems with how we live today is that so often we need to have an apparently valid reason for everything, and it has to be a reason that would stand up to scrutiny from those around us. It's not unusual for people to believe that unless there is a tangible and fairly immediate justification for doing something, it must somehow be a waste of time.

It's a situation not unlike the state of affairs described in Chapter 6: people not wanting to do nothing and requiring constant stimulation, and in this case just doing something, apparently for the sake of it, is often viewed as downtime. Then, to add to that, the most common reasons for getting fit and healthy are usually vanity-based, and also involve admitting you'd been getting something wrong in the first place.

This is why so many young(ish) men's only physical exercise is playing sports, because it makes obvious sense as to why they are doing it. Or they go running, because aiming to do a 10K or a marathon or something has a far greater sense of purpose to it and there's absolutely nothing vain or girly about it, thus it can be talked about without becoming the butt of anybody's jokes. It is, as Gideon Remfry said earlier, men in their thirties and forties who take up fitness for fitness sake, because, by that age, they are more aware of what is happening to them and are far less concerned with what is being said

B

Best investment: runner's backpack These marvellous pieces of kit have extra, cleverly positioned straps that hold the bag tight to your back, meaning there's a minimum of movement while you run, while cutaway sides allow your arms to pump unhindered. As a result, you can run to or from work and either have clothes to change into. or not have to leave your regular clothes on the back of your chair. The better models are waterproof, sturdily constructed with plenty of closable internal compartments to stop the contents shifting around, have an easily accessible pocket for a water bottle use breathable fabric where it is held against your body. Although they will cost around three times the price of an everyday backpack, you will soon claw that back with the amount you save in fares. Even if you are not a runner, having a backpack

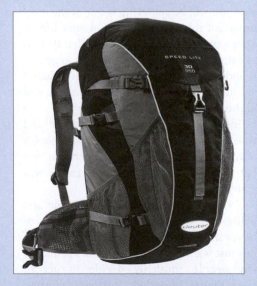

this figure-hugging will be much easier on your back than a regular model.

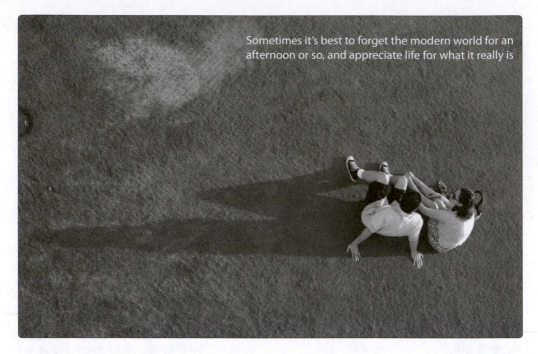

Sometimes it's best to forget the modern world for an afternoon or so, and appreciate life for what it really is

about them. Also, practically all of their peers are in the same state.

Again, it's a matter of mind over body, and it is important to acknowledge that although the motivation may be essentially superficial, what you will be achieving is one of the most important things you can do in your life. In other words, it has to be realized that there is no better way to spend your time than getting fit and healthy, if for no other reason than it will ultimately give you more time to spend on the "important" things in life.

Effua Baker, a personal trainer and fitness consultant, talks of most people's motivation being essentially superficial, but that shouldn't be allowed to get in the way of anything:

"I don't get people coming to me and saying they want to raise their VO^2 max or they want to improve how their heart beats; they just want a better body. That's primarily why people suddenly decide to get fit when they're into their thirties or forties. So many of them don't even want to know how it all works, just as long as they're losing the pounds.

Which is fine. It doesn't really matter why they're doing it to start off with, because once they start looking better they also realize how they feel better too and they'll probably have got into the habit by then and will keep it up. It shouldn't matter why you start as long as you do."

Engaging a personal trainer when you start your fitness programme can do wonders for your motivation, and should keep you on course until it's become a habit. This is because a personal trainer will not only gee you up at every opportunity, but if he/she is good, you will not want to fail him/her and you definitely won't want to have wasted the money you've spent on him/her.

But if even getting as far as the gym is a problem, then a good way to start might be to turn your routine into exercise: start cycling or walking to work. You can buy a runner's backpack (see box on previous page) to put your regular clothes in. Or mix things up: get to work by your usual method of transport in the morning, but run home from work a couple of evenings a week. You'll quickly notice how much money you save, and will probably find cycling or jogging to be a much less stressful, and much more fulfilling way of getting from A to B.

Will our lifestyles be the death of us?

The idea that twenty-first-century stress is running us down has been discussed in several places in this book, in different lifestyle situations, with phrases such as "these days" or "as part of the modern lifestyle" cropping up again and again. While modern times aren't killing us, they are making it much easier for us to slowly do ourselves in. Or at the very least, providing every opportunity we need to make ourselves unhealthy, overweight and miserable.

The problem is, we've evolved beyond our needs. Unlike every other animal we share the planet with, we can adapt our surroundings to suit us, rather than adapting to fit what happens to be there. Which means although we are still creatures of instinct to a degree, we are creating environments that are at odds with those instincts, to the detriment of what is actually best for us. So much of how we live today is because of the world we have created. We are almost serving it instead of the other way around.

There are straightforward physical elements to this, and the most obvious manifestation is in our recent eating habits, and how they were developed to save us time – rather than to nourish ourselves. Then there is the lack of the exercise we need to keep ourselves functioning efficiently. We have simply evolved it out of ourselves: nobody walks anywhere any more and physical labour is being progressively replaced with jobs in call centres, all in the name of progress. Then those of us sitting at

Sort your life out

There's nothing wrong with getting fit simply for the sake of it: don't view it as time wasted, because although there might not seem to be any immediate gain, it will affect every aspect of your life. You will feel so much more energized.

Accept you are going to have to work at changing some of your habits. This might include habits you may not even have realized are doing you any harm.

Don't take the easy option. Cooking real food from real ingredients, or walking to work rather than getting the bus, may seem like an imposition to start off with. But stick with them and they will become interesting and fun in themselves.

Think positive. Read up on mindfulness, a technique of "living in the moment" and recontextualising outside influences. (The books by writer and physician Dr Jon Kabat-Zinn are a good place to start.) It gives you the best chance of finding something good in every situation.

Act your age and you will get on in life much more successfully, and ultimately be much happier.

Remember that anything worth having is worth waiting for. Therefore, with something as worthwhile as getting fit and healthy, it is definitely going to be about the long game.

Don't forget it's not going to be all right all the time – things will go wrong. You just have to roll with it and carry on.

Realize you might not be paying your partner quite enough attention: when you put it in the perspective of the rest of your life, this will probably become obvious.

Cheer up!

computer screens all day are dehydrating and going down with several different RSIs.

These physical states of affairs can be dealt with, as the last three hundred or so pages have been explaining, but less palpable is the effect they are having on us mentally. And this is even more insidious as it stops us performing in the way we need to if we want to do anything about our physical health.

Being sad is okay

One of the reasons so few of us are getting everything we can out of life is because we have worked so hard to manage our moods that much of what we need to personally progress is lacking, and our appreciation of the lives we are living is being compromised. Dr Sandra Scott believes this is due to our obsession with engineering out anything we might not like, and refusing to feel unhappy about anything. Here's what she has to say about it:

"It's all right to feel sad. In fact you're supposed to. Having a low mood is a perfectly normal experience – if something bad happens, you feel bad about it. In fact, if something bad happens and you don't feel bad about it, that's when something can be wrong. Western societies today encourage a quick-fix attitude. We are surrounded by techniques, pills and gadgets to remove negative stimuli as quickly as possible. Thus, the subliminal message is that we should not have to put up with it. We should not even try to. And this has led many people to have a very low tolerance of negative stimuli of any sort, when the correct response is actually that we should tolerate it. More than that, we should accept it and learn to cope.

Because we can always get instant gratification for hunger or pain, we don't have to put up with them any more and now we have that sort of response to our sadness:

'I don't want to go through it, I don't want to tolerate it. I want it to go away *right now*.' We want a quick fix for it, but this is storing up problems for the future, as when sad things happen the normal response is to be sad. You have to endure that sadness, learn to live with it, accept it and it will pass. And that's an important part of the human condition. We need to learn these coping skills, as without this inner resilience we can become dependent on external escape routes such as illicit drugs, legal drugs, alcohol, television etc and find ourselves turning to them automatically every time we are a bit blue. All of these escape routes invariably come with a negative price tag, which gets greater with time and usage.

Experiencing sadness is important for your state of happiness – you can't fully appreciate the good parts of your life unless you accept and experience the bad parts. If you're really thirsty and somebody gives you an ice-cold drink, you appreciate it much more than if you were not thirsty in the first place. Food tastes better after working up a ravenous appetite with a taxing workout. Finally completing a difficult and exacting task gives a wonderful sense of achievement.

Sadness is happiness's twin – they're yin and yang. It's by experiencing the negatives that you fully appreciate the positives, and if you refuse those bad experiences, it actually reduces your ability to fully experience happiness. People would generally feel a lot better if they went along with their emotions a bit more and stopped trying to shut them off."

Reasons to be cheerful

Dr Liliana Risi, a GP, believes that many people who come to see her would be much better off – and in her surgery less often – if they just cheered up. One of the overwhelming assumptions about modern living is that it is guaranteed to be stressful; and that we all have endless pressures on us and things to worry about. This isn't really the case, according to Dr Risi, who believes we are no better or worse off now than we ever were, and this state of mind is contributing to a general feeling of malaise.

"It would be naive to say that everybody's lives were perfect, and that there was nothing to worry about. But so many people don't look at the positives and what they have to be happy about. Too often this state of unhappiness – the so-called stresses of life – are simply down to what is going on around you, that you have little control over or that won't really be adding to your life.

Mindfulness is the practice of being aware of what is happening in the present, at that moment. And focusing on that and everything that is positive about it. It allows you to slow down and realize that happiness is about what you make of your life at that time: it will let you discover what there is to be happy about. It can promote better health because it can relieve chronic stress and all that goes with that."

Mindfulness is based on ancient Buddhist teachings, and has gained a lot of ground among the Western healthcare professions as having a usefulness in the treatment of depression and stress. In the UK, Bangor University is host to the non-profit Centre for Mindfulness Research and Practice, and the university's website provides plenty of information: bangor. ac.uk/mindfulness

Be happier with your partner

You can improve your home life by taking a very simple piece of advice from Sarah Hedley, who maintains there's absolutely no reason why men and women shouldn't get along much better. Providing we put a bit more thought and effort into it.

"It can get difficult for men to work out what they're meant to be. We say that in a relationship we want a best friend but a lover as well – which is very difficult, because as a best friend you will be non-sexualized. It's difficult to keep a relationship erotically charged and still be able to talk to him about your period problems. And finding both those roles in the one person is difficult.

It all boils down to keeping that erotic side of the relationship going once you've established that best friendship and that trust. Maintain that erotic side, and to do that you need to spend time creating that erotic space and that erotic time. You have to literally work on your relationship, especially if you've got kids.

You need to give it the same amount of planning as you do to your career and your hobby. Draw a bar chart of your time on any given week and fill in how much time you have devoted to each aspect of your life, and I'll bet that in every single case the bit dedicated to sex or intimate time with your partner would be tiny. And I'm not talking just about doing it, but planning it, preparing it, thinking about what you will do. Spending time on it. The only effort people do put into this sort of activity is in the early parts of their relationship, so you should think back to then and use that as a model.

We spend time on our jobs, on our children, on our hobbies and with our friends, but we underestimate what sex actually means to us. Then every time we have to think about it in these sorts of terms we tend to start thinking about it as a chore, but go back to the benefits. True, you don't get any money for it, you don't get a bigger house, but it'll make life much more enjoyable for you and your other half. I'll bet she won't have it any other way."

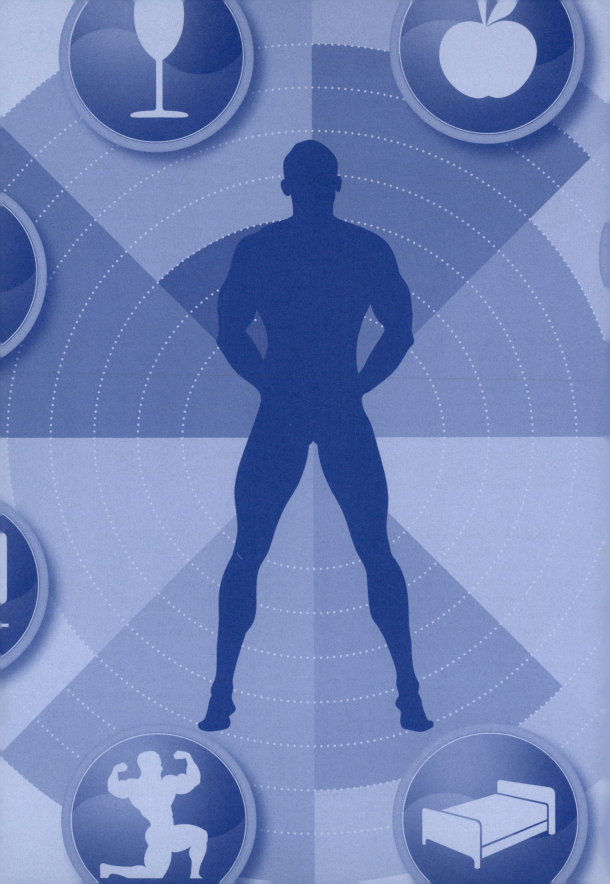

PART 3
REFERENCE

How bad could it be?

The list of ailments that afflict the modern man is a long one, but most of them aren't too serious and can be dealt with at home – usually it's simply a matter of giving up smoking and changing your diet. Here is a handy A–Z of what is most likely to strike you down.

A

Acne
An outbreak of blackheads or whiteheads, creating eruptions from under the skin.

Causes
An excess of sebum (oil) produced by the skin, brought on by the surge in male sex hormones, combining with the protein keratin and the clogging up of hair follicles. It can also be the result of internal toxins not being efficiently processed (for instance, as a side-effect of constipation or an inefficient liver).

Symptoms
A multitude of spots on your face, sometimes merging together into an angry-looking rash.

Treatment
Over-the-counter treatments include chemical facial masks, which dry out the top layer of skin to remove it and release trapped oil. Antibiotics may be prescribed.

Self-help
Don't squeeze the spot, as this will disperse some of the oil back under your skin; instead gently stretch the skin around it to create an opening big enough to slowly manipulate all the oil out. Large doses of zinc (3 x 30mg per day) and vitamin B complex have been shown to reduce acne, while beetroot juice, kale or celeriac will cleanse the liver and boost its performance.

Prevention
Regular washing of the face with light, unscented soap will keep oil levels down, but over-washing will irritate and inflame the skin. Cutting down on processed foods – particularly sugar and saturated fats – will help.

AIDS
Acquired Immunodeficiency Syndrome is the last, potentially lethal, phase of the Human Immunodeficiency Virus (HIV).

Causes
HIV has invaded the body and multiplied to destroy enough of the body's immune system (CD4 lymphocytes) to render it useless. This may take weeks, months, years or even decades.

Symptoms
Initially there are none, then fatigue, swollen

lymph nodes, loss of appetite, weight loss, increasing susceptibility to infections and viruses and purple lesions on the skin.

Treatment

There is no cure for AIDS, although antiretroviral drugs can successfully maintain the immune system for much longer than would have been thought possible in the 1980s and 90s. The infections that come about because of a compromised immune system can be treated with drugs just as they would be otherwise.

Self-help

Keep yourself as healthy as possible, and follow your doctor's orders and antiretroviral prescriptions.

Prevention

Practise safe sex, and do not, if at possible, allow yourself to receive a blood transfusion in a high-risk country. Needless to say, injecting any recreational illegal drugs is a very stupid idea.

Alcoholism

Psychological dependence on alcohol, leading to uncontrollable continued use, regardless of adverse effects. Alcoholism is classified as a "chronic disease".

Causes

As with any drug, the root cause of the addiction is likely to be psychological, but physical dependence on alcohol comes about after prolonged heavy drinking.

Symptoms

Needing rather than merely wanting a drink; drinking to feel "normal" rather than intoxicated; drinking regardless of the appropriateness of the time or place; losing interest in activities that don't involve drinking; ignoring – or simply being unaware of – the problems your drinking is causing in the rest of your life. Physical symptoms of advanced alcoholism include: damage to the liver, which can affect the rest of your system as it will process toxins less effectively; gastric problems, as alcohol damages the stomach

Ageing (the effects of)

The symptoms of getting on in years include a general slowing down, getting weaker, organs not functioning as efficiently and skin looking drier and wrinkly. While there isn't that much you can do to stop this – your body was only designed to last about eighty years and will start to wear out a couple of decades before that – you can minimize the effects by tackling the different manifestations individually.

Cardiovascular exercise will keep your heart from stiffening up and make sure it beats with strong strokes, and it will also maintain the lung capacity that is naturally starting to shrink. Strength and flexibility training staves off the decrease in muscle strength, the toughening of muscle fibres and stiffening of the joints. If your includes an impact exercise such as running, it can help keep the bones strong to guard against osteoporosis.

Maintaining a healthy diet will be vital, as your body will not be able to cope with processed foods as well as it used to, plus you will need every bit of nutrition you can get. In later life, the amount you are eating will have gone down, but you will need the same amount of nutrients, so you may need supplements. Drinking plenty of water is crucial, as is dietary fibre, because the likelihood of constipation increases with age, and the antioxidant vitamins A, C and E will slow down cell damage by free radicals, which contributes enormously to the ageing process.

Keep your brain in shape too, with daily workouts such as crossword puzzles, quizzes or sudoku. And don't stop thinking about things.

lining; general nutrition issues, as you will not be absorbing vitamins and minerals properly; heart disease, as your blood pressure will be raised; and diabetes, because alcohol impedes the release of glucose into your system from the liver.

Treatment

There are residential treatment programmes available for the more seriously addicted. These involve detoxification periods, treatment of the different alcoholism-induced conditions, psychological support and therapy addressing the compulsion to drink. In severe cases, there is drug treatment which will prompt severe reactions to alcohol such as vomiting or headaches.

Self-help

Be aware that you might have a problem. If you do accept it, then you can work to do something about it, by contacting a support group such as Alcoholics Anonymous.

Prevention

If you find you are drinking on your own on a regular basis, cut down. Have a look at how many units per week are considered safe. Think seriously about whether you might have a problem.

Allergies

Physical reaction or sensitivity to an ingested food or a substance breathed in or brought into contact with the skin.

T

Tip: Research in the USA discovered that nearly every allergy-sensitive subject benefited hugely by switching from drinking tap water to bottled mineral water. Allergy-sufferers may wish to consider getting a filter tap system fitted to their kitchen sink.

Causes

Pollen, pollution, food additives, pesticides, wheat, dairy, animal fur, nuts, shellfish… the list of substances that bring out an allergic reaction in somebody is pretty much endless in the twenty-first century. Allergies are very likely to be passed on down the generations.

Symptoms

Sneezing, runny nose, rashes, coughing, breathing difficulties, watering eyes; severe allergic reactions may trigger anaphylactic shock which is potentially fatal, as it can cause a massive drop in blood pressure and difficulty breathing because of bronchial constriction.

Treatment

Allergies are usually determined by skin testing, in which a minute amount of various substances is injected into marked areas of skin with reactions observed and recorded. There is a range of drugs used to inhibit the actions of many allergens – these include cortisone, antihistamine, hydrocortisone and adrenaline – or immunotherapy may be used. This introduces progressively larger doses of the allergen to the system in order to build up antibodies, much like vaccination.

Self-help

As regards food allergies, there is some evidence to show that maintaining healthy gut flora, through probiotic supplements, will reduce susceptibility.

Prevention

Avoid whatever it is you are allergic to. Those at risk of severe anaphylactic shock should always carry injectable epinephrine (adrenaline) with them.

Alzheimer's Disease

A progressive, irreversible disease that destroys brain cells.

Causes

Old age, but there is also increasing evidence of genetic disposition. In a proportion of people over the age of 65, some brain cells stop working properly, which affects their communication with others. Internal circuitry starts to break down and without the stimulation cells die.

Symptoms
Alzheimer's is the biggest single cause of senile dementia. It causes problems with long- and short-term memory and thinking in general.

Treatment
There is currently no cure for Alzheimer's, although there are drugs available to strengthen the connections between brain cells and so lessen the effects of the initial stages.

Self-help
Ultimately you have to trust those around you to look after you.

Prevention
Alzheimer's cannot be prevented, but can be slowed down in some cases.

Anaemia
A deficiency in haemoglobin – which can either be qualitative or quantitative – the oxygen-bearing molecule inside red blood cells.

Causes
Insufficiency of iron or the nutrients needed to absorb it into the system – such as folic acid, vitamin B12 and vitamin C. Anaemia

F

Fact: The average man has around 25 trillion red blood cells in his body, which make up about one-third of his total cell count. They have a surface area larger than other cells in order to maximize oxygen absorption, yet are flexible enough to squeeze into the tiniest blood vessels.

can also be caused by internal bleeding from gastric ulcers or within the colon.

Symptoms
Fatigue, pallor, inability to concentrate, irritability, brittle nails. Gastrointestinal bleeding will cause black or bloody faeces.

Treatment
A blood test will determine whether you are anaemic – your doctor can do this – and it will be addressed with iron or nutrient supplements; if it is the result of internal bleeding those causes will be treated separately.

Self-help
If you think you might be anaemic, step up your intake of iron, folic acid and vitamins B12 and C with a course of supplements. However, be careful not to overdo the iron, as this can cause constipation and in severe cases damage your liver.

Prevention
Make sure your diet includes plenty of leafy green vegetables, wholewheat flour and wheatgerm, red meat and liver. Avoid excess black coffee and tea, as it inhibits the absorption of iron into your system.

Angina
A symptom of coronary artery disease becoming established.

Causes
Due to a narrowing of the arteries, the heart muscle is not getting enough oxygen-rich blood and attacks will often be brought on by physical exertion when the oxygen requirements increase.

Symptoms
Pain in the centre of the chest, feeling like a weight pushing down on it or a band squeezing it. This pain may spread upward to the neck and it will often be accompanied by breathlessness, dizziness and sweating. If you have such an attack, seek medical attention immediately.

Treatment

Glyceryl trinitrate, as a spray or tablets, is used to relieve attacks as it immediately relaxes the blood vessels, increasing blood flow; cholesterol-lowering drugs may be prescribed to help clear your arteries.

Self-help

Taking an aspirin every day reduces the blood's stickiness, to allow it to flow more easily; root ginger and freshly ground black pepper improve the circulation; garlic and omega-3 fatty acids thin the blood.

Prevention

Avoid cholesterol-rich foods, do not smoke (it thickens the blood) and eat plenty of fibre, which will help regulate your cholesterol levels.

Anorexia nervosa

An eating disorder manifesting itself in excessive self-imposed restrictions on food and an irrational fear of gaining weight. Often accompanied by a distorted body self-perception. Not as uncommon among men as you might think – an estimated ten percent of cases are male, which means around nine thousand in the UK every year.

Causes

There may be a number of psychological reasons, but low self-esteem, wanting to be thin (and therefore "good looking") are common among sufferers. There is a theory that a sufferer could be genetically predisposed to the condition, and some evidence that, because the condition is so self-harming, the area of the anorexic's brain that regulates metabolic function may be faulty.

Symptoms

Radical loss of weight, fatigue, hair loss, erratic sleep patterns, irritability, withdrawal, constipation, low blood pressure, renal failure, depression.

Treatment

Weight gain is most important in the treatment of anorexia, then therapy or counselling to address the causes of the problem. Hospitalization may be necessary for advanced cases.

Self-help

Admitting you might have a problem is the first step. Doctors say the biggest hurdle to treating anorexics is that they refuse to believe there is anything wrong.

Prevention

Try to accept yourself and your body shape as being exactly what it should be. The most important thing is that you are healthy. If you think you do need to lose weight, see your doctor.

Anxiety attacks

Also known as panic attacks, they are sudden episodes of intense alarm or fear.

Causes

The system is reacting to what it perceives to be a threat, and releases adrenaline to prompt our body's fight-or-flight mode. But because there is nothing to physically react to – the cause of an anxiety attack is often irrational – the adrenaline is not used up and its internalization causes the physical symptoms.

Anorexia and bulimia

Both result in a dangerously low body weight. Anorexia sufferers avoid eating and exercise obsessively; bulimics eat either normal or abnormally large amounts of regular food then induce vomiting before it is digested. Bulimics will also take laxatives and diuretics, but generally do not lose weight as radically as anorexics.

Symptoms

Accelerated heartbeat, breathlessness, difficulty swallowing, raised blood pressure, dizziness, chest pains and blurred vision. Anxiety attacks will often be followed by spells of melancholy.

Treatment

Therapy or counselling will establish the root cause of the attacks, then work to understand and eliminate the anxiety caused.

Self-help

Relaxation techniques can assist you being less anxious in general; breathing exercises will help if an attack comes on. Reminding yourself that panic attacks are a very common occurrence among all sorts of people, that they are temporary, and not symptomatic of any real physical danger, will significantly help.

Prevention

Addressing the psychological cause of the panic is the only way to stop the attacks; merely avoiding their triggers will only put them off.

Apnoea

Obstructive sleep apnoea is the temporary cessation of breathing while sleeping.

Causes

Hypopnoea; fatigue.

Symptoms

The muscles of the throat relax so much during sleep they collapse inwards causing a complete blockage of the airways; hypopnoea is a partial blocking of the airways that reduces airflow by around fifty percent. Breathing stops for around ten seconds at a time, resulting in fractured sleep patterns as this will be enough to bring you out of deep sleep into lighter sleep or briefly wake you up completely.

Treatment

Turning to sleep on your side can help.

Self-help

Avoid alcohol within two hours of going to sleep, as it will overly relax the muscles in the throat. Smoking during the evening will contribute to increased mucus production, which in turn will contribute to the blocking of the throat.

Prevention

Lose some weight: if you are obese, you are much more likely to suffer from OSA.

Appendicitis

An infection of the appendix, which is an apparently pointless side-turning of the intestinal system.

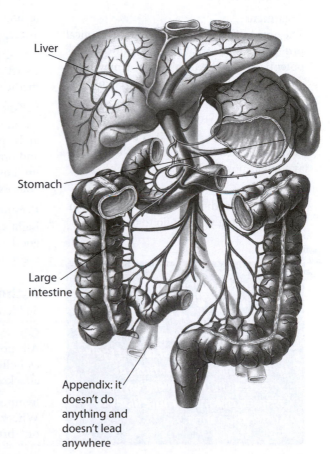

Liver

Stomach

Large intestine

Appendix: it doesn't do anything and doesn't lead anywhere

Arthritis: osteo vs rheumatoid

Osteoarthritis is by far the most common form of arthritis in the West and is a degenerative condition; rheumatoid arthritis is a chronic disease in which the body's own immune system starts eating away at joint tissue.

Causes
Either a bacterial infection in the appendix, or a piece of digestive waste that has become lodged in it.

Symptoms
An early sign, often missed, is a mild ache in the lower stomach. This then develops into a sharp, persistent pain in the lower right abdomen, accompanied by accelerated heartbeat and mild fever. Advanced symptoms include a visible swelling in that area.

Treatment
The appendix has to be removed by surgical procedure. Untreated appendicitis is potentially life-threatening, as it may burst and expel poisonous faecal matter into the abdominal cavity.

Self-help
There is little you can do if you suspect you have appendicitis, other than get to casualty as soon as possible.

Prevention
Because appendicitis is entirely random, there is nothing you can do to prevent it.

F

Fact: In the UK over half of those over the age of 65 suffer from arthritis, with a third of adults exhibiting some form of arthritic symptoms in at least one of their joints. This includes those as young as in their twenties, and women are much more likely to suffer than men.

Arthritis (osteo)
Stiffening and degeneration of the body's joints, particularly the load-bearing ones such as knees, ankles and fingers.

Causes
The regeneration of the joints' cushioning cartilage can no longer keep up with its breaking down, so it becomes thinner and less flexible.

Symptoms
Stiffening of the joints and the likelihood of feeling pain when they are flexed.

Treatment
Anti-inflammatory drugs may be prescribed to arthritis sufferers, and the pain will be medicated.

Self-help
Avoid acid-forming foods – processed flour and sugar, alcohol and coffee – while tomatoes and oranges can cause the condition to flare up. Losing weight will reduce the strain on your joints.

Prevention
Light exercise and stretching – yoga is very good – keeps the bones healthy and prevents the joints stiffening.

Asthma
Sudden constriction of the bronchial tubes.

Causes
Air pollution and airborne allergens such as pollen, dust or fur can trigger asthmatic attacks, as can sudden incidences of stress.

Symptoms
Wheezing breathing and shortness of breath. Severe attacks leave the

sufferer unable to speak and with a feeling of being suffocated, and this will be accompanied by a quickening pulse and sweating.

Treatment
A bronchial inhaler will reopen the airways during an attack, and a course of inhaled anti-inflammatory treatment can reduce any underlying swelling.

Self-help
Sit upright during an attack as this will ease breathing, while daily deep breathing exercises will keep your bronchial tubes in better condition.

Prevention
Don't smoke and avoid secondary smoke, drink plenty of water to keep mucus production to a minimum and, using a process of elimination, try to identify anything you may be allergic to.

Athlete's foot
Fungal infection of the feet – not restricted to athletes.

Causes
The fungus can be transmitted from other people – the damp floors in changing rooms are notorious – or picked up from micro-organisms in the soil. It then thrives in warm, dark, dank conditions – i.e. your socks and shoes.

Symptoms
Itchy, cracked and flaking skin between the toes and on the soles of the feet.

Treatment
There are numerous anti-fungal creams and sprays available over the counter.

Self-help
Eat garlic and onions as they have anti-fungal properties, while live yoghurt will help if it is a problem starting in your gut. Avoid anything fermented or sugary.

Prevention
Dry your feet properly, put talcum powder in between your toes; change your socks; go barefoot as much as possible.

B

Bad breath (halitosis)

Causes
Bad dental hygiene, in which insufficient attention paid to brushing and flossing has resulted in a plaque build-up and infections in the mouth. Or a slow digestive system means food is putrefying in the bowel, and toxins are being reabsorbed into the

Back pain

Eighty percent of all adults will, at some point in their lives, suffer from back pain serious enough to inhibit something they are doing: in the UK, over 20 million working days a year are lost to back pain, in the US that figure is nearer 250 million. There are probably as many different causes and specific types of pain as there are sufferers, and although people in general seem more aware of how to lift correctly and assume the correct posture at their desk, these figures show no sign of going down.

The underlying problem is that our bodies were never really designed to walk upright. Thus after thirty or forty years of doing so your back will start to complain, and before it does you should get it looked at. Every man over the age of thirty should visit an osteopath for maintenance, repositioning and advice on what you might be doing wrong. It will save so much grief and pain by the time you get to be fifty.

blood to reach the lungs where they create a rotten smell.

Symptoms
Your breath smells bad. If people keep their distance while you're talking, you might like to ask a straight-talking friend if you have halitosis.

Treatment
Clean your teeth after every meal and before you go to bed, and stop smoking, as it dries the mouth out, meaning there is less saliva available to combat bacteria. Stay away from processed foods, caffeine and sugar, which will all serve to slow down your digestion, and if you can't speed your digestion up by changing your diet and lifestyle, have an enema.

Self-help
Parsley, coriander and mint have an anti-bacterial effect in your mouth so freshen your breath; leafy green vegetables are rich in chlorophyll, which will freshen your breath while aiding your digestion.

Prevention
Visit your dentist and oral hygienist at least twice a year and change your toothbrush regularly. Eat smaller meals as this is less likely to overload your bowel.

Bleeding gums

Causes
Overenthusiastic brushing – this will be more likely among older men – or gum disease, prompted by a build-up of plaque.

Symptoms
Blood in the toothpaste you spit out, or blood on your pillowcase in the morning.

Treatment
Try a softer toothbrush and a less vigorous brushing technique; the gum disease may be the result of a vitamin C deficiency, so an increase in your intake may stop it and if that doesn't clear it up visit your dentist.

Self-help
Fresh sage makes an effective mouthwash for healing bleeding gums or soothing inflamed tissue inside the mouth – chop a handful of leaves and steep in a cup of boiling water, allow to cool and use as mouthwash, then keep what is left in a closed container in the fridge.

Prevention
Particular attention must be paid to brushing, flossing and rinsing, while you will need regular dental checkups and visits to the oral hygienist.

Body odour

Causes
Poor hygiene, leaving a build-up of bacteria on your skin, or toxins being expelled through the skin.

Symptoms
Nobody is keen to stand next to you!

Treatment
Washing away the sweat that feeds the bacteria, paying particular attention to the groin, armpits and feet where the most sweat is produced, and thoroughly washing your clothes. Speeding up the digestion to remove toxins from the system quicker.

Self-help
Drinking a large amount of water to flush out toxins, spraying armpits with an antibacterial spray before applying deodorant.

Prevention
Regular washing, changing your clothes and underwear, cutting down on constipation-inducing, low-fibre foods and drinking plenty of water to flush toxins out of the system.

Boils

Causes
A bacterial infection causing a blockage of a hair follicle. Regular outbreaks of boils are a sign that you are generally very run-down and your immune system isn't functioning properly.

Symptoms
Angry-looking, tender spots, probably a fair bit bigger than your everyday blackhead.

Treatment
Goldenseal root applied to the boil will kill the infection; apply tea tree oil once it has been drained.

Self-help
Take zinc to stimulate the immune system and vitamin A to keep the skin in good condition. Drink plenty of water.

Prevention
Eat plenty of fibre to avoid constipation; stay away from processed foods and hydrogenized fats; exercise to keep the metabolism moving.

Brain tumour

A growth of abnormally formed cells on the brain tissue or the membranes surrounding it.

Causes
Metastatic brain tumours are a cancer spread from somewhere else in the body; primary brain tumours originate in the brain and their cause is not known.

Symptoms
Headaches, blurred vision and confusion. Then, depending on which part of the brain they are in, they can affect coordination, speech, memory or any of the senses.

Treatment
If the tumour is near the surface of the brain it can be removed by conventional surgery; if it is deep within the folds then it will be treated with laser surgery or radiation therapy. There may be chemotherapy involved in either case.

Self-help
Curcumin – found in turmeric – has tumour-inhibiting properties, as it boosts the immune system and prevents the growth of blood vessels within the tumour, thus stopping it expanding.

Prevention
Get checked regularly for all cancers, and eat organic food, as it reduces the amount of cancer-friendly toxins you may be ingesting.

Bronchitis

Inflammation of the bronchial tubes – the narrow airways leading from the trachea to the lungs – resulting in excess mucus production which further obstructs the pipes.

Causes
The most common cause of bronchitis is smoking, but it is also caused by bacterial and viral infections and airborne pollutants.

Symptoms
Persistent hacking cough bringing up cloudy mucus – at its worst first thing in the morning – fever, breathlessness.

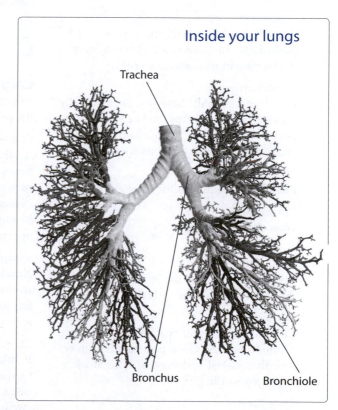

Inside your lungs

Trachea

Bronchus

Bronchiole

Treatment

Antibiotics will be prescribed for the infection, while cough medicine will suppress the cough and help you sleep.

Self-help

The steam from taking a hot shower will help loosen mucus deposits; drink plenty of water to keep the mucus as thin as possible. Papaya and mango are very good for your lungs.

Prevention

Give up smoking, if you smoke; keep your immune system in good shape.

Bunions

Bony growth on the outside of the joint where the big toe meets the foot.

Causes

Shoes that are too tight across the toes, as the pad of bone grows to protect the toes from being squashed.

Symptoms

Apart from the growth, the big toe will be pushed inwards, often under the toes next to it, resulting in pain and tenderness.

Treatment

Bad bunions will have to be surgically removed and the big toe (and perhaps the toe next to it) realigned. It's a relatively simple, local anaesthetic, outpatients operation.

Self-help

Pads fitted inside the shoe to ease pressure.

Prevention

Wear shoes that fit properly.

Bursitis

The inflammation of the bursae – the sacs of fluid that lubricate the insides of your joints.

Causes

Continued jolting of that joint – it is very common in sportsmen, particularly runners – or the general bashing that housework or labouring would give it.

Symptoms

Pain and stiffness in the affected joint;

Fact: Perhaps unsurprisingly, ten times as many women than men suffer from bunions.

particularly bad if it has remained immobile for some time or first thing in the morning.

Treatment

Your doctor may prescribe anti-inflammatory drugs, or even draw fluid from the bursae with a syringe.

Self-help

Wrap a tight bandage around the affected joint, apply an ice pack and sit down with that limb raised.

Prevention

Be careful of your joints, try not to leave them bent at a sharp angle for long stretches of time.

C

Carpal tunnel syndrome

Afflicts the median nerve, which runs from the palm of the hand to the wrist.

Causes

As this nerve passes in between the wrist bones (the carpals) it is pressed upon by the surrounding bones and tissue. This can be caused by repeated unnatural or awkward bending of the wrist – RSI – such as when operating a computer mouse.

Symptoms

Numbness and pain in the fingers and hand; weakness in the fingers; the fingers will feel as if they are swollen when they do not appear so.

Treatment

Painkillers, repositioning of hands while working to avoid the strain, and, in severe cases, diuretics may be prescribed to reduce swelling around the carpals.

Cancers

Cancer occurs when a group of cells within one area of the body starts growing uncontrollably due to genetic mutations in their DNA. There are over two hundred different types of cancer. Most are named after the organ or cell type in which they originate and most cause tumours from the mass of unwanted cells they produce. These tumours are either self-contained – benign – which means the cancer cannot spread to other parts of the body, or they are malignant, meaning it will invade other tissues. Benign tumours can usually be surgically removed; malignant cancers require chemo- or radiotherapy. Cancers are the biggest single killers in the world, with lung, breast, bowel pancreatic and prostate cancer being the most deadly.

Self-help
Take breaks from repetitive tasks and gently flex the wrists.

Prevention
Ergonomic wrist supports for typing or computer work. Several brands manufacture a "vertical" computer mouse, which allows your hand to stay in a "handshake" position, rather than unnaturally flat.

Cold sores
Sores caused by the herpes simplex virus.

Causes
A viral infection that can lie dormant in your body but which activates itself when you feel stressed or are run-down – or which can be triggered by excess amounts of the amino acid arginine, found in nuts and chocolate.

Symptoms
Clusters of small, painful sores in and around the mouth, swollen glands, sore throat, headaches, nausea, fever.

Treatment
Antiviral creams will speed the sores' healing,

while prescription antiviral tablets will clear up the virus. Regular use of an antiseptic mouthwash will help fight sores inside your mouth.

Self-help
Organic lean meat and poultry, fish and soya products are all rich in the antiviral amino acid lysine.

Prevention
Stay well-nourished and keep your immune system working efficiently; if you have cold sores don't fiddle with them as that will spread the infection.

Common cold
Infection of the upper respiratory system, inflaming the mucus membranes inside the nose and throat.

Causes
Infection by one of the many cold viruses – because there are so many of them and they are constantly mutating, it has proved impossible to find a cure that will deal with all of them.

Symptoms
Sore throat, nasal congestion, runny nose, coughing, fever, chills, headache, fatigue, muscle ache.

Treatment
Bed rest, plenty of fluids, keep warm; take paracetamol to bring your temperature down.

T

Tip: If you suffer from persistent cold sores, go and see your doctor for a full examination as they might be symptoms of a compromised immune system.

F

Fact: You don't catch cold from getting cold or going out with wet hair. In this case, your mum didn't know what she was talking about.

Self-help
Echinacea or vitamin C will shorten the duration of a cold; garlic and onion will fight the infection.

Prevention
Keep your immune system in tip-top condition.

Constipation
Inability to have bowel movements.

Causes
Lack of fibre in the diet; not drinking enough water; stress.

Symptoms
Lack of bowel movement or the necessity to strain; painful bowel movement; hard, compacted stools.

Treatment
A warm drink first thing in the morning will stimulate the colon; vitamin C powder dissolved in water with magnesium will soften your stools; psyllium husks with plenty of water act as a super-fibre.

Self-help
Early morning exercise prompts the colon to work more efficiently during the day.

Prevention
Avoid processed foods and opt for a diet that is high in fibre. Drink plenty of water.

Coronary artery disease (CAD)
An advanced form of angina, whereby the artery becomes completely blocked.

Causes
Extensive narrowing of the arteries that feed oxygenated blood to the heart, caused by smoking, high cholesterol or lack of exercise. A family history of CAD will mean you are more susceptible.

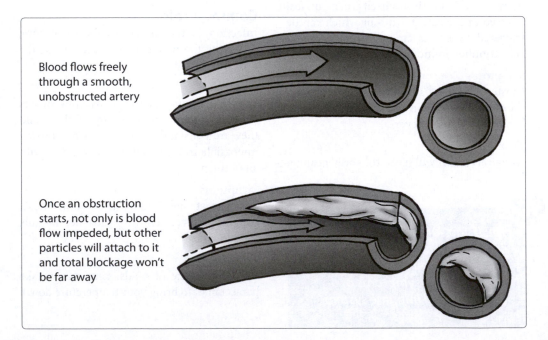

Blood flows freely through a smooth, unobstructed artery

Once an obstruction starts, not only is blood flow impeded, but other particles will attach to it and total blockage won't be far away

Symptoms
Angina is a symptom caused by your arteries clogging up, but they only complain during exertion. With CAD the chest pains, breathlessness, dizziness and sweating will happen when you are at rest too.

Treatment
Hospitalization will be required, and maybe a bypass operation to flow blood around the blocked bits. Nitroglycerin tablets administered at the start of an attack may expand the blood vessels.

Self-help
Daily doses of vitamin C and lysine (an amino acid) will, over time, reduce the congestion within the arteries.

Prevention
Lead a healthy lifestyle, avoid food that is high in cholesterol or saturated fat, and don't smoke.

Cramp
A contracted muscle that goes into spasm and will not relax.

Causes
Fatigue, dehydration, salt deficiency, restrictive positioning of the muscle to compress nerves or blood supply.

Symptoms
Sharp pain in affected muscle and an inability to straighten it.

Treatment
Massage, gentle stretching and rehydration.

Self-help
Maintain mineral levels, especially during sports or in hot weather.

Prevention
Exercise sensibly and remain hydrated.

D

Dandruff
The flaking of dead skin from the scalp.

Causes
Excess of skin oil (sebum) secretions, encouraging the growth of the malassezia fungus that feeds on it and causes accelerated cell turnover – hence the large amount of dead skin.

Symptoms
Clearly visible flakes of dead skin falling from the scalp.

Treatment
Anti-dandruff shampoo. But these are not all the same and will carry out different functions – combat the fungal infection, prevent oil build-up or scrub away dead skin. Talk to the pharmacist to find out which is best for you, then only use as directed.

Self-help
Maintain a healthy diet – zinc and the B vitamins work well against dandruff – and get some sun on your head: not too much, but a little sunlight will help prevent the fungus getting a hold.

Prevention
Daily washing of hair with a gentle shampoo will prevent excess sebum on the scalp and remove any dead skin. Regular application of tea tree oil will combat infection.

Deep vein thrombosis (DVT)
Causes
A blood clot forms in one of the large veins deep below the surface – usually in the legs – the most common cause is lack of movement slowing down the blood flow in your veins and inviting it to clot. Long-haul airline passengers are particularly susceptible.

Symptoms
Swelling, redness, sharp pains and the skin in that area feeling warmer than what is surrounding it.

Don't ignore DVT

The most dangerous aspect of deep vein thrombosis is the risk of a chunk of the clot breaking off to form an embolus, which will then travel through your bloodstream. Because the veins deep in the leg have such a large diameter, even part of a clot formed in them can be enough to totally block a smaller artery.

An embolus will be transported to the heart, and from the heart to the small arteries of the lungs, at which point it becomes a pulmonary embolism, which can do serious damage. A small clot might pass through causing little more than chest pains; a medium-sized embolism could partially block the artery. If it's sufficiently large it will block the blood flow to the lungs, which will probably be fatal. Around one in ten of the people who don't get DVT treated suffer a pulmonary embolism severe enough to hospitalize them, or worse.

Treatment

Anticoagulant medicine will be administered to prevent clotting or dissolve a clot that has formed.

Self-help

Compression stockings that squeeze the calf to increase blood pressure in the veins in your lower leg reduce the risk of clots forming in the most vulnerable area.

Prevention

Don't stay in your seat for long stretches of time; the obese and smokers are far more vulnerable to this condition as their blood flow will not be all that it should be.

Depression

A pervasive and persistent lowering of the mood.

Causes

The causes are manifold, and can be genetic, or a chemical imbalance in the brain, or outside factors such as situation or environment.

Symptoms

Constant feelings of sadness, worthlessness or hopelessness; an inability to make decisions or concentrate; chaotic sleep patterns; loss of appetite.

Treatment

Psychotherapy or drug treatment (antidepressants) or a combination of the two. Electroconvulsive therapy may be used in the most extreme cases.

Self-help

St John's Wort will reduce anxiety and assist sleeping, and eating foods containing tryptophan (turkey, avocados, bananas, cottage cheese) will raise your serotonin levels, which will help to lift your mood.

Prevention

Alcohol is a depressive and prolonged use can precipitate depression, while regular exercise releases endorphins, which will make you feel better about yourself.

Diabetes

The body either produces too little insulin (type 1 diabetes) or it is producing too much and has become resistant to it (type 2 diabetes).

Causes

Type 1 is a lifelong condition, because the pancreas is not functioning properly; type 2 is the ultimate result of a sustained poor diet.

Symptoms

Thirst, frequent urination, fatigue, increased appetite, tingling in the feet and hands; dangerously low levels of blood sugar could lead to collapse or coma.

Treatment

Type 1 requires daily insulin injections on strict timetables, and dietary regulation

The sugar trap

Taking a world average, adult males eat over 30kg (66lb) of sugar per year, and, according to the World Health Organization, this is one of the reasons they expect the number of diabetics in the world to more than double from 140 million to over 300 million during the next 25 years. And the vast number of these cases will be type 2 diabetes, which is rising because of the shift in lifestyle towards a sugary, processed diet and a decline in the amount of exercise we take. In the UK, nine out of ten diabetics are type 2, and three-quarters of them are obese. Type 2 is the fourth biggest killer of men.

that keeps fat and salt to a minimum; type 2 will be treated with medication to reduce insulin resistance, strict dietary controls and an exercise regime; it may also require insulin injections.

Self-help
Cinnamon reduces blood glucose levels and foods with a low glycaemic index (GI) – green vegetables, fresh fruit, wholewheat products – will produce the smallest blood glucose fluctuations.

Prevention
There is nothing you can do to prevent type 1 diabetes, but eating oily fish, raw fruit and vegetables, regular exercise and dumping the sugary junk food will lessen the likelihood of type 2.

Diarrhoea
Fluid is not being absorbed into the body through the intestinal walls.

Causes
Food poisoning, viral infection, large amounts of alcohol, adverse reaction to certain food additives and tap water that has not been thoroughly treated are frequent causes.

Symptoms
Liquid stools, frequent and uncontrollable bowel movements, stomach cramping, dehydration.

Treatment
Anti-diarrhoea medicine is available over the counter, but try not to take it immediately, as the diarrhoea may be the result of the system trying to rid itself of bacteria. Drink plenty of water as you will have been dehydrating since the attack began. After it has cleared up take probiotics to make sure your gut flora has not been compromised.

Self-help
Camomile tea four or five times a day will settle your stomach.

Prevention
Be as careful as you can with what you eat and your food preparation.

E

Epilepsy
The electrical impulses in the brain operate devoid of control; it affects around one in two hundred men in the UK.

Causes
Epilepsy's causes are identified in only about half of the diagnosed cases, and it is then usually traced to an accident or disease that affected the brain tissue in some way.

Symptoms
Because epilepsy is due to disrupted signals within the brain, epilepsy can affect virtually any aspect of brain activity and symptoms can include blacking out, uncontrollable twitching, jerking limbs, loss of speech and confusion.

> **T** Tip: You can pick up the bacteria that cause diarrhoea from hands, cutlery or crockery. It doesn't have to be the food itself.

> **T** Tip: To establish if erectile dysfunction is psychological or physiological, before going to sleep place a thin strip of paper around your flaccid penis and secure the ends with a small piece of adhesive tape – do not put the tape all the way around. This band should be tight enough not to fall off, but not restrictively so. If you have an erection during the night, and most men do, the paper ring will have broken, proving there is nothing mechanically wrong.

Treatment

In most cases seizures are successfully prevented with medication, which, after two or three years of regular dosing, usually leaves the sufferer free from future attacks. Some cases will be treated surgically, but that is only when the abnormal activity is confined to one small part of the brain.

Self-help

Keep a record of your seizures to more accurately inform your doctor of what needs to be addressed.

Prevention

Get plenty of rest – lack of sleep is very likely to trigger seizures.

Erectile dysfunction

Also known as impotence.

Causes

Fatigue, stress, anxiety, advancing years, depression, alcohol, hormonal problems lowering testosterone levels, cold weather.

Symptoms

The inability to raise an erection or to maintain one during sex.

Treatment

Talk to your partner about what might be the problem, and if it persists visit your doctor, who may recommend therapy.

Self-help

Try not to worry about it, as that will make it worse.

Prevention

Don't drink too much. Give up smoking. Keep in good physical shape.

Eyes – dark circles under them

Causes

Lack of refreshing sleep, allergies, food intolerances (particularly wheat), iron deficiency, kidney problems.

Symptoms

Er, dark circles under the eyes.

Treatment

A good night's sleep is the most obvious step. If that doesn't work cut wheat out of your diet for a week or take a course of iron tablets.

Self-help

Foods rich in vitamin K (seaweed, lentils, leafy green vegetables) will reduce the discolouration; carotene nourishes the eyes.

Prevention

Get enough rest, and eliminate any allergens.

Not a dry eye in the house

If you suffer from dry eyes as a result of air-conditioned buildings, long-haul flights, smoky atmospheres or long days in front of the computer screen, use natural or organic eye drops for instant relief. To prevent your eyes drying out, avoid diuretics such as coffee or alcohol, and don't eat foods rich in saturated fats – they prevent your natural oils from lubricating your body and so speed up dehydration. Eat foods rich in carotene (carrots and leafy green vegetables), which boost the eyes' overall health, drink more water and keep up your vitamin B intake.

F

Food poisoning

Causes
Contaminated or undercooked food – reheated dishes are a common source.

Symptoms
Diarrhoea, vomiting, stomach cramps, fever, chills, headaches.

Treatment
Usually nothing, as the vomiting or diarrhoea will be ridding your body of the toxins, but be careful not to dehydrate. If it lasts longer than four or five days, see your doctor who may prescribe antibiotics.

Self-help
You may need to top up your gut flora when the symptoms have passed.

Prevention
Pay attention to food hygiene; always wash your hands before and after handling food; don't risk eating anything questionable.

G

Gallstones
A small solidified mass in the gall bladder.

Causes
Hardened excess cholesterol produces over three-quarters of all gallstones; the others are produced within the bile itself by a chemical imbalance.

Symptoms
Although most gallstones produce no symptoms, the bigger ones, and they can be the size of apricots, will block the bile duct from the gall bladder to cause sharp pains in the right-hand side of the abdomen.

Treatment
In more serious cases the gall bladder will be surgically removed, otherwise non-surgical procedures involve medication, sound waves or chemicals introduced via a catheter to dissolve the stones.

Self-help
Take extra vitamin C, as this will turn cholesterol into bile in the gall bladder.

Prevention
Don't put on too much weight and keep your cholesterol levels down.

Gout
It isn't only an aristocrat's complaint.

Causes
Elevated levels of uric acid in the blood, forming crystals that collect in the joints. This is brought on by too much rich, hard-to-

F

Fact: Over 25 percent of men currently have gallstones, but fewer than 20 percent of sufferers will ever notice them. Women are twice as likely as men to develop them.

digest food. The obese are more susceptible and it is much more common among men than women, although the rates among women are rising rapidly.

Symptoms
Painful swelling and discolouration in isolated joints, usually the big toe.

Treatment
Resting in bed, anti-inflammatories and painkillers.

Self-help
Pineapple speeds the body's excretion of uric acid, while anything rich in bioflavonoids (blueberries or blackberries) will reduce residual levels.

Prevention
Lose weight and eat sensibly – but be careful to avoid oily fish and other high-protein foods as they can prompt uric acid production.

Glandular fever

More common among men under thirty, but often misdiagnosed merely as fatigue.

Causes
It's a viral infection.

Symptoms
Swollen lymph nodes in the neck, armpits and groin, sore throat, fever, general tiredness.

Treatment
Antibiotics don't work, and there is no cure as such – rest and healthy eating will clear it up, but it might take a month. Because the symptoms are flu-like and sufferers will seem much better after a week or so's rest it's often assumed to have been a bout of flu that has cleared up, but if it is glandular fever it likely to recur.

Self-help
Completely cut out processed food and go on a wholefood diet that is rich in protein to boost your immune system.

Prevention
It can't be prevented, but if your immune system is in good condition you will be able

to fight it off more quickly.

Groin strain

Stretching or tearing of the muscle at the top of the inside of the thigh – where the thigh bone connects to the pubic bone.

Causes
Lateral overstretching of the leg.

Symptoms
Pain in that region when the leg is moved upwards or outwards, tenderness on the inside of the thigh.

Treatment
Rest. Ice. Compression. Elevation. And no sport or exercise until it is fully recovered.

Self-help
Don't attempt to run this one off or you will make it much worse. Stop immediately.

Prevention
Warm up and stretch the muscle out properly before exerting it.

H

Haemorrhoids

Inflammation of the blood vessels in the anus (external haemorrhoids) or rectum (internal).

Causes
Straining during a bowel movement – the likelihood of this increases with age.

Symptoms
Very tender swellings either inside or outside the anus, up to the size of grapes.

Treatment
Wash anus with a soft cloth and warm soapy water after bowel movement and pat dry; over-the-counter creams are available to ease the pain and in serious cases your doctor may prescribe anti-inflammatory ointment. Usually, though, they clear up by themselves.

Why hay fever is worse in cities

Despite its name, levels of hay fever are higher in urban environments than they are in the countryside. This is because the large amount of residual pollution in cities keeps nose membranes slightly inflamed as a default setting. As a result they are on high alert and when something extra like pollen comes along they immediately switch into allergic mode as a defence. This is why hay fever has become more prevalent in recent years as pollution levels, rather than the pollen count, rise.

Self-help
Ice packs will reduce the swelling, while sitting in a warm – but not hot – bath will soothe the pain and itching.

Prevention
Avoid constipation, and keep stools soft by eating enough fibre and drinking plenty of water.

Hay fever

Causes
Allergic reaction to pollen or house dust, usually during the spring or summer.

Symptoms
Sneezing, blocked or runny nose, streaming, itchy or swollen eyes.

Treatment
Antihistamine sprays or tablets, or steroid sprays, minimize the symptoms.

Self-help
Bioflavonoids in dark berries will reduce

T

Tip: A spoonful of organic local honey once a day from early spring onwards can stop mild cases of hay fever as the small amounts of pollen in the honey can develop your immunity. This is why it has to be local honey because it will contain the same pollen you will be exposed to.

membrane inflammation; stop smoking and avoid smokers too, as this will aggravate the condition.

Prevention
Serious sufferers might try immunotherapy, take antihistamines, or even stay indoors, on days when the pollen count is high.

Heart attack
Part of the heart muscle ceases to function because it is deprived of oxygen through the bloodstream.

Causes
A sudden blockage in one of the coronary arteries supplying oxygenated blood to the heart – usually caused by a blood clot.

Symptoms
Crushing chest pain, difficulty breathing, dizziness, nausea, clammy and pale skin, possibility of collapse and the feeling that you are about to die.

Treatment
Call the emergency services immediately you suspect yourself or somebody else to be having a heart attack. Clot-busting drugs may be administered to clear the blockage, while post-attack treatments include medication to reduce the viscosity of your blood, beta-blockers to reduce strain on the heart and cholesterol-lowering drugs. If the heart has been seriously damaged it may require surgery.

Cardio-pulmonary resuscitation (CPR) – it may save somebody's life

CPR is a method of "buying" a short amount of time for a heart attack victim by artificially stimulating their breathing and heartbeat with a combination of mouth-to-mouth resuscitation and robust heart massage. Give two good breaths into the victim's lungs, then place one of your palms on their heart, and the other on top of that, and push down thirty times in quick succession. Repeat the cycle of two breaths and thirty chest compressions until the emergency services arrive. This may be enough to keep the sufferer going until the paramedics get there, so it is vital it is applied immediately to anybody who is not responding to people around them, or is breathing fitfully, or not at all.

Self-help

If you experience angina or other heart disease symptoms go and see your doctor immediately, as these may be overtures to an impending heart attack.

Prevention

Stop smoking, lose weight, take regular exercise, and make sure your cholesterol levels don't get too high.

Heartburn

An acute form of indigestion that has nothing to do with the heart.

Causes

Stomach acid escaping up through the valve at the top of the stomach and back into the oesophagus where it burns the lining – acid reflux. Excess stomach acid or eating too fast or too much in one go are the most likely culprits.

Symptoms

Burning sensation behind the breastbone; sometimes it feels like food or liquid is coming back up as far as your mouth.

Treatment

Antacid tablets or liquid.

Self-help

Liquorice, fennel or camomile will soothe restless stomach acid.

Prevention

If it occurs regularly, avoid rich food, black coffee or fried food, and increase your intake of raw fruit and vegetables.

Hepatitis

An inflammation of the liver, it is divided into five main types – Hep A, B, C, D and E.

Causes

It is a viral infection. A and E are typically caused by contaminated food or water; B, C and D are spread by bodily fluids – usually contaminated blood; B is most frequently transmitted by unprotected sex.

Symptoms

Yellowing of skin and eyes, fatigue, fever, nausea, brown urine, chronic stomach pain.

Treatment

Except for Hep C, the virus usually clears up by itself after a few weeks of rest, good nutrition and no alcohol. About twenty percent of Hep C sufferers will recover naturally, but the vast majority will carry it, and remain infectious, for the rest of their lives.

Self-help

Green tea has powerful antiviral powers, while vitamin B will boost your liver.

Prevention

Take all necessary precautions as regards sex and needles, especially in developing countries; it is possible to get vaccinated against both strains.

Hernia

An organ or tissue pushes out from behind a weakened area of muscle, usually the groin.

Causes

Heavy coughing, ill-advised lifting technique, straining during a bowel movement or while urinating.

Symptoms

Soft lump under the skin, which may cause pain or not hurt at all.

Treatment

Hernias are usually treated with minor surgery; trusses are rarely used for anything other than comedy sketches.

Self-help

Even if it doesn't hurt it should be dealt with as untreated hernias get bigger and will eventually interfere with your regular life.

Prevention

Don't strain yourself.

High blood pressure

Also known as hypertension, it is when your blood pressure is persistently measured at more than 140/90 – 120/80 is normal. (See box above for explanation of figures.)

Causes

If high blood pressure is not a reaction to medication or a symptom of an illness (secondary hypertension) then what causes it has yet to be identified – this primary hypertension accounts for around 95 percent of all cases. Lifestyle issues – weight, lack of exercise, smoking, drinking, stress, bad diet – are believed to contribute.

Symptoms

Heart palpitations, breathlessness, persistent headache, nausea, dizziness.

Treatment

If you are young enough and healthy enough, your doctor will recommend lifestyle changes as the initial treatment. For older people or those with very high blood pressure there are a number of drugs that can lower it. These are usually prescribed as a last resort because once you start on them you will probably have to continue taking them for the rest of your life.

Self-help

Potassium-rich foods like bananas or celery lower blood pressure.

Prevention

Stay away from stimulants – legal and otherwise – and reduce the amount of salt in your diet, as it increases your blood volume.

I

Indigestion (dyspepsia)

Disturbance in the upper abdomen.

Causes

Acid from your stomach gets into the oesophagus (acid reflux or heartburn) or the upper part of your small intestine and attacks the lining; a bacterial infection.

Symptoms

Stomach pains that could be a dull ache or a sharp stabbing or anything in between, an uncomfortable feeling of being full, gas attacks, nausea.

Blood pressure: what do those figures mean?

The two figures given in a blood pressure measurement – 120 over 80, for instance, written as 120/80 – refer to, respectively, the systolic pressure while the heart is contracted and actually pumping blood, and the diastolic pressure when the heart is at rest between beats. The numbers refer to millimetres of mercury (mmHg), which is a unit of pressure measured by the movement of a precise column of mercury.

Treatment

Antacids provide immediate relief, while for chronic indigestion your doctor may prescribe drugs to reduce the residual acid levels in your stomach. If it is a bacterial infection prescription medication will also be required.

Self-help

Tea made from grated root ginger steeped in boiling water aids digestion, as does fresh pineapple.

Prevention

If you are overweight, you will be putting pressure on your stomach, and losing weight will reduce the likelihood of acid being pushed out. Eat smaller meals and consume them less quickly.

Infertility

Inability to produce enough sperm (or enough mobile sperm) to fertilize your partner's egg.

Causes

Men can have a naturally low sperm count or produce sperm with little mobility. Testicular infections can affect sperm production (both quantity and quality), as can the side effects of anabolic steroids, some anti-inflammatory medication and chemotherapy. An unhealthy lifestyle can also contribute.

Symptoms

Failure to conceive – 85 percent of couples with no fertility problems will

F

Fact: Although no definite figures exist, infertility is not uncommon. In approximately half the cases treated it is female infertility, in around one-third it is male, and in the remaining seventeen percent the causes are unknown.

conceive within a year of having regular, unprotected sex.

Treatment

Surgical procedures can help if the problem is a blockage, and there is medication available to increase sperm count.

Self-help

Zinc is a sperm count booster, as are nuts and whole pulses and grains.

Prevention

Stop smoking and cut down on the drinking, as both hugely reduce levels of healthy sperm, as does chronic stress.

Influenza (flu)

A viral infection of the lungs and respiratory tract.

Causes

The flu virus is highly contagious and spread on saliva through coughing and sneezing, which is why epidemics are not uncommon.

Symptoms

Coughing, sneezing, aching muscles, fatigue, high temperature, chills, loss of appetite, nausea.

Treatment

Get plenty of sleep, drink plenty of fluids and take over-the-counter medication. This should clear it up in about a week or so. In severe cases you may be prescribed antiviral medicine.

Self-help

Vitamin C and echinacea are both highly effective in protecting against the flu virus.

Prevention

Annual flu vaccinations are widely available and very effective.

Insomnia

The inability to sleep restfully.

Causes

Stress, alcohol, eating too late at night, stimulants, depression, exercising late at night, not exercising enough, anxiety.

Symptoms

Regularly having trouble falling asleep, waking after a couple of hours and having difficulty getting back to sleep, general fatigue during the day.

Treatment

If the cause is psychological, counselling may help you get around that, and you should only take sleeping medication as a temporary measure. Don't lie there willing yourself to go to sleep as this will activate your brain and make dropping off even less likely.

Self-help

Tryptophan-loaded foods like turkey, chicken, wheatgerm and cottage cheese will help you produce more serotonin, which will help relax you. Valerian root prevents chaotic sleep patterns.

Prevention

Eliminate as many of the possible causes as apply, and make sure your bedroom is as sleep-friendly as possible.

Irritable bowel syndrome (IBS)

The most common gastric complaint among men in the Western world.

Causes

The muscles that line the intestine and ripple to push food in its various broken-down stages through the digestive tract go into spasm and move it through to the bowel either too quickly or too slowly. It may be brought on by high-fat foods, excess of dairy products, undiagnosed food allergies or even stress.

Symptoms

Nausea, stomach pains, excess gas, constipation, diarrhoea, abdominal cramps.

Treatment

Modify your diet, eat smaller meals and don't rush them. If diarrhoea is a symptom you may be depleting your nutrient reserves so you will need to replenish them.

Self-help

Linseeds or linseed-oil tablets taken daily will help regulate your bowel functions and return them to normal.

Prevention

Reduce fat and increase fibre intake, address any causes of stress and, if IBS persists, get tested for food allergies.

Jet lag

Causes

Travelling across different time zones faster than your body can adjust.

Symptoms

Disrupted sleep/wake cycle, fatigue.

Treatment

Don't dehydrate; stay up as long as you can in the new time zone; engage in some light exercise as soon as you arrive.

Self-help

Boosting your tryptophan levels with foods such as turkey or cottage cheese, or with supplements that will help you relax into a new sleep cycle.

Prevention

Make sure you have had a good night's sleep before travelling, eat with a view to maintaining even blood sugar levels and don't get drunk on the flight.

K

Kidney stones

Hard pieces of waste matter forming in the kidneys and passing into the ureter.

Causes

Minerals being filtered out of the blood to be passed out of the body in urine collect in the kidneys and solidify. Low volumes of urine can cause these deposits – nearly all kidney stones are mostly solidified calcium or uric acid.

F

Fact: Kidney stones are more common in the summer because you will be more dehydrated, and therefore your urine will be less in volume but of greater concentration.

Symptoms
Pains in the lower back that are sometimes very sharp; difficulty urinating; dark or cloudy urine; nausea.

Treatment
Small kidney stones pass out of the body through urination, and water intake should be increased to encourage this – this may happen without you noticing, or could cause considerable pain, depending on the size of the stone. Larger deposits may require painkillers and muscle relaxant medication to get them on their way, and stones capable of completely blocking the ureter will be broken up using sound waves then passed out with urine.

Self-help
Hydrangea root has long been used to dissolve kidney stones, while lemon juice taken every day will smooth the painful jagged edges of the stones.

Prevention
Drink plenty of water to flush minerals out of your kidneys before deposits can build up.

L

Laryngitis
An inflammation of the larynx.

Causes
Usually it is a viral infection, and occasionally it is bacterial. It can also come about through straining the vocal cords.

Symptoms
Sore throat, difficulty swallowing, croaky or weak speaking voice.

Treatment
Viral laryngitis will clear up by itself; take it easy and don't talk, but write things down to give your vocal cords a complete rest; drink warm, soothing drinks and ease the pain with over-the-counter throat lozenges. Antibiotics will only be prescribed if the infection is bacterial.

Self-help
Steam inhalation, maybe with a menthol infusion.

Prevention
Don't smoke and try not to strain your vocal cords.

Low blood sugar
Also known as hypoglycaemia.

Causes
The liver does not release enough glucose into the system, which can prompt increased adrenaline production.

Lactose intolerance

The inability to digest milk or dairy products is a common situation that has been diagnosed far more readily during the last couple of decades. It is the result of a body's insufficient production of an enzyme called lactase that is needed to break lactose down into a digestible form. Unmetabolized lactose can cause abdominal discomfort, bloating, gas and diarrhoea. It is far more common among those of African, African-Caribbean, Asian or Native American descent than in Caucasians, and the only remedy or means of prevention is to remove dairy produce containing lactose from your diet.

T

Tip: If you have laryngitis don't make any vocal sounds at all, especially not whispering as rather than saving your vocal chords, it actually puts more strain on them than shouting does.

Symptoms

Fatigue, irritability, lack of concentration, dizziness, hunger, headaches, anxiety, the shakes; severe hypoglycaemia can bring on partial paralysis.

Treatment

Eating a sugary snack or drinking a fast-acting carbohydrate like fruit juice or a sports drink. If it is a lasting condition brought on by diabetes or liver disorders, the sufferer should keep sugary products on hand for emergencies and make sure people know to administer them if they are having a serious attack.

Self-help

You should consult your doctor about managing your hypoglycaemia. Regular dosages of magnesium will help to keep blood sugar levels stable.

Prevention

Eat regularly and healthily, and don't skip breakfast.

M

Meningitis

Inflammation of membranes covering the brain.

Causes

It is a bacterial or a viral infection, and highly contagious.

Symptoms

Severe headaches, confusion, fatigue, fever, sensitivity to light, stiff neck.

Treatment

Bacterial meningitis will be treated with antibiotics, while viral meningitis usually clears up by itself after a period of bed rest

---

Liver disorders

The hardest working and only self-renewing organ in your body, your liver is far from immune to the punishment it takes as it filters toxins out of your system and regulates the flow of vital substances. Traditionally, the most likely cause of liver complaint has been cirrhosis, from drinking too much, as the effort involved in dealing with the toxins introduced by the alcohol destroys the liver's cells and replaces them with non-functioning scar tissue. Eventually this leads to liver failure as it no longer has the capacity to carry out its duties, but while it slowly shuts down you will experience fatigue, jaundice, loss of appetite, weight loss and nausea.

Cirrhosis is irreversible. The only way to stop its advancement is to stop drinking completely and switch to a healthy diet, and in severe cases a liver transplant might be necessary. You don't have to be a heavy drinker to adversely affect your liver – regular light drinking or two or three consecutive nights on the lash can start to overload it and make you feel tired and weakened. Make sure you have a couple of non-drinking days every week to give it time to recover.

More recently though, as the obesity crisis deepens, nonalcoholic fatty liver disease is gaining ground – it is currently affecting around twenty percent of American adults. It is caused by a build-up of fat in the liver as poor diets lead to such an ingestion of fat and cholesterol the organ cannot process and clear it away quick enough. When this occurs the liver functions far less efficiently, resulting in weakness and fatigue and, in advanced cases, chronic abdominal pain.

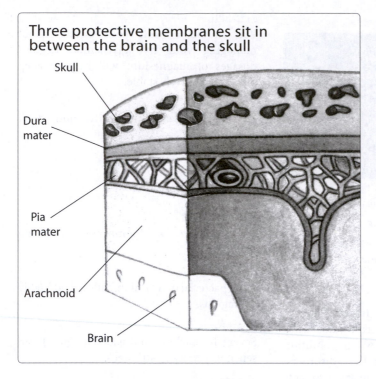

Three protective membranes sit in between the brain and the skull

Skull

Dura mater

Pia mater

Arachnoid

Brain

sleep/wake rhythms, as well as blood pressure and temperature control, which affect the desire to be active. These changes can be the aftermath of a previous infection, hormonal disturbance or even hereditary.

Symptoms
Fatigue after any form of exertion, lack of energy, aching joints and muscles, low blood pressure, headaches, fitful sleep patterns, lack of concentration.

Treatment
There is no cure for ME, although medication will be used to treat the symptoms. There is a commonly applied therapy called pacing, which encourages the sufferer to undertake physical and mental tasks within their limited capabilities, then gradually increases the amount of effort needed.

and good nutrition. The symptoms of the latter may be treated individually to ease discomfort.

Self-help
Homeopathic remedy Belladonna (deadly nightshade) may assist your recovery after the antibiotics have done their job or while you are getting over viral meningitis.

Prevention
You can be vaccinated against meningitis and this is recommended if travelling to a high-risk area or if you are an AIDS sufferer.

ME (myalgia encephalomyelitis)
Also known as chronic fatigue syndrome, a neurological disorder that affects around 0.3 percent of the UK population and 0.5 percent in the US. It is twice as likely to occur in women than in men.

Causes
Changes in the hormonal and chemical balance of the brain, disrupting the internal

Self-help
Don't attempt to combat any feelings of tiredness with caffeine – especially energy drinks that may have very high levels – as ultimately caffeine will compromise your immune system, disrupt your blood sugar levels and interfere with your adrenal gland.

Prevention
Apart from maintaining your immune system there is little to be done to prevent ME, although the majority of sufferers also have previously undiagnosed food allergies, so it may be worth exploring that avenue.

Migraines
Intense headaches, a condition that affects one in twelve British men on a regular basis

– the figure for women is three times as high, so she may really have a headache.

Causes
Low levels of serotonin can send blood vessels in the brain into rapid contraction and expansion mode, creating the conditions for a migraine, which can then be triggered by a number of factors. These can be emotional (stress, shock, depression), environmental (bright or flickering lights, loud noises, airless rooms) or physical (tension, fatigue, dehydration, food and food additives), and will be unique to everybody.

Symptoms
Severe headache, lack of coordination, problems speaking, heightened sensitivity to light or sound, visual oddities – vivid lights or patterns in your vision – numbness in shoulders or limbs, nausea.

Treatment
There is no cure, as such, for migraines. However, you can get over-the-counter preventative drugs. Painkillers may treat the headache and lying down in a cool dark room may help relieve other symptoms. In some cases, doctors may prescribe triptan, a medicine that stabilizes the blood vessels in the brain.

Self-help
If the blood vessels in your brain have gone into spasm, ginkgo biloba will stop them constricting.

Prevention
Avoid dehydration, maintain stable blood sugar levels (hypoglycaemia can bring migraines on) and learn to recognize the signs and avoid your particular trigger points.

Multiple sclerosis (MS)
A degenerative condition of the nerve cells in the brain and spinal column.

Causes
The causes of MS are unknown.

Symptoms
Loss of mental and physical control – balance and coordination difficulties, slurred speech, bladder control problems, mood swings, confusion, lack of concentration, memory loss, muscle weakness and stiffness, blurred vision, partial paralysis.

Treatment
There are medications to limit the severity and frequency of the attacks, but no actual cure, and the symptoms will be addressed individually.

Self-help
Keep cool – avoid hot environments, and attacks may be relieved with a cool shower or resting in a cool room.

Prevention
There is no way to prevent MS.

O

Obesity
Dangerously excessive fat accumulation.

Causes
Bad diet, lack of exercise, glandular disorders.

Symptoms
A body weight of over twenty percent more than it should be for your height, which can lead to heart disease, diabetes, liver failure, strokes, exhaustion, strain on every part of your body, decreased life expectancy.

Treatment
About two percent of obesity is a glandular problem (usually of the thyroid or the adrenal gland) and that can be medically treated. Otherwise it's a matter of lifestyle changes or such drastic measures as stomach stapling or gastric banding to limit your food consumption.

Self-help
Work out a coordinated diet and exercise plan tailored to you and your shape: getting professional help will be invaluable. Your

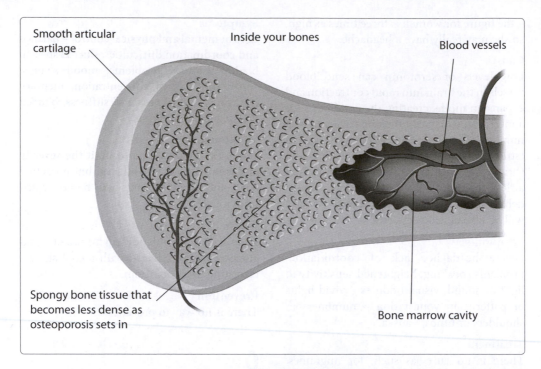

Smooth articular cartilage

Inside your bones

Blood vessels

Spongy bone tissue that becomes less dense as osteoporosis sets in

Bone marrow cavity

local doctor's surgery may well have a specialist clinic/session for this.

Prevention

If you are concerned about your weight, and think it might be verging on tipping into obesity, seek the advice of your doctor and look into whether there are any local dieting/counselling groups you could attend.

Osteoporosis

Weakening of bone density and strength.

Causes

Old age, calcium deficiency, lack of exercise.

Symptoms

Propensity to bone fractures, progressively stooping posture, chronic lower back pain.

Treatment

Your doctor may prescribe medication that assists the body's processing of calcium (bisphosphonates), or even recommend calcium supplements.

F

Fact: Due to the hormonal changes that take place during the menopause, women are four times as likely as men to suffer from osteoporosis.

Self-help

Regular weight-bearing exercise – running is very good – will keep your bones strong.

Prevention

Maintaining levels of calcium and vitamin D in your diet as you get older will keep your bones healthy, and don't smoke or drink to excess, as this will affect the production and utilization of calcium in your body.

P

Peptic ulcer
Ulceration in the stomach or digestive tract.

Causes
Infection, massive excesses of stomach acid, side effect to some medication, especially long-term use of anti-inflammatories.

Symptoms
Stomach pains, often immediately after eating, nausea, weight loss, black or bloody stools and sharp pain are the signs of a perforated ulcer and emergency treatment should be sought.

Treatment
Ulcers usually heal themselves within a couple of months, but it will ease the pain and assist healing if you take an antacid. More serious or persistent cases may require prescription medication to reduce stomach acid or combat infection.

Self-help
The bark of the slippery elm tree, brewed into tea soothes the intestines and speeds internal healing.

Prevention
A healthy, fibre-rich diet will keep your digestive system moving, preventing bits of food hanging about to irritate the walls.

Pneumonia
Inflammation of the lungs.

Causes
A viral or bacterial infection of the lungs, or caused by inhaled foreign bodies or poisonous gases. Pneumonia can also result from other conditions such as bronchitis, asthma, diabetes or leukaemia, and AIDS sufferers are particularly vulnerable.

Symptoms
Breathlessness, chest pain bringing up opaque phlegm, coughing, fever, fatigue.

Treatment
Antibiotics or antiviral drugs will be prescribed to treat infection; bed rest and in severe cases oxygen may need to be administered to assist breathing.

Self-help
Pneumonia is a serious condition, and you should follow your doctor's medical advice. A regular supplement of magnesium may contribute to keeping your lungs healthy.

Prevention
Don't smoke as it irritates the lungs; don't snort cocaine as you will be putting all sorts of pollutants directly into your lungs; maintain a healthy immune system.

Prostatitis
Inflammation of the prostate gland.

Causes
What causes it is not known, but it is believed to be sexually transmitted bacteria – it is far more common among young men with patterns of risky behaviour.

Repetitive strain injury (RSI)
Any injury to the joints, tendons, muscles, nerves or ligaments that is caused by the repetition of an action that is causing unusual strain. This can be occupational – operating machinery, equipment vibrations or a computer mouse – or as the result of a leisure-time activity – regular golfers and tennis players frequently suffer RSI. Carpal tunnel syndrome and bursitis, covered earlier in this chapter, are the most common examples of RSI. Others include rotator cuff syndrome (inflammation of the shoulder) and trigger finger (inflammation of the tendons in the index finger or thumb).

Symptoms

Painful urination, blood in urine or semen, lower back pain, bladder still feeling full after urination.

Treatment

Antibiotics, bed rest.

Self-help

Coffee should be avoided, as the diuretic properties will irritate your symptoms.

Prevention

Practise safe sex.

S

Schizophrenia

A psychotic disorder that tends to appear much earlier in men (teens and twenties) than in women.

Causes

The cause is unknown, but it is thought to have a genetic element to it. Brain damage can contribute, and although excessive drug use may produce schizophrenia-like episodes, it will not cause the condition.

Symptoms

Paranoia, delusions, hallucinations, erratic

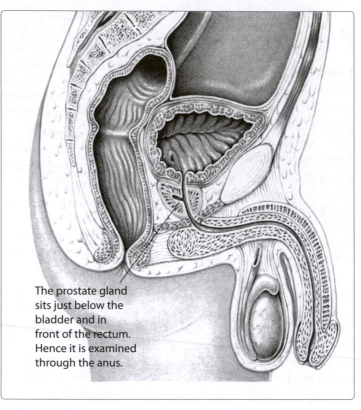

The prostate gland sits just below the bladder and in front of the rectum. Hence it is examined through the anus.

and inappropriate behaviour; obsessive and compulsive behavioural patterns.

Treatment

Antipsychotic drugs will be prescribed, combined with psychotherapy.

Self-help

Seek help as soon as you realize you may be a sufferer and work to trust those who will be trying to help you.

Prevention

Although schizophrenic episodes may be controlled with antipsychotic medication, there is no way of preventing the condition occurring in the first place.

Seasonal affective disorder

Also known as SADS (the last "S" standing for "syndrome"), this is a lowering of the mood that tends to coincide with the coming of autumn and persists through winter.

(T) *Tip: Frequent ejaculations will go a long way towards keeping your prostate gland healthy – tests have shown that men who either have sex or masturbate at least three times a week have far fewer prostate problems than men who come less often.*

Causes

When there is less sunshine and daylight, the pineal gland produces more melatonin, which disrupts the internal sleep/wake rhythms. This is believed to be a hangover from a primeval hibernating past, but can make some people feel very under-energized both physically and mentally – suicide rates are considerably higher in countries that have very little daylight in the winter.

Symptoms

Feeling down for no apparent reason, lack of energy, difficulty concentrating, irritability, weight gain.

Treatment

Get out in the daylight as much as possible.

Self-help

Full-spectrum light bulbs in your home will help to approximate sunlight. Tanning beds, however, are not the answer.

Prevention

Exercise to generally boost your system and eat serotonin-promoting foods such as avocados and bananas.

Sexually transmitted diseases

Genital herpes, gonorrhoea, non-specific urethritis, syphilis, HIV, pubic lice, thrush and others.

Causes

Unprotected sex with an infected partner.

Symptoms

Different infections will have different symptoms, but any of the following should prompt you to get checked out at a sexual health clinic: burning sensation during urination; discharge from penis; itching around or inside penis opening; blisters or sores in genital area; rashes, redness or swelling around the end of the penis; tiny black deposits in your underwear.

Treatment

Antibiotics or antiviral drugs, and don't have sex again until you are sure it is cleared up.

Self-help

In terms of recovery from a minor STD, doing as much as you can to boost your immune system will help.

Prevention

Practise safe sex. Always use a condom and, if you are making a commitment with a partner, don't be shy of diplomatically suggesting the pair of you both get checked out for STDs by a doctor or at a clinic.

Slipped disc

One of the cushioning discs in between the vertebrae slips out of place.

Causes

Incorrect lifting or chronic bad posture. The obese are much more likely to suffer slipped discs as their excess belly weight puts enormous strain on the lower back.

Symptoms

Progressively building pain if the disc is slipping out gradually, then sharp pain, which will be accompanied by increasing immobility; sudden excruciating pain if it just pops out, and the back will often lock.

Treatment

Painkillers and physiotherapy.

Self-help

Vitamin C aids collagen production to assist with the healing, and has anti-inflammatory properties.

Prevention

Glucosamine supplements help to keep all joints healthy and protected.

Snoring

Excessively loud breathing through the mouth while asleep.

Causes

Airways obstructed by internal collapse causing tissue in the throat to noisily vibrate against itself.

Symptoms

Resonant, rumbling sounds created by breathing.

Treatment

Try to avoid sleeping with your mouth open, which usually comes about through sleeping on your back; there are several devices on the market to keep it closed.

Self-help

A couple of drops of eucalyptus oil on your pillow will ease nasal congestion, which may be why you are sleeping with your mouth open.

Prevention

Don't smoke close to bedtime, as this inflames airways, while drinking will relax the throat muscles; check you are not allergic to the feathers in your pillow or duvet.

Stroke

Part of the brain is deprived of oxygen and those cells cease to function and start to die.

Causes

A blood clot in the brain or in one of the arteries that supply blood to the brain or a burst blood vessel in the brain.

Symptoms

Partial paralysis or numbness, coordination and muscle movement problems – this may manifest itself in speech or walking difficulties – blurred or obstructed vision, intense headaches.

Treatment

Blood-pressure lowering or anti-clotting drugs will be administered immediately, and stroke victims may require physical therapy to restore muscle activity and control.

Self-help

There is very little you can do, as this is a medical emergency and must be professionally treated as soon as possible to prevent lasting brain damage.

Prevention

Address the three major risk factors, which are high blood pressure, high cholesterol and smoking.

T

Thrombosis

See Deep Vein Thrombosis. It is the same condition, only it occurs in veins that are not so deep in the body.

Tinnitus

Not only the preserve of rock stars and roadies.

Causes

Usually it is the result of prolonged exposure to loud noise, but it can also be the result of a bacterial infection, a side effect of age-related hearing degeneration, or caused by a head injury or partial ear blockage.

Symptoms

Ringing or buzzing in the ears when there is no corresponding external sound, partial hearing loss, disrupted sleep.

Treatment

Antibiotics will treat an ear infection; there is no cure for noise-induced or degenerative tinnitus, though there are many therapies that can minimize the worst symptoms in non-extreme cases.

Self-help

Vitamin B12 helps reduce the ringing, and ginkgo biloba increases blood flow generally, including to the ears.

The demon drink

It might seem as if the cure or prevention for nearly everything that could be wrong with you is to pack up drinking. At the risk of sounding like a killjoy, this is the case to an extent. And not because anybody connected with this book has got anything against having a drink either; simply that alcohol is a poison. To take in even the responsible amounts will interfere with your healing process, because your body has to be functioning at the peak of its powers to give it its best chance. To have to deal with even a small amount of self-induced toxin will detract from that.

Prevention
Taking a discreet pair of earplugs (available from the better-stocked chemists) to concerts and clubs where you suspect music will be hyper-loud is a good idea. Every time you've been left with your ears ringing after a loud night out, you have damaged your hearing to some degree. Too much time listening to loud music on headphones will also lead to tinnitus.

V

Varicose veins
Patches of veins visible through the surface of the skin, almost uniquely in the legs.

Causes
Defective valves within the veins disrupt blood flow and allow de-oxygenated blood to pool. Standing for prolonged periods of time, lack of exercise and being overweight contribute to the condition.

Symptoms
Swollen and discoloured veins, swollen and aching legs and ankles.

Treatment
They are not a serious health risk, but look unsightly and can be easily surgically removed. Raising your legs above the level of your hips when going to sleep will help with circulation.

Self-help
Rosehip tea contains a bioflavonoid called rutin, which helps to maintain strong, healthy veins. It is also present in apple peel.

Prevention
Avoid standing for long periods, maintain a healthy weight and exercise regularly.

What's the problem?

With this handy, easy-to-use guide, you can give yourself a basic diagnosis. It features a list of man's most common ailments: find your cause for complaint then follow the row from left to right – in some cases you will need to read down a particular category to further define it. This should offer a selection of subsidiary symptoms, in different combinations, which will bring you to what is most likely to be wrong with you. The following column provides basic treatment advice. It must be stressed that this is no replacement for an assessment from a healthcare professional; it is merely an initial guideline.

Appetite, loss of

Visit your doctor if loss of appetite persists for more than a couple of weeks.

Accompanying symptoms	Condition	Treatment
Anxiety, irritability, lack of concentration, fatigue, sleeplessness, loss of appetite	Stress	Try to address aspects of your life that might be causing you agitation; talk to friends, family and/or colleagues about anything that might be troubling you; take a break from work
Fever, chills, fatigue, aching muscles, headache, nausea, excess mucus production, sore throat	Flu	Rest in bed, plenty of fluids, over-the-counter medication
Fever, chills, fatigue, aching muscles, headache, nausea, brown urine, yellowing skin, abdominal pain	Viral hepatitis	See your doctor. It usually clears up by itself: rest and a healthy immune system will speed recovery
Weight loss, constipation and infrequent urination	Possible early signs of cancer	Visit your doctor
Fatigue, pallor, inability to concentrate, irritability, brittle nails	Anaemia	Iron, folic acid, vitamin B12 and C supplements
No other symptoms	Side effect of prescription medication	Consult your doctor